BIOETHICS

Issues and Perspectives

Susan Scholle Connor
Hernán L. Fuenzalida-Puelma

Editors

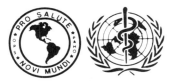

Scientific Publication No. 527

PAN AMERICAN HEALTH ORGANIZATION
Pan American Sanitary Bureau, Regional Office of the
WORLD HEALTH ORGANIZATION

525 Twenty-third Street, NW
Washington, DC 20037, USA

Pan American Health Organization
   Bioethics : Issues and Perspectives. —
Washington, D.C. : PAHO, c1990.
   250p.
   (Scientific Publication ; 527)

   Published also as special issue of the
Bull. Pan Am. Health Organ., v. 24, no.4
   Bibliography at end of chapters
   ISBN 92 75 11527 3

   1. BIOETHICS   2. ETHICS, MEDICAL
   I. Title   II. (Series)
   NLM   W50.MP2

                   Published also in Spanish (1990) with the title:
                        Bioética: Temas y perspectivas
_to_   ISBN 92 75 31527 2

ISBN 92 75 11527 3

© Pan American Health Organization, 1990

Contents

Commentaries

APPENDICES

Preface

Leafing through a major newspaper in any country of the Region will undoubtedly turn up an article that reports on bioethical concerns. The discipline of bioethics has advanced rapidly during the last 30 years in developed countries, and intense interest in it has awakened in the rest of the world. As the influence of technology and politics on medicine increases, public discussion of health and medical issues is also expanding. This expansion is due at least in part to the information and communications revolution that allows news of scientific advances to be disseminated from one country to another almost instantaneously. Many breakthroughs—in such fields as genetic engineering, organ transplantation, and human fertility—pose new moral dilemmas. In democratic and pluralistic societies, where the demand for equity and efficiency in health services is growing, open debates are taking place over who should be responsible for decisions that have a profound impact on the quality of life and on dignity at the time of death. Bioethical reflections provide a philosophic and moral framework in which to resolve these questions in an orderly and just manner, with respect and tolerance for diverse professional and personal ethics and beliefs in different societies.

In its effort to supply its Member Countries with the best possible technical cooperation, the Pan American Health Organization tries not only to respond to requests and concerns but to anticipate them. A popular and effective medium for in-depth examination of critical current topics from an international perspective are special publications like the present volume. This book, the first produced in the international health system on the theory and practice of bioethics, is also the first analysis of this field in the Americas as a whole. It is our hope that the works presented here will bring to mind the precious principles on which Western medical tradition and our ethics as health professionals are founded—the duty to treat, respect for the patient, confidentiality, concern, and humanity: "I urge you not to be too unkind. . . . And if you have occasion, especially provide care for someone who is a foreigner or who is poor, for where there is love of man there also is love of art" (*Precepts* 6, Hippocratic Corpus). On recalling these ideals, our compassion and dedication cannot help but be restored.

Medicine and health are today and always will be social practices with deep and undeniable links to humanistic and moral considerations. As our capacity to intervene in the course of an individual's life or a society's development is amplified through science and technology, the need also grows to scrutinize their use in the light of ethical reasoning. This current challenge will become even more important in the future.

Carlyle Guerra de Macedo, Director
PAN AMERICAN SANITARY BUREAU

Introduction

Susan Scholle Connor and Hernán L. Fuenzalida-Puelma
Editors

The introduction to the *Encyclopedia of Bioethics* defines bioethics as ". . . the systematic study of human conduct in the area of life sciences and health care, insofar as this conduct is examined in the light of moral values and principles . . .

"Bioethics encompasses medical ethics and extends beyond it. Medical ethics in the traditional sense deals with value-related problems that arise in the physician-patient relationship. Bioethics is more inclusive in four important ways:

- ☐ It embraces the value-related problems that arise in all health professions, including the 'allied' professions, mental health professions, and so forth.
- ☐ It extends to biomedical research and behavioral research, whether or not that research has a direct bearing on therapy.
- ☐ It includes a broad range of social issues, such as those associated with public health, occupational health, international health, and the ethics of population control.
- ☐ It extends beyond human life and health to embrace issues involving animal and plant life, e.g., in matters relating to animal experimentation and to competing environmental claims."[1]

Within the realm of the biologic sciences, the inquiry of bioethics is very similar to the moral inquiry arising after World War II and the creation of nuclear weapons that could obliterate mankind, regarding the limits that society should impose upon science and technology. Interest in this field has increased following successes in deciphering the human genetic code and the emergence of new possibilities for scientific manipulation of nature. Such diverse matters as the role of biomedical sciences in war, release into the environment of compounds derived with recombinant DNA technology, compulsory population control policies, the dehumanization and institutionalization of medical care, and research on children, sexual ethics, and suicide all fall within the scope of bioethics.

This presentation is far more limited in scope, dealing in an introductory fashion with only the traditional ethics of medicine and allied health professions and the ethics of research involving human subjects (both "microethics" issues), and the philosophic bases for allocation of resources in a health care system (a "macroethics" issue). From the viewpoint of the editors, this work is a logical extension of our previous collaboration on human rights in health. The microethical questions raised here involve the individual human rights of privacy, dignity, and integrity, while the macroethical question addresses the nature and extent of society's human right to health.

In North America, bioethical reflection has achieved a full flowering and maturity, and is being taught at schools of medicine, philosophy, theology, and law. More than 220 journals in the English-speaking world alone are devoted in whole or in part to bioethics. In Latin America, the field can be considered as just emerging; materials in Spanish are scattered and less abundant, although here also important work is being done.

Within this context, the purpose of this book is twofold. One aim, that of providing an intro-

---

[1] W. T. Reich (ed.), *Encyclopedia of Bioethics*, The Free Press, Macmillan, 1982, p. xix.

ductory overview of the above mentioned "microethics" and "macroethics" issues, is served by three initial sections (which deal with bioethics theory, practice, and application from a microethics standpoint) and the Round Table section (in which three presentations treat the macroethics issue). The second aim, that of showing where particular countries stand in terms of policy and development of programs related to bioethics issues, is achieved through the contributions in the "Regional Panorama" section.

A word of caution: While all the contributors are esteemed intellectuals and most are recognized international bioethics leaders, many of the chapters were written over a year before publication of this volume. In particular, some of the presentations on individual countries may be slightly out of date—an all but inevitable occurrence where the exigencies of translation and multilingual editing invariably cause delay.

In the *Theorema* section, the contributing authors give theoretical and historical background to modern perspectives in bioethics and discuss relationships with other spheres of inquiry including philosophy, religion, law, and technology. The meaning and interrelationships of the bioethics "trinity" of autonomy, beneficence (including nonmaleficence), and justice are brought out in these chapters.

Diego Gracia's contribution, from his recently completed *Fundamentos de la bioética*, defines the field, reviews the historical bases for the modern approach to it, and shows why—quite aside from high technology—developments relating to pluralism, democracy, and human rights have created a need for review of bioethics.

Edmund Pellegrino, considered by many as the godfather of bioethics, explores the search for virtue and beneficence in the doctor-patient relationship, suggesting that the legalistic term "autonomy" be replaced with the more humanistic term "integrity" and stressing that both integrity of persons and autonomy depend on the physician's being a person of integrity.

Hans-Martin Sass, a noted philosopher, an-alyzes the relationship of bioethics and philosophy, examining their historical connections, the philosophic nature of medicine, and the principles of modern bioethics. Among his conclusions: "Ethics without expertise can never be efficacious, while expertise without ethics is unlikely to serve the patient's good."

Francisco Vilardell underscores the ethical conflicts inherent in technologic advances—conflicts involving technologic abuses, unrealized public expectations, and social cost. He suggests that cost-benefit reviews be conducted before introducing new technologies, especially in developing countries.

The undeniable impact of religious perspectives on bioethics and the importance of religious narratives for recognition of moral issues is discussed by theologian Courtney Campbell, who also briefly considers how three religious perspectives (Orthodox Jewish, Roman Catholic, and Protestant) can influence approaches to the bioethical issue of death and dying.

The *Practicum* section explores several techniques developed to apply bioethics principles to concrete moral problems. James Drane leads off this section with an analysis and review of the leading methodologies of clinical ethics. He expresses the view that a European and Latin American approach may be less technical and more philosophically sophisticated than the approach generally used in the United States and Canada.

A number of realistic cases involving ethical problems in nursing are described and analyzed by M. Angélica Piwonka. The author concentrates on the point that health care must be based on humanistic recognition of the overall dignity of the individual, especially in view of the dehumanizing factors present in modern society.

The history and varied functions (clinical, scientific, and deontologic) of hospital ethics review committees are summarized by Juan Carlos Tealdi and José Alberto Mainetti, who also give insight into their own experiences in Argentina and make valuable recommendations about formation of such committees in Latin America.

María del Carmen Lara and Juan Ramón de la Fuente explore the basic concept of informed consent. They explain its derivation from the concepts of autonomy and dignity, point out theoretical and practical difficulties with it, note the principal differences between consent to treatment and consent to experimentation, and provide suggestions based on their own extensive experience in Mexico.

The *Applicatum* section, unfortunately not as broad as initially planned, deals with the application of bioethics in four sensitive areas—organ transplantation, the act of dying, the reporting of AIDS cases, and research on human subjects.

One of the editors, Hernán Fuenzalida-Puelma, reviews the issues involved in organ transplantation from a legal perspective. The matters discussed include donor consent, determination of death, conflicts of interest, recipient selection, donor compensation, and commerce in tissues and organs for transplant. Extensive annex tables provide an important source of information about laws on organ transplants in Latin America.

The "new form of dying" and its various ethical problems are given thoughtful humanistic treatment by Alfonso Llano Escobar, S.J., who reminds us that God must continue being God, and man, however technical and wise, must be conscious of his limitations and of his role as an instrument in the hands of God for the good of humanity.

Key legal and ethical aspects of AIDS, matters of great concern to PAHO and WHO, are described by Ronald Bayer and Larry Gostin. The authors masterfully underscore the need to respect the fundamental values of liberal society in designing a public health policy on AIDS that "at once protects the public health and the rights of the vulnerable."

Diana Serrano LaVertu and Ana María Linares, both in the PAHO Legal Office, explore circumstances and problems that researchers from the developed world may encounter when undertaking research involving human subjects in the developing world.

A fourth section, "Regional Panorama," brings together a collection of articles dealing with current controversies in diverse countries. For the purpose of obtaining this collection, we asked eminent national scholars to give a brief overview of the situation in their countries and suggested the following possible topics: (1) regulation of biotechnology; (2) education in bioethics; (3) ethics review committees; (4) research involving human subjects; (5) regulation of reproduction (family planning, abortion, defective newborns, surrogate mothers, artificial insemination, genetics research); (6) death and dying (definition of death, "do not resuscitate" orders, withdrawal of life-support systems, withdrawal of artificial feeding, and participation by the patient, family, physician, hospital, and judicial system); (7) organ transplants (regulation, prevention of disease transmission, national registry, allocation of resources, commerce); and (8) AIDS (testing, confidentiality, third party notification, reporting).

We were astounded at the depth and sophistication of the analyses received. Many authors, besides addressing these specific topics, also gave a full description of bioethics principles and related activities in their own countries. The result is a rich mosaic of national perspectives from nine countries, as follows:

Argentina: Justo Zanier and colleagues review the postgraduate course in bioethics at Mar del Plata University, the international bioethics symposium held in that city in 1988, and formation of the Inter-American Group for Bioethics.

Brazil: Hélio Pereira Dias, Legal Counsel to the Ministry of Health and foremost Brazilian health lawyer, discusses the legal and ethical provisions relating to control of the health professions, family planning, research, euthanasia, organ transplants, abortion, and medical confidentiality.

Canada: Bernard Dickens, professor in the Faculties of Law and Medicine at the University of Toronto, provides a brief but complete overview of virtually all the suggested topics, citing references to important Canadian texts and detailed policy descriptions.

Chile: Fernando Lolas, noted professor of

psychophysiology at the University of Chile, briefly outlines the Chilean health system and the various bioethics activities carried out by the Colegio Médico de Chile, focusing on the professional ethical practices of physicians relative to other physicians, the public, and the State.

Colombia: Fernando Sánchez-Torres, professor of medicine and President of the Colombian Institute for Bioethical Studies, presents a frank overview of the state of bioethics in his country, devoting particular attention to limitations, possibilities, and the institutions involved in applying bioethics principals.

Mexico: José Kuthy Porter and Gabriel de la Escosura draw on extensive clinical experience to summarize principles of bioethics commonly observed in Mexico. The authors also discuss creation of research, ethics, and biosafety committees and touch on many of the eight suggested topics.

Peru: Roberto Llanos Zuloaga, professor of psychology at Cayetano Heredia University, touches on all the suggested topics, bringing to his discussion a realistic awareness of the cost and public nature of many of decisions involved—on matters such as euthanasia, abortion, and artificial insemination.

Spain: Francesc Abel, S.J., Director of the Borja Institute of Bioethics, furnishes an insightful overview of Spain in transition since the end of the Franco era, highlighting the influence of the Catholic Church, increased secularization since adoption of the 1978 Constitution, and bioethics work performed by Spain's medical schools, a variety of authors, and several centers of bioethics.

United States: The complex 30-odd years of bioethics' history in the United States are succinctly described by Daniel Callahan, Director of the prestigious Hastings Center, who suggests that the leading current bioethics issues in the U.S. involve (1) patients' rights and autonomy, (2) the sanctity of life versus the quality of life, (3) interventions into nature, (4) alloca-

tion of resources, and (5) the role of public decision-making.

The next section, a "Round Table" presentation, deals with a difficult and universally important question: What is a just health services system and how should scarce resources be allocated? No specific answers are attempted. Rather, differing philosophic perspectives and traditions, both historic and current, are described by three leading bioethicists (Gracia, Drane, and Mainetti) whose additional individual contributions appear elsewhere in this publication.

Finally, a documentary Appendix provides reprints of selected international codes of ethics, research codes of ethics, patients' bills of rights, and international texts relating to health as a human right. Unless otherwise specified, inclusion of these documents in this work does not imply or constitute their endorsement by PAHO or WHO.

This publication, while not exhaustive, is designed to serve as an introduction to bioethics in the Americas. Of course, we have not worked alone on this effort. In addition to the writings, encouragement, and dedication provided by the contributors, we have received extraordinary assistance from three people without whom this work simply would not have been produced. These are, first, Diego Gracia, the teacher, scholar, physician, and humanist who helped us design the work and gave unstintingly of his experience and contacts in the Spanish-speaking world; second, the theologian, philosopher, and teacher James S. Drane who provided invaluable expertise and technical insight, and whose commitment is such that he has dedicated his sabbatical leave to PAHO, where he is serving as our first resident bioethicist; and third, our Director, Carlyle Guerra de Macedo, who with customary imagination and foresight has supported and encouraged this foray by PAHO (and its Legal Office) outside its traditional areas into this rich and provocative field of the future.

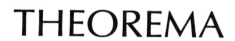

THEOREMA

Medical Bioethics[1]

Diego Gracia

Since the beginnings of Western medicine, which is to say from the time of the writings which tradition has ascribed to the Greek physician Hippocrates of Kos, medical ethics has made use of a "naturalistic" criterion to distinguish good from bad. This criterion, irrespective of whether it has involved what has been known since the start of this century as the "naturalistic fallacy," has customarily identified good with the "natural" order, while considering any departure from that order to be bad. Nature is the work of God, said the Christian theologians of the Middle Ages, and so the natural order is essentially good.

This explains why medieval culture revolved around the idea of "order," which embraced not only those things we customarily call natural but also men, society, and history. In the area of medicine, any disordered or unnatural use of the body or any of its organs was considered bad; and it was also felt that the physician-patient relationship, like other social and human relations, had to conform to a certain order.

This order was not univocal, since within it the physician was considered to be the subject agent and the patient the subject patient. The physician's duty was to "do good" for the patient, and that of the patient was to accept this. The morality of the physician-patient relationship thus had to be a characteristic "morality of beneficence."

What the physician was attempting to achieve was an "objective" good, the restitution of the natural "order," for which reason he had to impose this order on the patient, even against the patient's own wishes. It is true that the patient might not consider what the physician was advocating to be good, but this was due to a "subjective" error which, obviously, could not be expected to possess the same merits as the objective truth.

As a result, within the bounds of the physician-patient relationship the physician was not only a technical agent but also a moral one, while the sick person was a patient in need of both technical and ethical help. The one possessing knowledge of the natural order, in the case of disease, was the physician, who was both able and obliged to proceed on the basis of this knowledge, even in opposition to the patient's desires. It was the essence of "paternalism," a constant in all medical ethics of the natural "order."

Few literary documents show this as clearly as Plato's *Republic*, which has shaped Western political thought for more than a millennium. According to Plato, any well-constituted political society must consist of several types of people, as follows:

One type includes those within the city who dedicate themselves to the cultivation of the so-called servile or mechanical arts (agriculture, manufacturing, carpentry, blacksmithing, masonry, etc.). As a consequence of their work, Plato says, such people are deformed in body and ignoble of spirit. In them there is no possible health or morality. For this reason their political status cannot be that of free persons, but instead must be that of serfs or slaves. They are thus without political or civil liberties.

The opposite is true of other men who dedicate themselves to cultivation of the liberal or

[1]Originally published in Spanish as an introductory essay to the author's book *Fundamentos de Bioética*, Ediciones de la Universidad de Madrid, Madrid, 1989.

scholarly arts (arithmetic, geometry, music, astronomy), upon whom Plato confers the estate of guardians. These must fulfill two functions within the city, that of defending the city from external threats (for which purpose they must be healthy and strong of body), and that of imposing order and peace upon internal disputes (something that cannot be accomplished except through a good moral education coupled with an exquisite sense of the four cardinal virtues: prudence, justice, fortitude, and temperance). If the artisans are considered to be of diseased and low moral condition, the guardians, in contrast, are considered healthy in body and soul. They can thus be free men and can enjoy liberties.

From the best of the guardians come the governors, who Plato feels represent the category of perfect men. From this derives the fact that the rank of philosopher, together with mastery of the highest science, dialectics, is inherent to the Governor of the Republic.

Through dialectics the philosopher is able to differentiate the true from the false, the good from the bad, the just from the unjust, and to convey it, inasmuch as he is the monarch, to the community. In this manner the platonic governor "imposes" values on the other members of the social body. He is an absolute and absolutist sovereign, the polar opposite of a democratic governor. Human beings, the inhabitants of the city, are not the prime holders of rights and political liberties, some of which they delegate to the sovereign; on the contrary, the governor by nature is the prime holder of these things, and the liberties enjoyed by the citizens are imposed upon them from above.

In concrete terms, the moral order seen by Plato is derived from the privileged view that the monarch has of the world of ideas, above all the idea of goodness. And the governor's function is none other than that of mediating between the world of ideas and the world of men. However strange it may appear, then, the moral order does not derive from free acceptance but from imposition. It is well known that in the Socratic tradition such imposition does not conflict with freedom, since whoever sees the good cannot fail to yearn for it. What is free is not in opposition to what is necessary. Compelling his subjects to comply with the imposed moral order, the platonic governor in fact promotes the freedom of each and every individual.

Such is the moral justification of political absolutism. And if the term "physician" is substituted for "monarch" or "governor," and the term "patient" for "subject," one arrives at a strictly faithful image of the traditional enlightened despotism of the physician. The physician has always been to the body what the monarch has been to the republic—an absolute and absolutist sovereign until the democratic revolutions of modern times, one perpetually oscillating between the paternalism of family relations and the tyranny of slave relations.

This intellectual universe did not undergo any substantial change until the modern world was well established. Indeed, if the Protestant Reformation sought and obtained something, it was the substitution of the idea of "autonomy" for that of "order," and of the "moral" order or order of freedom for the "natural" order. From this arose the second major moral paradigm of Western history, whose origins are intertwined with the progressive discovery of human rights from Locke's time to the present.

As this way of thinking was taught, the old human relationships established in conformity with the medieval idea of hierarchic order came to seem excessively vertical, monarchic, and paternalistic. As an alternative to these relationships, others of a more horizontal, democratic, and symmetrical nature were proposed. The great democratic revolutions of the modern world—first the English Revolution, then the North American, and then the French—were carried out in this spirit.

It is impossible to understand the meaning of medical bioethics in isolation from this context. Bioethics is a necessary consequence of the principles that have been molding the spiritual life of the Western countries for two centuries. If since the Enlightenment there has been affirmation of the autonomous and absolute nature of human individuals, in both the religious order (through the principle of religious freedom) and the political order (through the principle of democracy), it is logical that this should have led to what we might call the "principle of moral freedom," which can be formulated as follows: All human beings are autonomous moral agents, and as such should be respected by all those who hold distinct moral positions. Just as religious pluralism and political pluralism are human rights, so too should moral pluralism be accepted as a right. No morality can be imposed on human beings against the dictates of their own consciences. The sanctuary of individual morality is inviolate.

Pluralism, democracy, and civil and political human rights have been leading achievements of the modern era. The same is true of ethics in the strict sense, that is, of the moral in contradistinction to the physical. For this reason it should not seem strange that the development of ethics has been linked to the development of democracy and human rights. Indeed, all of the democratic revolutions, those which have taken place in the Western world since the eighteenth century, were mounted to defend these principles.

Nevertheless, there is a curious circumstance—that this pluralistic and democratic movement, which was already established in the civil life of Western societies centuries ago, only reached medicine very recently. The relationship between the physician and the patient has obeyed the guiding principles set forth by Plato more than it has obeyed principles of a democratic cut. Specifically, within the framework of the physician-patient relationship the patient has been considered both physically and morally unfit, making it necessary for his physician to lead him in both areas.

In general, the physician-patient relationship has traditionally been paternalistic and absolutist. Pluralism, democracy, and human rights—in other words, ethics, understood in the modern sense—have not touched this relationship until recently. It was only during the 1970s that patients began to be fully aware of their status as autonomous moral agents, both free and responsible, who had no wish to establish parent-child relationships with their physicians, but who instead sought adult relationships based on mutual needs and mutual respect. Since then, however, that awareness has caused the physician-patient relationship to be based upon the principle of autonomy and freedom for all the participating subjects, including both physicians and their patients.

Notice what this signifies. When all the mature human beings who make up a social group live as autonomous adults, it is highly probable, not only in the world of politics but also in the world of morality and religion, that they will maintain different positions. This has two results. The first is that a society based on the liberty and autonomy of all its members must by necessity be plural and pluralistic; in other words, its members will not only have distinct views in the areas of politics, religion, morality, etc., but will also commit themselves to respect the views of others, on condition that these others do likewise. And the second is that besides maintaining pluralism, the society will have to be secularized, since it will be practically impossible to achieve uniformity in religious matters.

Let us now return to medical ethics. During the many centuries in which the Greek philosophy of the natural order prevailed, a philosophy that was subsequently Christianized by the theologians, medical ethics was drawn up by moralists and applied by confessors. The physician was presented with everything in completed form and asked—or required—to comply with it. Nor was there any clear understanding that specific cases could provoke grave and substantial conflicts, since once the general, immutable principles had been established, the only things that might vary were the circumstances.

Expressed in other terms, over the course of all those centuries there was no true medical ethics, if by this is meant the moral autonomy of physicians and patients. What existed was something else, in principle heteronomous, which we might call "ethics of medicine." This explains why physicians have not generally been competent in questions of "ethics," their activity having been reduced to the sphere of "asceticism" (how to educate the good or virtuous physician) and of "etiquette" (what standards of propriety and civility should govern the practice of medicine). The history of so-called medical ethics offers effective proof of this.

Nevertheless, the current panorama is quite different. In a society where everyone, in lieu of evidence to the contrary, is an autonomous moral agent with distinctive criteria of good and bad, the medical relationship, being an interpersonal relationship, may involve inherent rather than accidental conflict.

For instance, consider one of the most typical examples. A Jehovah's Witness is in an automobile accident and arrives at the emergency room suffering from severe hypovolemic shock. On seeing this, the emergency room physician makes a decision, based on the deeply rooted moral criterion of beneficence, to give the patient a blood transfusion. The patient's wife, who is at his side, informs the physician that her husband is a Jehovah's Witness and that he has on repeated occasions said that he does not wish to receive blood from other persons, even if this endangers his life.

In expressing her husband's views, the patient's wife is asking that his moral criterion be respected; she shares it, the doctor does not. Faced with the moral criterion of beneficence wielded by the physician, the wife in our example defends the criterion of autonomy, according to which all human beings, unless there is evidence to the contrary, are considered autonomous moral agents fully responsible for all their actions.

Here one can see how the simplest medical relationship, the one established between a physician and a patient, has been transformed into one that is autonomous, pluralistic, secularized, and characterized by conflict.

The potential intensity of this conflict is increased by the fact that others besides the physician and patient (nurses, the hospital administration, the social security agency, the patient's family, etc.) may intervene in the health relationship. However, all of these agents in the physician-patient relationship can be reduced to three: the physician, the patient, and society. Each of these participants plays a particular moral role. By and large, the patient is guided by the moral principle of "autonomy," the physician by that of "beneficence," and society by that of "justice." Naturally, the patient's family is guided by the principle of beneficence relative to the patient, and in this sense acts morally in a way quite similar to that of the physician; while the hospital administration, health insurance representatives, and judges have to look above all to safeguarding the principle of justice. Hence, these three dimensions are always present in the physician-patient relationship, and this is a good thing. If the physician and the family were to shift camps from beneficence to justice, the health relationship would suffer irreversibly, as would also happen should the patient cease to act as an autonomous moral subject.

But the fact that these three elements are essential does not mean they must always be complementary, and thus never in conflict. The actual situation is more the reverse. It is never possible to completely respect autonomy without causing beneficence to suffer, or to honor beneficence completely except at the expense of justice, etc. From this arises the need to keep the three principles in play, weighing their importance in each specific situation. As David Ross would say, those three principles work like primary obligations, which must be weighed in each specific situation. Only then will it be seen how they might best articulate with each other, giving way to specific or effective duties.

Thus, for example, despite the fact that all of us feel it necessary to scrupulously respect personal autonomy, we believe that in the case of a just war the State may compel individuals to give up their lives (that is, their autonomy) for others. Here it can be clearly seen how a primary obligation, respect for personal autonomy, may fail to coincide with the concrete and effective obligation, precisely as a consequence of the need to honor another primary obligation, justice, which in this specific case seems to be of a higher order.

Medical ethics has to do whatever is possible to scrupulously and simultaneously honor autonomy, beneficence, and justice. There is an obligation to act in this way, even though the objective is very difficult and at times quite impossible to achieve.

The situation being thus, it is evident that the urgency of specific and daily problems cannot free us from the prescribed exigencies. Rather, very much to the contrary, these problems force us to take the utmost precautions and to find the strictest possible foundation for our decision-making criteria. When the issues are of such gravity that they determine the lives of individuals and societies, as frequently happens in medicine, then rationality must be honed to its finest edge, and as much time as necessary must be dedicated to the problems involved in laying foundations.

In so doing, it is important to approach medical bioethics aided not only by logic but also by history, since human reason is simultaneously logical and historical. Hence, the history of bioethics should not be viewed as an erudite curiosity presented with no other purpose than to enlighten the reader. Rather, it should be seen as the best possible introduction to the study of bioethics, and as something that facilitates analysis of the problems involved in the laying of the discipline's logical and philosophical foundations. In this way it improves our ability to answer the question that serves as a kind of summary of all the other questions: What are the moral conditions that should attend upon what the Greeks called *téleios iatrós*, the Latins *optimus medicus*, and the Castilians *el perfecto médico*? This book aspires to no greater task, nor to any lesser one.

The Relationship of Autonomy and Integrity in Medical Ethics[1]

Edmund D. Pellegrino

"Integrity without knowledge is weak and useless, and knowledge without integrity is dangerous and dreadful."
Samuel Johnson (*Rasselas*, 1759)

In the last 25 years autonomy has superseded beneficence as the first principle of medical ethics. This is the most radical reorientation in the long history of the Hippocratic tradition. As a result, the physician-patient relationship has become more honest, open, and respectful of the dignity of patients.

This shift in the locus of decision-making is a response to the coalescence of sociopolitical, legal, and ethical forces that make it well-nigh irreversible. The central ethical question today is not whether patient autonomy will remain a predominant principle. Rather, the issue involves a critical assessment of patient autonomy's full impact on the relationships between physicians and patients. Does the principle of autonomy as now construed encompass the full meaning of respect for the dignity of persons? May the tendency to absolutize autonomy defeat some of the purposes for which it has been so vigorously propounded? Is there a deeper source for the principle of autonomy that more fully encompasses the special nuances required by authentic respect for persons?

In this essay I shall argue: (1) that autonomy as now construed has certain moral and practical limitations; (2) that these limitations can be ameliorated by linking autonomy to the principle of respect for the integrity of persons; and (3) that this move encompasses a more fundamental and richer safeguard for the dignity of both patient and physician than current interpretations of the principle of autonomy.

I shall attempt to advance these propositions by examining the following: (1) the origins and nature of the concept and principle of autonomy and its expression in today's paradigm for ethical decision-making; (2) the concept and principle of integrity, its relationships to autonomy, and the distinctions between integrity and autonomy; and (3) the relationship of the principles of autonomy and the integrity of persons to the virtue of integrity.

Autonomy: Its Origins and Nature as a Concept and Principle

Autonomy, despite its universal usage in medical ethics, is too often simplistically interpreted, as Faden and Beauchamp have so cogently pointed out (1). For example, they make a sharp and valid distinction between the autonomous person and the autonomous action, preferring in their treatment of informed consent to emphasize the autonomous act, rather than the autonomous person. While agreeing with their distinction, this essay will place more emphasis on the autonomous person and on the relationship of that concept to the concept of the integrity of persons which underlies it.

Autonomy, in keeping with its Greek etymol-

[1]Based on an address originally presented at the Third International Congress on Ethics and Medicine, Karolinska Institute, Nobel Conference, Stockholm, Sweden, 13 September 1989. Reprinted with the author's permission.

ogy, literally means self-rule. In today's parlance, autonomy has variously been interpreted as a moral and legal claim or as a right, duty, concept, or principle. For purposes of this essay, I shall take it to be a capacity for self-rule, a quality inherent in rational beings that enables them to make reasoned choices and take actions based on a personal assessment of future possibilities weighed in terms of their own value systems. In this view, autonomy is a capacity that flows from the fact that humans can think and feel and make judgments about what they deem to be good.

The universal existence of this capacity in rational beings does not guarantee that it can or will function fully or at all. Both internal and external constraints can impede autonomous decisions and actions. Internal constraints include such things as brain damage or dysfunction induced by disordered metabolic states, drugs, injury, lack of mental competence related to infancy and childhood, mental retardation, psychoses, obsessive-compulsive neuroses, etc. In these instances the physiological substratum requisite to the exercise of the capacity for autonomy is impaired—sometimes reversibly, sometimes not.

Or else autonomy, while unimpaired internally, may be prevented from operating by external events like coercion, physical and emotional deception, or deprivation of essential information. In these cases the person has the capacity for self-rule, but that capacity cannot be realized in an autonomous act, i.e., an act that gives evidence of "autonomous authorization" (2). (An autonomous act satisfies the criteria for informed consent. It is a decision and act free from internal or external constraints, informed as fully as the situation requires, and consistent with the person's evaluation at the moment of choice of that person's own value system.)

The existence of the capacity for self-rule is so deeply embedded in what it means to be a human being that it constitutes a moral claim, a claim which generates a duty of respect in other persons. This claim is expressed as the principle of autonomy: i.e., so act in relationships with others that their capacity for autonomy (and thus their moral claim) can be exercised as fully as circumstances will permit.

Social and Political Sources

The recent shift in the locus of the decision from physician to patient, while seemingly abrupt, had been developing in the Western world since the birth, in the eighteenth century, of the modern idea of a participatory democracy. This article is not the place to review that history. We need only enumerate the sociopolitical forces that coalesced in the mid-1960s to place autonomy in the forefront of medical ethics legally and philosophically: the Nuremberg trials; the worldwide spread of participatory democracy; mistrust of authority in general and technical expertise in particular; the expansion of public education; the civil rights movement; the intrusions of law, economics, and commerce into medical decisions; and the challenges of biotechnology that had to be faced in a progressively pluralistic society that could muster little moral consensus.

These forces converged to engender both mistrust of the physician's traditional paternalism and a demand for self-determination and informed consent in medical relationships. "Autonomy" has become the watchword that symbolizes the moral and legal claim of patients to make their own decisions without constraint or coercion, however beneficent the physician's intentions might be. The sociopolitical claim to autonomous decision and action was reentered by the legal concept of privacy and by the philosophic principle of autonomy.

The Legal Basis for Individual Autonomy

Though still debated among legal scholars, the legal basis for the claim to autonomy is usually grounded in the right to privacy (3). Such a right is not specifically stated in the United States Constitution, but has been derived in a series of Supreme Court decisions as a "penumbra" of several amendments of the Bill of Rights (4). This right to privacy has been applied in practical terms to the right of personal decision regarding the education of children, choice of a marriage partner, religious preference, access to contraceptive devices, and termination of pregnancy (5). This same right has been explicitly invoked to protect a patient's right to refuse medical treatments (6).

In the last two decades, the legal right to self-determination has been progressively extended from the patient to his or her surrogate, from mechanical respirators to food and fluid, from terminal to nonterminal patients, and from the patient himself to his or her living will.[2] This legal right to self-determination and privacy has acted as a powerful restraint on the traditional benevolent paternalism of the physician. It has also given impetus to the doctrine of informed consent.

The Philosophic Roots

The principle of autonomy has several sources in moral philosophy. One is Locke's *Second Treatise on Government*, which held Man in the state of Nature to be free and equal so that none might have sovereignty over another except through a social contract freely entered into (7). Locke's arguments gave rise to the notion of "negative rights"—rights of a person not to be interfered with by others. These negative rights have come to be the foundation of liberal democracy for many people (8).

A second powerful and influential philosophical moral claim to autonomy is propounded in Kant's *Groundwork for the Metaphysics of Morals* (9). Here Kant argues that freedom is essential to all morality, that it is identical with autonomy, and that autonomy is "the ground of the dignity of human nature and of every rational nature" (10). Kant unites the idea of a rational being with dignity this way: ". . . a rational being himself must be the ground for all maxims of action *never merely as a means*, but as a supreme condition restricting the use of every means, that is, *always also as an end*" (11). "And the dignity of man consists precisely in his capacity to make universal law, although only on condition of being himself subject to the law he makes" (12).

A third source for a moral claim to autonomy is John S. Mill's essay *On Liberty*. Mill asserts that the only restraint on liberty is harm to others, not harm to self (13). This latter notion, joined with the Lockean idea of negative rights, is the major connecting link between the philosophic notion of autonomy and the legal notion of privacy. This link is most influential with the courts in America. It is the principle generally used to resolve conflicts about who should make the final decision in accepting or rejecting medical treatments. It is the dominant concept as well in the report of the President's Commission on withholding and withdrawing life-sustaining treatment (14).

This conjunction of the legal concept of privacy and the moral concept of autonomy has resulted in a widely accepted medical decision-making paradigm: Competent patients have the moral and legal right to make their own decisions, and these decisions take precedence over those of the doctor or the family. When patients are no longer competent (or have never been competent—e.g., patients such as infants or the retarded), their rights of decision are transferred to a valid surrogate or to some anticipatory statement by the patient (such as a living will, medical directive, or durable power of attorney), or in the absence of these to a legally appointed

---

[2]*In re Quinlan*, 70 N.J. 10, 355 A. 2d 647 (1976); *In re Eichner*, 52 N.Y. 2d 363, 420 N.E. 2d 64, 438 N.Y.S. 2d 266, *cert. denied*, 454 U.S. 858 (1981); *In re Conroy*, 98 N.J. 321, 486 A. 2d 1209 (1985); *Bouvia vs. Superior Court (Glenchur)*, 179 Cal. App. 3d 1127, 225 Cal. Rptr. 297 (Ct. App. 1986), *review denied* (Cal. June 5, 1986); *In re Jobes*, 108 N.J. 394, 529 A. 2d 434 (1987); *Brophy vs. New England Sinai Hospital, Inc.*, 398 Mass. 417, 497 N.E. 2d 626 (1986). One exception is the Missouri Supreme Court in *Nancy Beth Cruzan vs. Robert Harmon et al.* (#70813 Miss. Sup. Ct., Nov. 16, 1988), which expresses "grave doubts as to the applicability of privacy rights to decisions to terminate food and water to incompetent patients."

guardian. Some have so absolutized the principle of autonomy and the right of privacy that they would place no limits on its exercise. Others accept varying degrees of limitation on autonomy. We shall return to these exceptions later when we examine the links between autonomy and integrity.

The most concrete actualization of the principles of privacy and autonomy lies in the doctrine of informed consent that has become the central requirement of morally valid medical decision-making. For consent to fulfill the claims of human persons to self-governance, it must be based on sufficient information to make a reasoned choice and must be free of coercion or deception. The procedures surrounding informed consent are designed to facilitate the capacity of rational beings to make judgments of what they consider best rather than what the physician or any other person might consider best for them.

Deficiencies of Autonomy as a Moral Guide

There can be no question of the importance of the sociopolitical, legal, and moral emphasis on autonomy in protecting the patient's right of self-determination. But there are certain limitations to the concept of autonomy itself that may impede the fullest expressions of the respect for persons which autonomy is supposed to enhance.

For one thing, autonomy has come to have a strong legalistic quality centering all too often on invasion of privacy, assault, battery, and tort law in general. Such conceptions tend to moral minimalism, i.e., to fulfillment only of what is specifically prescribed. Documentary evidence and protection against lawsuit become almost obsessive concerns, rather than the moral quality of the consent process. This focus fosters the all-to-frequent view of the physician-patient relationship as a contract rather than a fiduciary relationship or a covenant. The fiction is encouraged that a contract is possible in a relationship in which one party is ill, vulnerable, and exploitable while the other holds the needed knowledge and power. In this contractual view, the procedures for making a valid informed consent, important as they are, come to take the place of the substantive moral issue itself.

A strong emphasis on self-determination also minimizes the physician's obligations of beneficence and effacement of self-interest. Some even see beneficence as antipathetic to autonomy—a false dichotomy I shall treat a little further on in this essay. Autonomy, when viewed as a legal right or even as a moral claim, can severely circumscribe the range of discretionary decisions—those unanticipated choices the clinical situation may force on the physician. Ordinarily the physician would feel free to act in the patient's best interests as he himself perceives them. For example, the proposed "medical directive," which consists of six pages of detailed instruction on how the physician should manage life-sustaining and other treatments, could easily lead to a paralysis of decision-making injurious to the patient (15). When patients are unable to spell out everything in advance, the physician may spend more time trying to figure out what the patient wishes than deciding what is in the patient's best interests.

Finally, the prevailing emphasis on autonomy generates a cult of moral privatism, atomism, and individualism that is insensitive to the fact that humans are members of a moral community. When autonomy is absolutized, each person is a moral atom who asserts his or her rights independently and even against the claims of the social entity to which he or she belongs. Conflicts between the rights of a community and the rights of its individual members raise serious questions of economic and social justice that demand a better balance between autonomy and the common good than now prevails.

Many of the moral shortcomings of the concept and principle of autonomy are ameliorated if we look to the more fundamental concept of integrity of persons—of which autonomy is a partial, but not a full, expression.

Integrity of Persons and Persons of Integrity

Etymologically, integrity is from the Latin *integer*, and it means wholeness, completeness, or unimpaired unity. It is a more complex notion than autonomy. Integrity encompasses autonomy, because loss of autonomy impairs acting as an intact and whole human being. But autonomy is not synonymous with integrity of the person, since integrity includes physiological, psychological, and spiritual wholeness. Autonomy is a capacity of the whole person, but not the whole of a person's capacities. As Karol Wojtyla puts it, "integration is an essential condition for the transcendence of the person in the whole of the psychosomatic complexity of the human subject" (*16*). Gabriel Marcel puts it this way: "I want to run my own life" is "the radical formula of autonomy." Autonomy belongs to the order of *having*, to the things we possess, while true freedom belongs to the order of *being*, to what we *are*. In this view, freedom may paradoxically include even nonfreedom (*17*).

Integrity has two senses of significance for medical ethics. One sense refers to the integrity of the person, of the patient, and of the physician; the other refers to being a person of integrity. In the first sense, integrity is a moral claim which belongs to every human simply by virtue of being human. In the second sense, integrity is a virtue, a moral *habitus* acquired by constant practice in our relation with others. Integrity belongs to all persons as humans, but not all are persons of integrity. Each sense of integrity has important ethical implications in medical ethics.

Integrity of the Person

By the integrity of the person we mean the right ordering of the parts to the whole, the balance and harmony between the various dimensions of human existence necessary for the well-functioning of the whole human organism. The integrity of a person is expressed in a balanced relationship between the bodily, psycho-social, and intellectual elements of his or her life. No one element is out of proportion to the others. Each takes the lead when the good of the whole requires it. Each yields to the other in the interest of the whole. Integrity in this sense is synonymous with health. Disease amounts to disintegration, a rupture of the unity of the person (*18*). This rupture may occur in one or more of three spheres, each with its own ethical implications: the corporeal, the psychological, and the axiological.

Bodily integrity implies a physiologically well-functioning organism, a body that can serve the aims and purposes of the person efficiently and effectively with a minimum of discomfort or disability. With physical illness, corporeal unity is shattered. The body (or one of its organs) becomes the focus of attention and loses some or all of its capacity for work, play, or human relationships. There may even be loss of an organ or a function. The functional integrity of the whole organism is disrupted by a sick organ, organ system, or metabolic mechanism.

Illness may also assault the psychological integrity of the person in two ways. First, emotional illness is a form of disintegration in which anxieties, obsessions, compulsions, illusions, and other psychopathologic disorders assume control of existence. The resulting distortions of the balance and unity of the person interfere with that person's well-functioning as much as the rupture of corporeal unity.

Second, psychological integrity is the unity of the self in its relationship to the body. When illness afflicts a part of the body, we feel alienated from that part, we stand in some senses away from the offending body, and we sometimes reject it and resent it as an enemy. The image we have fashioned of our self-identity relative to our bodily integrity is threatened. We all live with a unique balance we have struck over the years between our hopes and aspirations and the limitations imposed by our physiological, psychological, or physical shortcomings. Serious illness forces a confrontation between that image and the impact of disability, pain, and death. It confronts us with the possibility of a substantially altered self-image or even nonexistence. A new image, new points of balance, and a new definition of what constitutes health must be established if we are to become "whole" again.

Another facet of the integrity of persons is axiological integrity, i.e., the intactness of the values we cherish and espouse. Each of us is in a real sense defined by the particular configuration of values we have chosen as our own. In illness these values may be in conflict with those of the physician, our families, or society. Our conception of healing reflects our personal assessment of what constitutes well-functioning. This is as much a value-determined conception as it is a physical or psychological one. In order for us to be cured or treated, our most cherished values must also become the subject of the physician's scrutiny and possible manipulation. Thus, our values are at risk of challenge or damage in the medical transaction.

The potential for the tripartite disintegration of the person, which is part of being ill, creates obligations for the physician—who is bound by covenant to heal and help. Healing means to make whole again, that is, to reestablish the wholeness that constitutes a healthy existence. To be faithful to this covenant the physician is obliged to remedy disease-inflicted disintegration of the person. In this view, restoration of the integrity of the person is the moral basis of the physician-patient relationship. That is why any morally authentic doctor-patient relationship must by definition be "holistic."

In illness the vulnerability of the patient's body, psyche, and values generates the obligation to enhance and restore the patient's autonomous capacity for decision-making. Autonomy is thus grounded ultimately in the integrity of the person. To usurp the patient's human capacity for self-governance is to violate that integrity. To ignore, override, repudiate, or ridicule the patient's values is to assault the patient's very humanity. This affront aggravates the disintegration of the person already there as a result of illness. Nothing could be further from a morally defensible healing relationship.

Paradoxically, however, in order to repair the disintegration produced by disease the integrity of the person must to some degree be violated. The physician lays hands on the patient, peers into every orifice, inquires into the details of the patient's social relationships and psychological responses. This is a licit invasion of integrity to which the patient gives assent. But consent cannot obviate the exposure of integrity to serious risk attendant upon medical treatment. Such risk is another source of moral obligation that binds the physician, in exercising the right to invade the integrity of the patient, to do so with the utmost care and sensitivity.

The Limits of the Patient's Claim to Autonomy

However fundamental, the patient's moral claim to respect for his integrity and autonomy is not absolute. There are several limitations that arise when the patient's moral claim conflicts with the equivalent claim to integrity made by other persons.

One such limitation is the claim of the physician, as a person, to his own autonomy. The patient cannot violate the physician's integrity as a person. If the physician is morally opposed to abortion, euthanasia, withdrawal or withholding of food or fluid, or artificial insemination, for example, he cannot be expected to comply with the patient's autonomy and suppress the integrity of his own person. This will become an increasingly important matter as morally debatable procedures such as voluntary and involuntary euthanasia become legalized or, eventually perhaps, become eligible for the benefits of health insurance. Both physician and patient are obliged to respect the integrity of each other's person; neither may impose his or her values on the other. Therefore, respectful withdrawal from the relationship may be necessary for the physician or the patient in order to avoid cooperation in acts that might compromise personal moral integrity.

Another limitation on a patient's autonomous decision occurs when action might produce a serious, definable, and direct harm to another person. An example here is the patient who is HIV seropositive and refuses to have that fact revealed to his or her spouse or sexual partner. In this instance the physician cannot withdraw, but instead has the obligation in justice to tell the person at risk, after first offering the patient the opportunity to do so. The same limitation applies to the patient who wishes to conceal some health problem that might compromise his or her capacity to fulfill a position of trust—e.g., as a pilot, surgeon, or cleric.

The autonomous decision of a valid surrogate must also be resisted if there is clear evidence of a conflict of interest that might lead to the overtreatment or undertreatment of an infant or incompetent adult. The physician's primary obligation is the preservation of the integrity of the person who is his patient. Under circumstances like these, the physician cannot withdraw but must take the measures available in a democratic society to protect the patient's interests. This protection may involve referral of the matter to an ethics committee, appointment of a legal guardian, or court intervention to limit the autonomy of the surrogates in emergencies, when the outcome is in doubt and when, in the absence of a specific instruction, the physician must act in the patient's best medical interests— at least until the patient's wishes are clear.

Finally, the patient may, on the moral strength of his or her own moral claim to autonomy, yield up his or her claim to autonomy. Sometimes the physician has made a sincere effort to involve the competent patient, yet the patient does not wish to participate as fully as others might. The patient might then ask that the physician should decide what is "best." Under such conditions, and only these, the physician has a moral mandate to decide for the patient—that is, to act in the patient's place and in the patient's interests. Not to do so is a form of moral abandonment. But the physician must never assume this mandate nor accept it too eagerly or lightly.

Carried to extremes, the morally justifiable claim to autonomy could erode the commu-

nality of human existence. Autonomy absolutized leads to moral atomism, privatism, and anarchy. Humans are social animals. They cannot be fulfilled except in social relationships, as Aristotle so wisely pointed out (19). The community within which the patient resides has moral claims as well. This communitarian dimension of biomedical ethics is in danger of compromise if the current drive for autonomy is not modulated and balanced against the moral claims of other persons and the community.

The community, too, has a claim to integrity, i.e., to the same kind of wholeness, completeness, and intactness to which the individual lays claim. The fabric of a society can be torn, and the existence of society itself threatened, if individuals retreat into private morality independent of the community. We are in some danger of this when individuals or groups with special interests irresponsibly use resources common to all. Economically, the entrepreneur threatens the integrity of society when he despoils the environment. To a certain degree so do physicians, patients, or families who demand and use scarce medical resources when treatment is futile or the benefits disproportionate to the costs.

Patients, therefore, owe a debt to the community for the lifelong benefits they derive from being members of human communities. They should feel some duty to limit their demands for expensive or marginally beneficial treatments and technologies that impose financial burdens on society and their families. Among other things, out of a sense of social justice, voluntary limitations should be placed on life-support measures that are futile or that merely prolong the act of dying.

Finally, if we look at autonomy as a derivative of the integrity of the person and not as an isolated ethical principle, the presumed conflict between autonomy and beneficence should disappear. Paternalism should not be equated with beneficence, as some authors propose (20). Paternalism involves the physician's usurpation of the patient's moral claim as a human being to decide what is in his or her own best interests. This action violates the integrity of the person and can under no circumstances be a beneficent act. Rather, to be beneficent, respect for the patient's values and choices is essential. As Thomasma and I have pointed out elsewhere, the physician holds beneficence in trust (21), a point I will enlarge upon a little later.

Autonomy and Integrity Contrasted

We may summarize the differences between autonomy and integrity as follows:

Autonomy is a capacity inherent in being a rational person. It is something we have or possess. If we have never developed our capacity for rational judgment we do not have autonomy, and we can lose our autonomy when we lose this rational capacity. We can have degrees of autonomy, however, depending on the interactions of internal and external impediments to the operation of our capacity for self-determined choices and actions. Under these circumstances our right to autonomy can be transferred to the decisions of a morally valid proxy or to a document like a living will, a durable power of attorney, or a medical directive. To transfer our autonomy is to violate an important part of our humanity, but it does not deprive us of our status as human persons.

Integrity, on the other hand, is a matter of being. It is an attribute possessed by all humans—competent or not, adult or not, conscious or not. It does not admit of degrees, nor can it be lost. Hence, integrity is not something we have but is part of our being. It cannot be transferred to someone else. To violate our integrity is to violate our whole being as humans.

Integrity of the Decision

The principle of respect for integrity can and does ameliorate some deficiencies of the principle of autonomy. For one thing, respect for integrity is inconsistent with the minimalistic view of some physicians—namely, that autonomy is reducible to a right to refuse treatment. In order

to truly respect the integrity of the person, we must strive to give integrity to his or her decision as well, to respect a wholeness that places that decision within the history and the background of the patient's life. A particular decision can never stand isolated from the whole narrative of the patient's life, the drama he or she has lived and is living, and the way he or she perceives self, family, and community in relation to the decision in question. All of these particulars must enter into the final choice if that choice is to have integrity in itself and be the act or decision of a whole or complete person.

Respect for the integrity of persons also moves the patient's decision from the level of simple assent or dissent to the level of consent—because it implies mutual and consensual arrival at a decision by the doctor and patient acting together. In this view, respect for the integrity of persons requires a positive effort to get not just a decision that is autonomous by external criteria but one that represents the common ground of knowing and feeling that exists between the doctor and patient. It is not a case of the patient assenting or dissenting as an isolated entity, but of the doctor and patient consenting—that is, acting together, with each respecting the integrity of the other's person.

The Person of Integrity

The law of privacy, the principle of autonomy, and respect for the integrity of persons are necessary but not sufficient to fully preserve the integrity of the sick person in the medical transaction. What is indispensable is the person of integrity, the person of moral wholeness, who can be trusted to respect the nuances and subtleties of the moral claim to autonomy. The physician, therefore, must be a person who exhibits the virtue of integrity, a person who not only accepts respect for the autonomy of others as a principle or concept but who can also be trusted to interpret its application in the most morally sensitive way.

The ultimate safeguard of the integrity of the

patient's person is the fidelity of the physician to the trust inherent in the healing relationship. It is the physician who interprets and applies the principle of autonomy. Much depends upon how the physician presents the facts, which facts are selected and emphasized, how much or how little is revealed, how risks and benefits are weighed, and how the fears and anxieties unique to the patient are respected or exploited—in sum, how the physician uses his or her "Aesculaean power." Every patient, the most educated and the most independent, is potentially a victim or a beneficiary of that power. As a result, the physician has a heavy responsibility to be sensitive to the dependent, vulnerable, frightened state of the patient and not to exploit that state, even if the physician deems it to be in the patient's best interests.

Clearly, no contract, law, or abstract ethical principle can eradicate the need for trust, just as trust cannot be eradicated from any other human relationship. The present emphasis on autonomy has served to reduce the grosser violations of the integrity of persons. But the physician's character remains the ultimate safeguard of the patient's autonomous wishes.

The physician is the pathway through which decisions, actions, and policies relating to the patient must pass. He or she is in a position to enhance and protect the patient's capacity for self-determination. This sensitive position does not give the physician privileges, but only a heightened responsibility to be a steward of the moral quality of the healing relationship and the integrity of the person of the patient. The physician must never forget that he or she is automatically a moral accomplice in any policy, act, or decision that endangers the patient's integrity and autonomy. The fiduciary relationship is never entirely eradicable from the medical relationship. The physician must therefore be a person of integrity and must cultivate the virtue of fidelity to trust. In fact, fidelity is perhaps the most fundamental of the virtues of the physician—as essential as beneficence and effacement of self-interest (22).

The relationships between autonomy, integrity, and trust that I have outlined for the medical relationship are of course not unique. But the nature of illness (what it portends physically and emotionally) and the invasions of the integrity of persons that are entailed in being healed—taken together—form a constellation of obligations rarely encountered in other kinds of human activity. To be sure, medical ethics is a part of general moral philosophy—but an exquisitely sensitive part, given the phenomenology of being sick, being healed, and offering to heal.

For these reasons, a formula for morally defensible decision-making appears to be this: The decision should not be made by the physician in place of the patient, nor by the patient in isolation from the physician or the community. Phenomenologically, these elements of a medical decision are inseparable from each other. The morally optimal condition is one in which the decision arises between doctor and patient. That is, the physician should make the decision for, and with, the patient—the "for" signifying not "in place of" but "in the interests of" the patient. This formulation preserves the legal right to privacy, the moral claim to autonomy, and the deeper moral claim to the integrity of persons.

References

1. Faden, R. R., and T. L. Beauchamp. *A History and Theory of Informed Consent.* Oxford University Press, New York and Oxford, 1986. See especially pp. 235–268.

2. *Ibid.,* p. 3.

3. *Ibid.,* pp. 39–43.

4. *Griswold vs. Connecticut,* 381 U.S. 479 (1965).

5. *Pierce vs. Society of Sisters,* 268 U.S. 510 (1925); *Loving vs. Virginia,* 388 U.S. 1 (1967); *West Virginia State Board vs. Barnette,* 319 U.S. 624 (1943); *Eisenstadt vs. Baird,* 405 U.S. 438 (1972); *Roe vs. Wade,* 410 U.S. 113 (1973); *Griswold vs. Connecticut,* 381 U.S. 479 (1965).

6. *Schloendorff vs. Society of New York Hospitals,* 211 N.Y. 125, 126, 105, N.E. 92, 93 (1914).

7. Locke, J. *Of Civil Government; Two Treatises.* J. M. Dent, London, 1924.

8. Reck, A. Natural law and the Constitution. *The Review of Metaphysics,* March 1989, pp. 483–511.

9. Kant, I. *Groundwork for the Metaphysics of Morals.* Harper and Row, New York, 1964.

10. *Ibid.*, p. 103.

11. *Ibid.*, p. 105.

12. *Ibid.*, p. 107.

13. Mill, J. S. *On Liberty.* J. W. Parker, London, 1859.

14. United States. *Deciding to Forego Life-Sustaining Treatment.* Washington, D.C. President's Commission for the Study of Ethical Problems in Medicine and Biomedical and Behavioral Research. 1983.

15. Emanuel, L. L., and E. J. Emanuel. The medical directive. *JAMA* 261(22):3288–3293, 1989.

16. Wojtyla, K. *The Acting Person.* Dordrecht, Reidel, 1979.

17. Marcel, G. *Being and Having: An Existentialist Diary.* Harper and Row, New York, 1965, pp. 172–173.

18. Pellegrino, E. D. Toward a reconstruction of medical morality: The primacy of the act of profession and the fact of illness. *J Med Philos* 4(1):32–56, 1979.

19. Aristotle. Politics. In: R. McKeon (ed.). *Basic Works of Aristotle.* Random House, New York, 1968, p. 1129.

20. Beauchamp, T. L., and L. B. McCullough. *Medical Ethics: The Moral Responsibilities of Physicians.* Prentice Hall, Englewood Cliffs, 1984, pp. 82–85.

21. Pellegrino, E. D., and D. C. Thomasma. *For the Patient's Good: The Restoration of Beneficence in Health Care.* Oxford University Press, New York and Oxford, 1988.

22. Pellegrino, E. D. Character, virtue, and self-interest in the ethics of the professions. *Journal of Contemporary Health Law and Policy* 5:53–57, 1989.

Bioethics: Its Philosophical Basis and Application

Hans-Martin Sass

Medicine and philosophy are not alien to each other. The questions arising from the cycles of birth, life, happiness, suffering, pain, and death are essential questions of human existence. They are dealt with professionally by different methods in philosophy, ethics, and medicine. Within this context, classic medical philosophy deals with metaphysical concepts of (a) Man's place in Nature, (b) his or her relationship to the Divine, (c) health and disease, and (d) epistemologic and methodologic concepts of diagnosis, classification, risk assessment, and treatment. Classic medical ethics deals with judgments regarding the patient-physician relationship, the patient's "best interest," and the set of virtues required of the good physician.

Traditional Interactions of Medicine and Philosophy, Ethics and Expertise

Pythagorean thinking in the West and Taoist teaching in the East nearly 2,500 years ago laid the foundation for a medical philosophy emphasizing the principles of harmony and balance. Health and happiness were understood to represent a cosmic balance or a goal of harmony in life. Disease resulted from something out of balance. The role of medicine was to reinstitute balance or harmony, to fight imbalances and disharmonies, and to accept and understand the limits of medical expertise as natural limits of human manipulation. Both the *Corpus Hippocraticum* and early Asian medical authorities such as Sun Simiao in China (1) stress the im-

portance of philosophic studies for mastery in medicine.

Today the practice of medicine is guided by ethical principles that in turn are rooted in philosophic concepts. Among these ethical principles are *nil nocere*, "do no harm," and *bonum facere*, "do good for the patient." Most classic medical texts point to limitations on the goals of medicine and times when medical expertise may not be used. Euthanasia, abortion, torture, and exercising power or manipulating people by means of medical intervention may be especially excluded from good and masterful medical practice by such limits to professional conduct. Traditionally, medical ethics and expertise belong together. Ethics without expertise can never be efficacious, while expertise without ethics is unlikely to serve the patient's good.

Progress in medical technology and the rise of pluralistic society have produced a combination of factors responsible for the particular set of priorities prevailing in medical philosophy and ethics as we approach the twenty-first century. Modern medicine allows us to prolong the lives of some patients in intensive care to a point where we have to ask ourselves whether or not such prolongation is mandated by the medical ethos and its proud tradition. "Organ transplantation," "*in vitro* fertilization," "intensive care," "resuscitation," and "psychopharmacopeia" are some of the new terms suggesting the increased moral responsibilities that arise from increased technical capabilities, while other terms like "teamwork," "medical specialists," "shift work," "sickness insurance," and "health care systems" point to organizational changes in the traditional physician-patient relationship. Within this context, terms such as "patient autonomy" and "informed consent" have emerged from trends toward a more "emancipated" lifestyle and individual self-understanding by the educated citizen.

Even the new term "bioethics" indicates that epistemologic and moral aspects of providing health care services can no longer be described in terms of the traditional parameters of the physician-patient relationship. Bioethics encompasses a field that is wider than just the relationship between the individual physician and the patient, one that includes a professional responsibility toward all forms of life as well as the specific ethos that must prevail in modern forms of institutionalized and organized medicine (2).

Among the numerous philosophic issues of bioethics, the following will be taken up in this article: (a) concepts of health and disease, (b) the principles of bioethics, (c) the physician-patient relationship, (d) lifestyle "medicalization" and related value issues.

Medical and Moral Uncertainty and the Models of Medical Science

Descartes, during the high days of rationalism, postulated that only those things would be true which could be perceived clearly and distinctly: "*illud omne esse verum quod valde clare et distincte percipio*" (3). However, if such a clear and distinct perception were required before any medical intervention, physicians would rarely be able to act.

Descartes' critics developed the NeoKantian theory of science, differentiating between the nomothetic sciences (natural science) and the idiographic sciences (the humanities) (4). Here again, the risky business of diagnosis, prognosis, and therapy did not fit the models, which were confined to setting laws or describing ideas.

Toulmin has suggested that the historical model proposed by Vico provides a better framework for analyzing medical science than does the Cartesian geometric model (5). After all, the human body, its health, the deterioration of its health, and accidents that pose risks to its health all have a history. This history, reconstructed in medical anamnesis, provides information for predicting possible future developments, with or without medical intervention.

Reviewing the various parameters involved, it seems clear that medicine is neither a science in the strict sense of the word (a "natural" science) nor a judgmental art. Rather, it is an expert method of assessing risks, handling uncertainties, and making prognoses in a professionally responsible manner based on experience, role models, and other factors.

The application of ethics in medicine follows the same rules as the application of technical expertise in medicine. Both require careful and differential diagnosis, a weighing of the options of intervention, and selection of the most beneficial option. Medical diagnosis follows the rules of interpretation, researching and assessing individual patients' stories of well-being and well-feeling; for just as life is a story that can be narrated, so are the changes, improvements, and deteriorations in life. But in contrast to hermeneutics (interpretation) in the humanities, medicine does not just interpret but acts on the results of hermeneutic procedures, dialectically intertwining interpretation and interaction, measurement and manipulation, theory and practice.

Clearly, medicine cannot be reduced to the parameters of a simple natural science. The professional responsibility for healing and comforting cannot depend exclusively on the results of blood tests or other scientific data. The patient's values are as important as such test results for diagnosis, prognosis, and deciding upon a course of therapeutic action.

Similarly, the values of the physician and the values incorporated into the health care environment are as important as the technical abilities of individual health care professionals, the technical capacity of the health care system, and the technical quality of the participating health care institutions. Of particular interest is the role professional organizations play in shaping, protecting, and developing the principles of professional ethics, paternalistically guiding both their members and their members' clients.

When it comes to patient care, it is important to be aware of the value-laden environment of medical intervention. This is the reason that checklists for nonscientific data have been developed—to help deal with personal and value issues in the physician-patient relationship and in the process of determining the "patient's best interest" (6, 7). Nevertheless, medical intervention should not be based solely on scientific data—because of the complex nature of medical explanation, because of essential uncertainties in diagnosis and prognosis, and because the aim of medicine is to treat the entire patient rather than isolated symptoms or diseases. Therefore, especially in this age of high medical technology, the history of medical science supports a demand for reappreciation of traditional humanist and ethical values that were a part of the "healing arts and sciences"; for in good medical practice the patient's axiogram is as important as his or her hemogram. The concepts of health, well-being, well-feeling, and happiness, as well as their opposites, involve more than laboratory data. Within this context, bioethics is the necessary complement of bioscience; for while bioscience is based on principles of natural science and risk assessment, bioethics is based on the moral principles developed during the history of general and professional ethics and their application.

Principles of Bioethics in the Modern World

Contemporary medicine involves a lot more than the growth of technologies that permit medical intervention in cases where no effective intervention was possible before. The technologic changes of the modern world have been accompanied by changes in social and cultural attitudes that emphasize the individual's impor-

tance as the prime decision-maker in value-related questions of life's style and goals. Indeed, modern society has been called pluralistic because it has developed a wealth of different sets of value-priorities for individuals and because it emancipates the educated citizen from formerly dominating and quite often indoctrinating ideational forces.

Educated citizens, both as clients and providers of services, have to communicate regarding the risks and the benefits that certain services entail—because the cultural and moral assessment of risk by different educated persons in a pluralistic society may not be the same. This new situation in a society rich in different individual value preferences requires concentration on the traditional mid-level moral principles of medical ethics—principles such as beneficence, nil nocere, justice, professional responsibility, patient autonomy, individual good, common good, pain care, and not prolonging the process of dying (8). These principles of bioethics have been and will continue to be recognized by a broad range of religious, philosophic, and ideologic viewpoints. As Jesus stressed in the study of the Good Samaritan (Luke, 10, 25ff), the mid-level principle of mutual aid to a neighbor can be supported by a variety of metaphysical or religious traditions.

Regarding the traditional principle of medical beneficence, it is comforting to note that this concept can be supported and indeed has been supported by traditions as diverse as Christian ethics of different denominations, the non-religious humanist tradition, British utilitarian philosophy, Kantian rigorisms of a Categorical Imperative, Marxist concepts of solidarity, even the anarchist concept of mutual aid proposed by Kropotkin. Other principles of bioethics that can be widely supported by various traditions in a pluralistic society include respect for patient autonomy, the principle of "doing no harm," and the idea that the individual patient's case should have priority over general political or economic considerations. As this suggests, it appears that certain mid-level principles are essential for good medical practice, regardless of the different cultural or historical circumstances in which medical services are rendered.

Other principles are harder to apply to specific cases, because people disagree about matters such as contraception, abortion, and withholding treatment from severely handicapped newborns or comatose or brain-dead patients. However, bioethics has developed a number of pragmatic principles for reducing moral risks that can help diminish or resolve some of the problems arising from different world views in pluralistic societies (9). Focusing on these mid-level principles instead of contending against others' basic beliefs can contribute to development of a peaceful society rich in diverse values. Among the principles:

☐ A leading principle of bioethics and all other applied ethical systems in a pluralistic society is that of respecting the individual citizen's priorities—so that no one is asked to perform acts that he or she cannot justify morally. Among other things, this means never asking someone to perform an abortion or to share blood or organs if that person feels aborting fetuses or sharing blood or organs is unjustifiable for religious, metaphysical, or other reasons.

☐ The century-old Thomist principle of subsidiarity holds that services that can be provided on a decentralized volunteer basis should not be handled by the central government or dealt with at the societal level. Such decentralization tends to reduce political pressure for central government institutions to accept responsibility in controversial areas, while simultaneously encouraging volunteer and decentralized groups to act according to their own specific moral priorities.

☐ In a similar vein, the individual patient's urgent needs should take precedence over general considerations of justice for all and also over considerations relating to the structure of the general health care system; this allows the physician to differentiate between his or her medical obligations as a professional and civic duties as a citizen.

☐ Another principle, that of human solidarity, requires that assistance and protection against suffering be given to a fellow human being despite profound individual ideologic or religious differences.

☐ Also, it should be noted that moral assessments in specific cases require micro-application of bioethical concepts in order to precisely target intended moral and medical goals. For example, informed consent must be applied this way in some particular form—such as proxy consent, presumed consent, educated consent, consent under pain, persuaded consent, or a living will. Similarly, the beneficent physician has to apply his or her good intentions this way in cases where there is a conflict between aims—so as to either reduce pain or provide aggressive treatment, prolong life or comfort the patient, and provide intensive care or palliative care.

☐ Finally, there are many times when more than one moral principle must be applied to the same case. This requires mixed application of principles in possible conflict with each other—such as respect for the patient's autonomy and a paternalistic sense of medical responsibility, or achieving reduction of pain with drugs that might pose severe risks for the patient's health or life.

The Beneficent Physician and the Patient's Good

Changes in the social and institutional delivery of health care services, as well as societal and cultural movement toward a more pluralistic society, have influenced the physician-patient relationship. In the days of Hippocrates—and indeed, up to the last century—the efficacy of medicine was rather marginal, and the doctor defined what was good for the patient. Today the definition of *bonum facere*—beneficence, doing what is in the patient's best interests—cannot be defined exclusively by the physician, for two reasons.

The first reason is that while medical options for intervention are abundant, the goal of intervention needs to be defined. Should one choose aggressive and intensive postoperative chemotherapy or radiotherapy, or should one choose palliative care? Which best serves the patient's "good"?

The second reason is that different people have different concepts of life and what they want from it. Some place strong emphasis on health, while others abide unhealthy "workaholic" habits or recreational drug consumption; some emphasize paying for health insurance or saving for old age, while others prefer spending to make life more pleasant now.

Pellegrino and Thomasma have found an unhealthy overemphasis on autonomy in contemporary bioethics and have called for restoration of the beneficence principle in the form of *beneficence-in-trust*, i.e., "that physicians and patients hold 'in trust' (Latin: *fiducia*) the goal of acting in the best interests of one another" (*10*). They hold that patients as well as physicians need to orient themselves according to specific sets of virtues; and they propose a "post-Hippocratic oath" that transforms basic Hippocratic principles, adapting them to the modern world of educated patients and to the sharing of decision-making between patient and physician.

The role of the physician in the post-Hippocratic era relates to at least three different models: (a) The Hippocratic model deals with the anthropologic and existential situation of urgent aid and urgent need; this is the traditional model, one that cannot be replaced so long as fellow humans suffer and are in need of moral and medical attention. (b) The contractual model sees the physician as the provider and the patient as the recipient of specialized services—such as specialized diagnosis and treatment, laboratory work, radiation therapy, anesthesia, and certain specialized kinds of surgery. This model envisions the patient as having full autonomy and the physician-patient relationship as being no different from other provider-client relationships. (c) The partner model makes the physician the patient's consultant and partner in managing long-term health risks or chronic diseases such as diabetes or hypertension. The patient is involved as the main gatekeeper of his or her balance of health, well-being, or well-feeling; the physician's role is to assist the patient's self-help efforts. More than the other two models, this one requires an educated patient ready to accept the major share of responsibility (*11*). All three models describe different physician-patient situations, which in specific cases can be found mixed together in varying degrees.

The Virtuous Patient and Lifestyle-related Health Risks

Bioethics has focused extensively on the physician's changing role and responsibilities, but has tended to neglect the educated citizen's role as patient, gatekeeper for good health, and preventer of health risks.

Traditionally, the only two virtues required of the patient were compliance and trust. Low levels of education and of means to assure good health kept the ordinary citizen from becoming involved in medical decision-making, prevention of health risks, or responsibility for health. There was classic nutritional teaching, which applied the wisdom of the Golden Rule by telling people to avoid the extremes in life and thereby reduce individual exposure to risk; but this was relatively bland and general compared to the concept that has replaced it—one that regards medicine as intervention to repair defects that could have been avoided in the first place.

Today, more and more diseases and health risks appear lifestyle-related. Within this context, we have a moral obligation to consider not only the citizen's right to good health care, but also the citizen's duty and responsibility for health care. This latter is primarily an obligation to safeguard personal health through proper nutrition, exercise, recreation, and avoidance of occupational and recreational health risks. Two reasons for this obligation: It is morally difficult to accept the idea that the benefits (if any) of lifestyles that pose a threat to health should accrue to the individual, while related health costs are shared socially. Also, it contravenes the concept of citizen and patient autonomy if the individual is disinclined to deal responsibly with personal health care matters.

Wherever public health care is readily available, some personal value conflicts will be dealt with indirectly by "medicalizing" feelings such as unhappiness, frustration, disappointment, and grief. Such action constitutes an abuse of medical knowledge and is actually counterproductive for purposes of confronting and mastering the personal crises and challenges of life.

Concluding Remarks

The future of medicine—and of health and happiness—will depend on good and prudent analysis, assessment and management of philosophic questions, and development of moral expertise related to health and well-being—just as over the last hundred years good and successful medicine has depended on careful analysis, assessment, and management of technical expertise. The future of bioethics, however, will depend on the progress that it can make in establishing and reaffirming both physician and patient ethics—the ethics of educated and responsible people who, as Aristotle maintained in a past age, are the most essential ingredients for a peaceable, happy, and culturally rich society.

The health of future individuals and future societies will depend upon the extent to which accumulated philosophic and ethical knowledge can be put into practice—first by the educated

citizen and thereafter by the medical community. This will also pose the ultimate test of whether autonomy, responsibility, and beneficence are merely words in oaths, declarations, and philosophy books, or whether they are part and parcel of our human nature—a nature that admittedly still needs refinement and cultivation, but one inclined toward genuine acts of beneficence, comforting, healing, and support.

References

1. Qiu, R. Medicine, the art of humaneness. *Journal of Medicine and Philosophy* 13:277–300, 1988.
2. Sass, H. M. *Bioethik in den USA.* Springer, Heidelberg, 1988.
3. Descartes, R. *Meditationes de prima philosophiae (III).* Paris, 1641.
4. Windelband, W. Präludien. In: *Geschichte und Naturwissenschaften (fifth ed.).* Mohr, Tuebingen, 1915, pp. 136–160.
5. Toulmin, S. E. *An Examination of the Place of Reason in Ethics.* Cambridge University Press, New York, 1950.
6. Batistiole, J. V. *Protocolo de Bochum para la Práctica de Etica Médica.* Zentrum fúr Medizinische Ethik, Bochum, 1988.
7. Mainetti, J. M. *Protocolo para la Práctica Eticomédica.* Zentrum fúr Medizinische Ethik, Bochum, 1988.
8. Beauchamp, T. L., and J. F. Childress. *Principles of Biomedical Ethics (second ed.).* Oxford University Press, New York and Oxford, 1983.
9. Sass, H. M. *Training in Differential Ethics.* Zentrum fúr Medizinische Ethik, Bochum, 1990.
10. Pellegrino, E. D., and D. C. Thomasma. *For the Patient's Good: The Restoration of Beneficence in Health Care.* Oxford University Press, New York and Oxford, 1988.
11. Wolff, H. P. *Arzt und Patient.* Zentrum fúr Medizinische Ethik, Bochum, 1989.

Ethical Problems of Medical Technology

Francisco Vilardell

The practice of medicine continually presents dilemmas of an ethical nature. Many conflicting alternatives compel the physician to make value judgments, choosing a path that respects the hopes and wishes of the patient while also respecting the dictates of politicians, who, in heeding the goal of Health for All by the Year 2000, incline more toward investment in society as a whole rather than in the isolated individual. This implies not only greater concern for primary, community, and family medicine, but also restraints—budgetary restrictions—upon the development of tertiary technology.

There is no doubt that these budgetary restrictions on tertiary care, which are the result of decisions taken by health authorities, conflict with the preference of broad segments of the population that have followed the technological advances of modern medicine and consider their proclaimed benefits to be valid and legitimate. Such technological advances range from spectacular forms of treatment—including organ transplants as well as biliary or renal lithotripsy using new and extremely costly equipment prototypes whose use is not yet well-defined—to methodologies used to obtain costly diagnoses, the most visible examples of which are imaging techniques (computerized tomography, magnetic resonance, etc.).

Despite the indisputable successes of these technologies in selected cases, their high cost renders medical care much more expensive, particularly if they are employed in the absence of precise and rigorous indications.

The desires of the patient, who wants to be examined or treated with the most advanced technology, are often in agreement with those of the physician. Indeed, as a matter of principle the physician favors technological development against the wishes of the health authorities, who see medical care costs rising well beyond all forecasts of inflation, without the technology involved appearing to offer compensatory benefits. Moreover, governments often feel powerless to halt a technological onslaught of this kind, whose successes cannot be ignored because of the publicity accompanying them, and which at times even appear to involve national prestige. Generally speaking, all this occurs with respect to any technological advance before proper cost/benefit studies have been conducted.

Technological Abuse

In recent years there have been many protests against the misuse of diagnostic tests by physicians—and not only with regard to advanced technology. A routine test erroneously prescribed for a large number of patients may incur losses as costly as those incurred by a sophisticated diagnostic test erroneously prescribed for a few patients.

A multicenter survey recently performed in the United States that examined the use of a series of preoperative diagnostic tests found that of the 6,200 tests performed on 2,000 patients, more than 60% were not warranted by the patient's clinical history or physical examination (1). Another multicenter survey in the same country showed that 17% of the digestive endoscopies performed were not specifically warranted (2), while other similar surveys have cited even higher figures (3). Perhaps more worrisome is the finding that some 17% of a series of 1,677 angiographies were not clearly warranted (2).

It is logical to suppose that if these discrepancies have been found at prestigious hospitals in the United States and other countries, then the discrepancies occurring in the realm of private practice, where much less control is exercised, are even greater. In this regard it is worth noting that both radiologists and analysts complain of the gradual increase in requests for analyses and diagnoses, many of them apparently unwarranted (4). And several interhospital meetings on these matters have confirmed that the use of diagnostic tests for the management of patients with the same disease varies greatly from one center to another (5).

Obviously, there are several ways in which diagnostic technologies may be used incorrectly (6). Tests may be performed when none are warranted; an excessive number may be performed, various of which are superfluous; or those performed may be less informative, less efficient, and more costly than other tests available for the same purpose. At present the available data lead to an inevitable conclusion—that many practitioners are unaware of the true usefulness of the tests they prescribe relative to others, with regard to either cost or possible value in different clinical circumstances (6).

Furthermore, beyond the realm of diagnostic tests are a whole host of more serious problems associated with incorrect use of therapeutic intervention. To cite only two examples, one study found that 32% of the endoarterectomies performed at several centers were unnecessary (6), while another yielded similar findings with respect to 20% of the pacemaker implantations performed at a Philadelphia hospital (7). Clearly, these matters demand attention.

The Relevance of Technology

The constant rise in medical service costs will no doubt lead to the development of surveys to investigate the use of both diagnostic and therapeutic techniques and their relevance to patient management. This relevance may differ from one country to another.

Unfortunately, advanced technology is often imported from a more developed country by a less developed one and used without taking account of local circumstances—including the organization of medical and technical personnel and the economic factors involved in use of the technology. Consequently, it is not surprising that maintenance difficulties arise, that the results are not entirely satisfactory or comparable to those obtained in the country of origin, and that the end result is a squandering of resources.

However, the rapid growth of technology that has led to this misuse, excessive consumption, and diversion of funds assigned to more pressing primary care needs appears to be uncontainable. The sensationalist influence of the mass media, whose information is far from objective, usually impels the public to demand use of "life-saving" technologies in which it has placed its often unfounded hopes. Since all too frequently the results offer nothing more than a precarious and pitiful quality of life, this combination of circumstances makes an already uncontrollable market grow substantially and press for development of costly technologies publicized via sales techniques similar to those usually employed to market everyday consumer goods—development of technologies that often goes unaccompanied by development of the trained personnel needed to make those technologies fulfill their promise.

Any comparison of the year-to-year costs of X-ray machines, ultrasound equipment, fiber-optic endoscopes, pressure monitors, etc. reveals that the prices increase each year far more rapidly than the cost of living. Moreover, high import duties are levied on such items—duties that paradoxically tend to be higher in the countries that need the items most. This constant escalation of prices is not necessarily accompanied by greater equipment yields or by any clear added patient benefit.

The situation is even more serious in countries with significantly aging populations, to which ever-increasing resources must be allocated. This contrasts with the fact that complete periodic examination of asymptomatic individuals requires relatively few tests involving no costly apparatus (8).

Causes of Technological Abuse

A serious problem emerges from the fact that technologies of the sort described may invade the health care market without having been subjected to careful scrutiny regarding possible risks, actual benefits, and superiority vis-à-vis other procedures customarily employed. This is evident in the case of heart surgery, whose benefits have been the cause of controversy for years, and in the case of heart and liver transplants, which, after many years of experimentation, only now appear to be providing hopeful results.

This lack of precise data in evaluating results only gives rise to substantial doubts when decisions must be taken regarding the suitability of intervention. A common consequence is overuse of interventions, since, in case of doubt, use rather than nonuse tends to be the rule, particularly if use is accompanied by financial benefit to the user.

John Farrar (9) has studied physicians' motivations for using new technologies. He has found the motivations to range from a noble desire to assist the patient all the way to desire for profit, desire for enhanced prestige in an academic or hospital setting, desire to experience the fascination or pleasure associated with performing a new procedure, and the simple desire for self-protection against possible legal action, particularly when facing the legal circumstances found in the United States.

Ethical Aspects of Medical Technology

Although it is not possible to subject new medical technology to quantitative analysis with respect to the foregoing concerns (10), the following questions must be answered: Is the use of a new technology warranted on the basis of its cost, results, and efficacy? Are the available personnel sufficiently trained to use it properly? Is the new technology superior to those in use, and does it offer economic advantages? Will it improve the quality of life of patients who use it? Will it be available for use by the general population, or will it be reserved for the privileged few? Have its short-term and long-term risks been identified? Have any studies been made of other options that could prove a better investment?

Although the costs and benefits of new technologies have been widely discussed in recent years, much less attention has been paid to the entrance of such technologies into medical practice and the mechanisms that are or should be required for their acceptance. For instance, What kinds of studies are required for their approval? What kind of consent should be obtained from patients before a new technology is applied? Do physicians have a special obligation to inform their patients that the benefits of a new technology are still uncertain? These are questions that demand clear answers (11).

During a 1976 symposium held in Budapest on the ethical problems of managing patients with digestive disorders (12), participants developed a list of variables for use in assessing the risks of diagnostic techniques. These variables, which are worth recalling when any new diagnostic technology is being considered, are shown in Table 1.

An opinion that has become increasingly prevalent is that introduction of new technology is akin to research and should consequently be subjected to controls similar to those used for evaluation of new drugs (11). In the United States such controls have been precisely defined by the National Commission for the Protection of Human Subjects of Biomedical and Behavioral Research, to the effect that all procedures or their variants—diagnostic, therapeutic, or preventive—that are used with the aim of obtaining a direct benefit for the health of patients and that differ from customary routine practice

Table 1. Factors influencing risk in diagnostic techniques.

Factor	Risk
Instrument	Inherent in the instrument (for example, flexible or rigid endoscopes)
	Defective maintenance of instruments
Technique	Preparation of the patient incurs risk (for example, intubation, enema, or allergy to contrast mediums)
	Risk of the technique itself (for example, hemorrhage or perforation)
	Delayed secondary effects (for example, thrombosis or infection)
Operator	Operator with insufficient experience
	Untrained auxiliary personnel
	Careless operator (for example, omission of routine precautions)
Interpretation	Technical defects (for example, defective sampling or poor-quality X-rays)
	Inexperience of the interpreter of the results
Patient	High-risk patient
	Uncooperative patient

Source: F. Vilardell (*12*).

should be subjected to a research protocol to determine their safety and efficacy (*13*).

The United States has been a pioneer in these evaluations, and several reports relating to them have been published (*14, 15*). Obviously, the basic problem is deciding whether modification of an established technique should be considered research or not, a situation that may differ from one hospital to another. The correct answer depends on careful review of the circumstances in the local environment by an ethics committee organized within the institution where the question arises, one that has been assigned the task of ensuring that no technique will be used in the institution that has not been previously evaluated (*13*).

In this same vein, an ethics seminar sponsored by the World Organization of Gastroenterology some years ago (*16*) prompted a noteworthy discussion, among other things, of the development, selection, and evaluation of new technical procedures. Although these procedures were related to the field of gerontology, the meeting's conclusions appear perfectly valid for any other field of medicine. These conclusions were as follows:

First, an important distinction was made between the advent of previously unproven techniques (that is, techniques being tested for the

first time) and the introduction of new techniques at a hospital center. The former clearly involves research and should adhere to the controls defined by the Declaration of Helsinki. All such unproven technology should be subjected to comparative studies with regard to the technology already in use—among other things so as to prevent its rapid introduction into practice, tacit acceptance, and dissemination from interfering with later objective evaluation.

Second, it was proposed that when a recently invented technique is adopted in a hospital, the hospital's ethics committee should evaluate it in order to establish the basis for a study ensuring that appropriate trained personnel will be available to manage it and that the advance consent of patients upon whom the new technique is to be used will be obtained.

Third, particular attention was given to the need for testing a new technique on volunteers (especially on medical, nursing, and other students recruited for this purpose) during the initial phases of its adoption (*16*). The use of coercive recruitment methods or ones involving academic remuneration are clearly to be avoided.

Finally, it was noted that introduction of new technology has commercial implications for industry, making it necessary to ensure that a technology being introduced receives appropriate evaluation by selected medical centers or societies. In no case should industry influence publication of the results of these evaluations.

Technology and Society

The President of the Royal College of Surgeons of the United Kingdom has classified technological medical advances into three categories: those that facilitate the prevention of disease and promote health with little expenditure; those that permit the cure of disease at moderate cost; and those that make it possible to maintain health and a reasonable quality of life but whose success depends on the expenditure of substantial material and human resources (16). As far as society is concerned, it is obviously the latter that create problems, since over the long run economic factors will decide whether or not the advent of a new technology is to have a direct impact upon a community by facilitating, limiting, or barring use of that technology.

In a certain sense this implies a rationing of health resources, which although indirect is nonetheless real (17). The fact that a technique is available does not necessarily mean it should be used, especially if resources are scarce and restrict its use. This is the situation prevailing in the case of heart or liver transplants, for example, because prolific use of these procedures could overwhelm all medical budgets and obstruct programs of more general interest. (In our own hospital we could vaccinate multitudes of employees at risk of contracting hepatitis B for the price of a single heart or liver transplant operation, regardless of its result—18).

Despite these objections, advanced technology, including transplant surgery, is a firmly entrenched if debatable medical and social reality. It is very difficult, if not impossible, to accurately determine its costs and benefits because the studies required are extremely complex in view of the extraordinary number of variables involved whose management gives rise to very diverse interpretations (6). Therefore, a sound balance between the absolutely necessary promotion of technical advances and the economic drain they may impose is hard to strike, especially in a society accustomed to renovation of what has come to be seen as obsolescence in other commonly used technologies (involving such items as household electrical appliances, sound systems, computers, etc.).

What this really means is that society or its representatives must demand that the introduction of new medical technologies be accompanied from the outset by systematic evaluation of their correct application and their benefits. If this were done, many of the current problems would be at least partially avoided—especially in the developing countries, which see themselves as being forced to adopt advanced technologies in order to dissuade numerous patients within their populations from going to other countries, often unnecessarily, to seek medical relief (19).

References

1. Kaplan, E. B., L. B. Sheiner, A. J. Boeckmann, et al. The usefulness of preoperative laboratory screening. JAMA 253:3576–3581, 1985.
2. Chassin, M., J. Kosecoff, R. E. Park, et al. Does inappropriate use explain geographic variations in the use of health care services? JAMA 258:2533–2537, 1987.
3. Kahn, K. L., J. Kosecoff, M. R. Chassin, et al. Use and misuse of upper gastrointestinal endoscopy. Ann Intern Med 109:664–670, 1988.
4. Fowkes, F. G. R. Containing the use of diagnostic tests. Br Med J 290:488–489, 1985.
5. Ashley, J. S. A., P. Pasker, and J. C. Beresford. How much clinical investigation? Lancet 1:890–892, 1972.
6. Jennet, B. High Technology Medicine: Benefits and Burdens. Oxford University Press, Oxford, 1986, pp. 53–74.
7. Greenspan, A. M., H. R. Day, B. C. Berger, et al. Incidence of unwarranted pacemaker implantation in a large medical population. N Engl J Med 318:158–163, 1988.
8. Oboler, S. K., and F. M. La Force. The periodic physical examination in asymptomatic adults. Ann Intern Med 110:214–226, 1989.
9. Farrar, J. Gastroenterology and the impact of the rise of technology in the United States. Ital J Gastroenterol 21:49–52, 1989.
10. Institute of Medicine, Committee for Evaluation of Medical Technologies in Clinical Use. Assessing Medical

Technologies. National Academy Press, Washington, D.C., 1985, pp. 154–160.

11. McMahon, L. F., D. Fleischer, and R. Levine. Emerging technology: Patient protection versus proliferation. *J Clin Gastroenterol* 9:258–273, 1987.

12. Vilardell, F. (ed.). Ethical problems in the management of gastroenterological patients. *Scand J Gastroenterol* 12(suppl):47, 1977.

13. United States, National Commission for the Protection of Human Subjects of Biomedical and Behavioral Research. *The Belmont Report: Ethical Principles and Guidelines for the Protection of Human Subjects of Research.* DHEW Publication (OS) 78–0012, 1978. U.S. Government Printing Office, Washington, D.C., 1978.

14. Kessler, D. A., S. M. Pape, and D. N. Sundwall. The federal regulation of medical devices. *N Engl J Med* 317:357–365, 1987.

15. Perry, S. Technology assessment: Continuing uncertainty. *N Engl J Med* 314:240–243, 1986.

16. Black, D. The paradox of medical care. *J R Coll Physicians Lond* 13:57–65, 1979.

17. Churchill, L. R. *Rationing Health Care in America: Perceptions and Principles of Justice.* University of Notre Dame Press, Notre Dame, Indiana, 1987.

18. Vilardell, F. Organ transplantations: Are they ethical? *World Health,* June 1988, pp. 20–21.

19. Woolhandler, S., D. U. Himmelstein, B. Labar, et al. Transplanted technology: Third World options and First World science. *N Engl J Med* 317:504–506, 1987.

The Moral Meaning of Religion for Bioethics

Courtney S. Campbell

Religion is inescapably concerned with questions of health, medicine, and disease. In the normative scriptures of the Judeo-Christian tradition, images of God as healer and physician are powerful and prominent. At the same time, religious communities have historically seen the existence of disease as confirming evidence of the presence of evil and sin in the world; indeed, the nature and extent of disease, as in the case of plague, for example, can present serious theologic questions about the moral character of the Deity.

Moreover, our very concepts of "health" and "disease" reflect values that are frequently influenced by religious presuppositions. Thus, whether an alcoholic is considered a sinner, a criminal, or a victim of genetic or environmental factors beyond his or her control involves evaluations that can be conditioned by theologic perspectives on free will, human nature, and appropriate social conduct. Similarly, the "suffering" caused by illness, while undesired, may not be considered meaningless from a religious standpoint. And an impaired newborn may yet be considered a "gift" of God with a special religious meaning, rather than an unwanted burden for its parents.

The complex ways in which religion encompasses and qualifies health, medicine, and disease help explain its multifaceted relation to bioethics. Regarding bioethics itself, tremendous technologic advances in the United States in the mid-1960s and broader moral concerns about individual self-determination and social justice converged to generate this very distinctive and innovative field of ethical inquiry. At that point theologians found themselves in the unique position of being able to give bioethics an initial impetus and substantive direction, because they brought to bear on its subject matter the substantial resources of the moral reflection, historic traditions, and practices of religious communities. Some very new questions about life and death could be put into context and more readily approached from the direction of already-formed convictions about respect for the individual's integrity and his or her body, care and treatment for the dying, a demand for equity in the provision of health care, and a concern for including the socially voiceless and vulnerable within the boundaries of the moral community.

This article will consider how religion has held and can hold moral meaning for bioethics and enrich it—both in a descriptive, empirical manner and in a normative, conceptual manner. It will also examine how one complex bioethical issue (whether available medical technology should be used to prolong life) might be approached from the standpoint of different religious traditions.

Religion and the Secularization of Bioethics

As a matter of simple historic evolution, it is safe to say that contemporary bioethics is substantially indebted to religion. The very concrete considerations that fall under the domain of bioethics, such as whether a particular person should be treated medically or allowed to die, are often rightly credited with prompting a major transformation in philosophic ethics from an abstract, analytical discipline to an applied one. By contrast, the religions of Western culture, embedded in practicing historic communities, have always had concrete dimensions of morality (as manifested in the imperative of neighbor-love) and spirituality; initially, therefore, their affinity for questions of bioethics was direct and not open to question.

This influence of religious perspectives, especially strong in the formative years of bioethics, is now no longer as extensive or as explicit in the United States, though it may be in many nations where bioethics has only recently begun to gain a foothold. Therefore, it is important to examine retrospectively what has been termed the "secularization of bioethics" in the United States as a way of possibly illuminating the prospective nature of the relationship between religion and bioethics in other countries.

One meaning of the term "secularization" is *removal* of central institutions (medicine) or values (health) from the influence of religious thought and practice. This has undeniably occurred to a significant extent in the development of bioethics in the United States. The field is now suffused with philosophic and legal paradigms, principles, and discourse; religion seems morally interesting only when a particularly difficult issue arises, such as refusal of medical treatment for a minor on religious grounds.

Part of the reason is that bioethics issues, much more than in the past, are vexing matters of *public* policy. Determination of death, for example, is no longer considered the exclusive preserve of medical practitioners, but one that needs public scrutiny, perhaps by a government advisory panel. The question of whether a particular patient should receive an organ transplant to prolong his or her life no longer involves simply organ availability and compatibility, but also the concern of legislators who believe the money spent on "rescue" medicine to save one life might be better spent on "preventive" medicine, such as prenatal care for expectant mothers, that will ultimately benefit many people.

This prominent public policy orientation of contemporary bioethics has worked against consideration of religious perspectives in a couple of important ways.

Religion in the United States is considered an essentially "private" matter. It must not be discriminated against—on grounds of respect for freedom of conscience—but neither can it be "established" or appealed to as a basis for public policy. Thus, in the very composition of a pluralistic society there is an inherent bias against conceptions of human goodness or welfare that are attributable to particular convictions, including religious convictions, that are not generalizable or shared by the entire society. Since all citizens are presumed to have a stake in "public" policy, the basis for policy on a controversial bioethics issue must reside in some common convictions, rather than on religious grounds that may prove divisive.

Also, from *within* theologic circles longstanding disputes worked to minimize the significance of religion for bioethics. In particular, theologians (as well as philosophers) questioned whether religious views really made any *distinctive* (that is, different from philosophic) contributions to bioethics debates, especially as these debates came to be directed at finding a suitable policy for the entire public. If they did not make a distinctive contribution, so the reasoning went, philosophic approaches could work just as well and were preferable because they were presumed to be less divisive in a pluralistic society.

But even if the differences of religion for ethics could be successfully articulated for a public audience, some theologic ethicists questioned whether this was an *appropriate* audience. They suggested that the primary vocational responsibility of a theologian is to respond to the spiritual and moral claims of his or her own religious tradition and practicing community; in speaking to a broader audience than one's tradition, or doing bioethics on behalf of a "public," the integrity of the vocation of theologian is compromised. These two *theological* constraints on an invigorating relation between religion and bioethics continue to persist and to present an important challenge for theologians in the United States and other countries.

But "secularization" can also mean that values and beliefs once explicitly affirmed as religious may command widespread acceptance, even if their religious grounds do not. Using this definition, the "secularization of bioethics" may mean that religion has an important leavening impact on bioethics even if its influence is not recognized as such. Religious concerns about the "sanctity of human life," human "stewardship" for nature, and protecting the vulnerable in the human community can support practices and principles of medical treatment, technology, and care that are presented publicly on secular or philosophic grounds. We can develop this aspect of secularization further by considering the relation between religion and the normative principles of bioethics.

Religion and the Bioethics Paradigm

The moral controversies of contemporary bioethics are typically analyzed with reference to what has been termed "the bioethics paradigm," which consists of a "trinity" of moral concepts—those of beneficence, justice, and autonomy.

Beneficence, at its minimum, requires moral agents to refrain from harming others; it can also involve positive obligations to do good to others and promote their welfare. Provision of medical treatment conforms to this principle because it typically benefits a patient.

The principle of *justice* obligates one to ensure that the benefits of health care (or in some cases the burdens, such as taxes for hospitals) are distributed fairly and equitably. For example, the benefits of experimental research on human beings can be inestimable for many people, but it is important that those subject to the risks of experimentation not be drawn unfairly from a particularly vulnerable class of people—such as children, prisoners, or the mentally retarded—or

be selected on the basis of nonmedical criteria such as race, ethnicity, or social class that can reflect discrimination.

The principle of *autonomy* obliges us to treat other people as ends in themselves and respect their freedom, liberty of action, and self-determined choices. Respect for autonomy is presupposed in moral positions and legal decisions that require patients' informed consent to treatment and that recognize patients' rights to privacy and to refuse medical treatment.

Each of these governing principles, while capable of defense and explication in the discourse of secular moral philosophy, is compatible with fundamental themes in religious traditions. The principle of beneficence, both historically and conceptually, is rooted in the commandment of neighbor-love. There is also implicit in this commandment a universalistic impulse that accommodates a shift in moral concern from the one to the many, thus encompassing the norm of justice.

In addition, major religious traditions of Western culture have affirmed that we share a common origin and destiny: We are created as social beings to live in community with other persons, so that the collective good and equality must be in the forefront of our moral universe.

Moreover, these traditions understand all human beings to be created in the image of God (*imago Dei*); and this *imago Dei* concept not only reinforces a sense of commonality and equality but also respect for individual autonomy. Thus, moral norms with profound meaning for religious traditions have served and can continue to serve as background presuppositions of the bioethics paradigm.

Nevertheless, these affinities should not be mistaken for identity. From within the perspectives of a religious community, the meaning and content of the normative principles of bioethics will be deepened and transformed. Neighbor-love does indeed encompass duties of refraining from doing harm and having at least minimal expectations of benefitting others; but in a religious context these expectations will typically be heightened to the extent that some degree of self-sacrifice will be required so that the good of others is pursued actively.

The principle of justice may also be vested with different meaning in a religious context. In some theologic traditions, such as that of the theology of liberation propounded by some theologians and priests in Latin America, justice is informed by a "preferential option" for the poor. That is, in considering social justice issues, including such things as access to quality health care, the needs of the society's most vulnerable members are given priority over strict adherence to equality. We do not all begin life with the same choices, resources, and capacities; and the "preferential" qualification of justice can be understood as an attempt to redress those natural and social inequalities that exist for reasons beyond our control, and that deprive some people of full participation in the life and benefits of society.

In a similar manner, the *imago Dei* concept transforms understandings of the meaning of autonomy. In contrast to an exclusive focus on autonomous choice and freedom of will, the *imago Dei* concept asserts that people are more than their wills; they are *embodied* selves; and so, just as much as their rational faculties, their physical, temporal bodies are deserving of moral respect.

This conviction has practical implications when the ethics of organ procurement policies are examined. Certain policies may be considered theologically suspect or even unacceptable because of their implicit disrespect for the body (in the case of routine salvage policies, for example) or commercialization of it (in the case of an organ market).

Moreover, autonomy frequently presupposes an excessively narrow, individualistic vision of moral life, a temptation limited by the solidarity and community with all other persons expressed in the *imago Dei*. The theologic concept therefore contains inherent limits on freedom and individual choice that may not be adequately conveyed by the normative principle of autonomy.

Religious traditions will therefore not consider the moral dimensions of bioethics to be exhaustively subsumed under the normative principles encompassed by the bioethics paradigm; indeed, an ethical model that proceeds on such an assumption is in fundamental respects limited and substantively deprived. This is not only because a religious perspective may alter and transform the meaning of these norms, but also because the paradigm itself presents a somewhat distorted picture of the moral life. Specifically, in focusing on "problem-solving" in bioethics, the paradigm fails to adequately reflect the narrative structure of our lives and the stories all persons use for "problem-seeing." Significantly, "seeing" and "setting" moral problems in bioethics often occurs against the background of religiously informed narratives.

Playing God and Good Samaritans

Perhaps the most prominent metaphor for understanding bioethics in popular culture is that of "playing God." That perception typically conveys a negative evaluation, in that it is considered pretentious for human beings to "play God" with respect to creating life (through reproductive technologies), terminating it (by withholding medical treatments), or determining what type of people there will be (through genetic screening or engineering). Yet both this perception and negative evaluation assume the significance of a religious narrative, that of Creation, for seeing and interpreting the particular moral question. Indeed, without this religious presupposition, the phrase "playing God" would be unintelligible. My point here is that irrespective of the impact of religion at the level of bioethical problem-solving, it can be indispensable at a *prior* stage for *recognition* of what the moral issues are.

Once we have grasped how religious stories can fundamentally shape the way bioethical problems are understood, we can then raise some very interesting questions. What, for example, does the metaphor of "playing God" convey morally that makes it such a commonly invoked expression in debates over reproductive technologies or genetic engineering? A partial answer is that it expresses a sense that human beings are taking control over, or usurping authority for, the process of creating life—in a way that at the very least prompts serious moral reservations. For we are in very important ways different from the nature of the Being presented and re-presented in theologic reflection. We have limited capacities for predicting the outcome of actions, controlling the courses of events that we initiate, or accurately evaluating the results of an action. The "playing God" metaphor, then, draws on a basic religious story to remind us of our finitude and fallibility, considerations that are of substantial moral significance when we contemplate "creating new life-forms."

In another context, however, the "playing God" metaphor may be invoked in a much more positive sense to prescribe, rather than critique, conduct. The story of God as one who is nonpreferential and indiscriminate in distributing resources necessary to life, who makes the sun and the rain to "fall on the just and unjust alike," provides a positive moral direction for many bioethicists confronted with the vexing issue of allocating scarce resources. That is, our allocation and rationing policies should likewise be nonpreferential and should affirm the fundamental equality of all human beings. This might, in contrast to the brave new world of reproductive technologies or genetic engineering, be construed as a "correct" way to play God in bioethics.

Another instructive example of how religious narratives can provide affirmative moral guidance in bioethics is presented by incorporation of the "Good Samaritan" image into the ethos of the medical profession. The Good Samaritan parable of Jesus has frequently been understood as the paradigm expression of the meaning of neighbor-love in the New Testament. It establishes expectations of self-sacrifice, care, and compassion on the part of moral agents toward anyone in need, even one who may be considered a stranger. Originally, of course, these ex-

pectations were established within a religious community. However, the story may well be used in other contexts, such as that of the medical profession, as a way of interpreting the profession's identity and moral meaning and articulating the responsibilities and commitments of physicians toward their patients. In this context the story does not function so much to resolve a moral problem as to set the moral and professional parameters within which the problem is then discussed.

Since our modern society has deep roots in a religious heritage, it should not be especially surprising that religious stories and narratives such as these (many others could be identified) provide a cultural perspective for understanding the moral problems found in bioethics. What is surprising is that this impact of religion upon bioethics is very seldom acknowledged. That is important, for we cannot know what conclusions to reach on a bioethical issue unless we have a clear idea of the questions formulated; and, I suggest, as often as not the questions formulated have been shaped by religious narratives.

Religious Perspectives on the Prolongation of Life

Up to now, this analysis has concentrated on very general ways that religious perspectives may influence, direct, and limit bioethics. The next point to be considered briefly is how different religious traditions—specifically Orthodox Jewish, Roman Catholic, and Protestant—approach one particular bioethics issue, the use of life-sustaining medical technology.

The theological premise of the *imago Dei* is prominent in each of these traditions and helps establish the moral parameters for discussion: Even in dying, and perhaps especially in dying, we are deserving of respect, care, and compassion. Also, each tradition has historically emphasized the sovereignty of God over life-and-death decisions, a fundamental theologic claim influencing our perspectives on the use of technology. Beyond these points of general convergence, however, themes particular to each tradition help shape distinctive positions.

In the tradition of Orthodox Judaism, life is sanctified as part of the work of the Creator and possesses absolute value. If life is threatened, it is deemed permissible in rabbinic reflection to violate all the laws of the Torah except the prohibitions against murder, idolatry, and adultery in order to save it. Thus, while the Orthodox Jewish tradition asserts God's ultimate sovereignty over life and death, it has also been open to technologic advances that hold promise for prolonging life. This has typically meant favoring all available means of life-support for patients who would die without life-sustaining treatment.

This strong commitment to the sanctity of life has also meant that Orthodox Judaism has been very reluctant to embrace technologic and medical developments that appear to risk shortening life. For example, the tradition has consistently opposed use of brain criteria to determine death, relying instead on traditional heart-lung criteria. This has meant a practical presumption against organ transplant, since organ procurement policies assume the validity of brain criteria for death. Even though an organ transplant may save the life of another, in a theologically real sense (informed by the Torah), the "donor" should not be considered "dead" until circulation and respiration cease.

In contrast, an historically important moral element in Roman Catholic reflection has been that while life is a fundamental and intrinsic value (because it reflects the goodness of the Creator), it is not an *absolute* value. Life is but the necessary condition for achieving greater human ends, which typically can be achieved only by an individual relating to a "community" of other human beings. Here the use of life-prolonging medical technology is considered a positive moral benefit to the extent that it maintains these relationships or sustains the individual's capacity to orient his or her life to the achievement of these greater ends.

In certain circumstances, however, the possibility of life in relation with others, the "quality of life," is very much diminished or altogether absent—as in the case of a permanently comatose patient such as Karen Ann Quinlan. In such cases, the Roman Catholic tradition has considered it permissible to withdraw or withhold certain forms of medical technology from dying patients; the reasoning commonly invoked by the tradition (which has been very influential in secular bioethics) has typically claimed that "ordinary" treatments are obligatory while "extraordinary" treatments are morally optional or discretionary.

The debate within the tradition then becomes which treatments fall into which category. For example, most Catholic moralists will accept that mechanical ventilation can be "extraordinary" treatment and can permissibly be withdrawn under appropriate circumstances; but there is much less consensus on whether it is permissible to withhold antibiotics or withdraw feeding tubes providing nutrition and hydration.

It is also possible that, in the course of a disease process, pain and suffering may become so excruciating as to permit only the most minimal modes of human interaction. The Roman Catholic tradition has historically prohibited suicide or assisted suicide, as well as active euthanasia, as unjustifiable killing and a usurpation of divine sovereignty. However, under the "rule of double effect" it has also asserted that it is permissible to provide substantial medication, such as morphine, for pain relief, even if the result is to hasten death. This would not be considered "active killing" in the Roman Catholic tradition, because the intent is compassionate, to relieve pain, even if death is foreseen as a "second effect" of the action. On the other hand, an actual intention to kill, by administering a lethal dose of medication for example, would violate the "rule of double effect" and would be considered unjustifiable.

The Roman Catholic tradition's emphasis on the relational quality of human life has enabled it to accommodate the idea of defining death by brain criteria much more than is possible in Orthodox Judaism. This in turn has provided a medical condition for organ transplant that is theologically reinforced by the theme of "community," for donated organs may save the lives of others who are part of a broader community or social whole.

Regarding the Protestant outlook, as is typical of Protestant theology in general, Protestant perspectives on life-prolonging medical treatment are very diverse. They range from a vitalistic commitment to the sanctity of life resembling Orthodox Judaism's, through a willingness to accept "quality of life" considerations in deciding whether to terminate treatment that is like the Catholic position, to a greater tolerance for even active euthanasia or medical killing to relieve suffering that overlaps with secular positions. This diversity itself reflects a fundamental Protestant theme—theologic commitment to the freedom of the believer. Yet this freedom, together with its implications for greater personal discretion in moral matters, can be limited in Protestant positions by both the *imago Dei* concept and that of "stewardship." The concept of "stewardship" (also present in Jewish and Catholic thought to some extent) asserts that we are entrusted by God with responsibility for our temporal lives and physical bodies, so that acting with disregard toward our lives or those of others is a violation of this trust. There are thus theologic resources within Protestant traditions that may establish presumptions against active euthanasia and in favor of organ transplants.

Conclusion

The significance of theologic perspectives cannot, as is so often the case, be considered of limited relevance to bioethics. Religious traditions and communities bring to these very difficult questions historically shaped substantive understandings of the nature and destiny of human beings and the moral norms they should live by. The value of religious understandings for bioethics is not that they provide answers that all must accept, but rather that they raise questions we need to confront.[1]

---

[1] J. M. Gustafson, *The Contributions of Theology to Medical Ethics*, Marquette University Press, Milwaukee, 1975, pp. 93–94.

PRACTICUM

Methodologies for Clinical Ethics

James F. Drane

Medical ethics is about decisions involving some element of difficulty. Existentialists remind us of the difficulty associated with the very act of deciding, given the effect choices have on the constitution of the self. Physicians and ethicists are aware of this difficulty, because each hard decision forces them to forego important possibilities and commit themselves and their resources to a certain option.

Decisions in a clinical setting can also be difficult because we may feel inclined to do something we know is morally wrong. Temptation is not something that occurs only outside the hospital. In fact, besides serving up its share of unusual temptations, the clinical setting sometimes intensifies and extends the ordinary ones as well.

Even more than in ordinary life, the clinical environment presents options and alternatives that make correct choice especially difficult. Many clinical cases are tragic—in the sense that the available alternatives seem wrong, and yet something has to be done. In many such cases the stakes are high, and the consequences are both hard to determine and difficult to accept.

One last difficulty peculiar to the clinical setting derives from the fact that each case is different and the right choice cannot be determined in advance. Therefore, in each new clinical situation a careful analysis of relevant data is essential.

Can Medical Ethics Be Anything but Relativistic?

The fact that modern medicine is wedded to powerful new technologies has created unprece-

dented new possibilities for treatment. Consequently, new moral problems abound. All these developments have been occurring in a period when secularization had previously undermined an older moral order based upon commonly held religious beliefs. Thus, not only has each new medical advance created new moral options, but choices from among these must be made in a climate of pluralism.

This situation has led some to despair about ethics. Those despairing tend to claim that any agreement about right and wrong in today's moral climate is impossible, and that radical subjectivism and relativism are inevitable.

However, this view seems unnecessarily pessimistic. Even when opposing views are based on seemingly incompatible belief systems, negotiation and compromise are possible. Different belief systems can lead to identical principles, and people of good will can come to agreement about what is right, even though they may disagree about ultimate meanings or the philosophic foundations of ethics. John Stuart Mill's utilitarianism is a long way from the ethics of Jesus, and yet Mill concluded that his ethics was basically the same as Jesus' Golden Rule. "In the Golden Rule of Jesus of Nazareth we read the complete spirit of the ethics of utility. To do as one would be done to, and to love one's neighbor as oneself, constitute the ideal perfection of utilitarian morality."[1] In fact, the tendency of

---

[1] J. S. Mill, *Utilitarianism*, Longmans, Green, London, 1987, Chapter 11, pp. 24, 25. The very same point was made by Thomas Hobbes, who is even further removed from religious foundations of ethics. Cf. T. Hobbes, *Leviathan*, in: Sir William Malesworth (ed.), *The English Works of Thomas Hobbes*, John Bohn, London, 1839, vols. 2 and 3, ch. 15, pp. 144–145.

different theoretical foundations toward a similar list of ethical standards (truth, sanctity of life, fidelity, autonomy, beneficence, justice, equality, respect for persons, reasonableness, etc.) gives solid grounds of hope for the prospects for overcoming radical relativism.

People of good will, including committed medical professionals, can come to agreement in most clinical situations. Given an all-important commitment to doing what is right and a fairly wide agreement about guiding ethical principles, the critical process becomes one of *competent moral thinking*: moving through certain intellectual steps before arriving at a decision.

Methodology and Discernment in Ethics

If love without strategy is little more than a fleeting feeling, the same is true of ethics. The passage from moral feeling to ethics is by way of a strategy for making moral evaluations. Committed professionals will not reach the same conclusion in every clinical case; but they will avoid the worst moral mistakes and come to defensible and respectful decisions more often than not, so long as they pursue an adequate evaluation process. Of course, even with broad general agreement about moral principles, applying such principles to a concrete case, or deciding which principle to apply when two or more are in conflict, is a difficult and delicate task. Therefore, while medical ethics can offer many things, one of its main tasks is to provide an appropriate moral strategy or methodology for making evaluations.

Not unlike science, medical ethics must weigh, assess, and analyze relationships shown by empirical data. But unlike many schools of philosophic ethics, the applied philosophy of medical ethics is grounded in concrete life situations where people do their living and dying. Consequently, the practicing clinical ethicist, like the scientist, must first be a fact gatherer, and then, again like the scientist, must proceed systematically to the analytic task at hand. Even in the initial fact-gathering stage, however, the competent clinical ethicist is aware of background assumptions and presuppositions; and so, while objectivity is a goal in medical ethics, it is an informed rather than a simple-minded objectivity, one that considers the subjective dimensions even at the early stages of observation and description.

Of course, no strategy or methodology can compensate for retarded ethical development or character flaws on the part of the decision-maker. People who are impulsive, antisocial, or narcissistic cannot distance themselves sufficiently from their own interests to make objective evaluations, let alone initiate actions for the benefit of patients. Therefore, the decision-maker in a clinical setting must have reached at least that stage of character development where response to principles and ideals is possible. This is a prime reason why physicians are expected to operate at an imprincipled level of development. Nevertheless, instances where people have attained high professional status without having attained a correspondingly high level of ethical development are legion.

An even more common obstacle to ethical discernment derives from a tendency to reach moral decisions without taking advantage of adequate methodology. When this happens, the personal capacity for discernment may be present, but clarity about how to make moral judgments is missing. Some professionals who rightly consider themselves decent and upstanding actually make decisions of great ethical importance in a willy-nilly fashion. Others, without a systematic strategy or reflective methodology, make their decisions in more pragmatic ways. Some rely on outside authority for their moral orientation; others are confident that they themselves have an intuitive grasp of what is right; and many make decisions according to group expectations. No adequate medical ethics can be based on these unreflective foundations. Truly professional medical ethics requires an ethical methodology that generates both moral discernment and consistently right judgments.

Such methodology provides an ethical decision-making framework which ensures that relevant data are considered. It also clarifies rights and responsibilities and reassures an ever-more-suspicious society that decisions important to patients and their families are made with proper deliberation. But good methodology does not ensure infallibility. The right decision will not always be made; but what can be done consistently, and this is important, is that the worst mistakes can be avoided.

It is also true that a given methodology's authority depends on the reasoned and respectful determinations derived from its use. Sometimes legal advice will be required before coming to an ethical decision, but most often the law is satisfied when persons rightfully involved in decision-making are careful and systematic about how they make decisions. This is something that a sound methodology can guarantee.

Historical Methodologies and Emphasis on the Situation

Recent strategies or methodologies of clinical ethics are not entirely novel. They were antedated by procedures for arriving at defensible choices that one finds in religious ethics. Catholic moral theology, especially, was interested in such strategies for guiding the decisions of spiritual directors and for use in a confessional context. And in fact these historic methodologies have had considerable influence on the most widely used current strategies of clinical ethics.

Every model or strategy has two phases, one that directs attention to the gathering of facts and another that applies evaluative standards. A separation between the two phases is usually explicitly reflected in the model itself. The classic methodology of St. Thomas Aquinas, for example, applied standard Christian guidelines, but only after extensive attention to factual elements. Aquinas went so far as to say that human actions were evaluated as right or wrong, depending on factual or circumstantial consid-

erations. "*Actionas humanae secundum circumstantias sunt bonae vel malae.*"[2]

St. Thomas considered the circumstances, or the factual dimensions of the case, to be neither accidental nor of secondary importance. Hence the judgment, as to whether an act was right or wrong, could not derive exclusively from the structure of the act or from the intention that informed it. This is because the factual dimensions of a human action, or the peculiar and particular circumstances in which it is performed, have everything to do with its being judged right or wrong. Thus, facts and circumstances are as important as evaluative standards or principles in determining the right thing to do.

What is true of classic moral theology is also true of modern medical ethics. Medical ethics emerges from clinical contexts, and every decision is linked to a particular set of circumstances called a "case." Some forms of ethics bask in generalities and abstractions, but this is not so of either classic theologic ethics or contemporary medical ethics. Indeed, every helpful modern methodology in medical ethics gives clear prominence to the explication of medical, human, and economic factors that shift and criss-cross in every clinical case.

Medical ethics is unavoidably situational, and a workable methodology must be useful for the explication of case particulars. But being situational is not the same as being a situation ethics. Neither classic Catholic theology nor modern medical ethics are situation ethics in the sense of being radically relativistic. Objective standards and agreed-upon main-line moral determinations exist in both traditions. But in both, an act that in one situation would be considered killing and wrong, in another situation may not be considered killing and certainly not wrong.

The evaluative elements (codes, statutes, precedents, ethical principles, group or individ-

---

[2]T. Aquinas. *Summa Theologica (parts 1 and 2)*, Question 18, Article 3.

ual experiences, rational arguments, cultural norms, authority, and faith) that interact with explications of factual or clinical circumstances are all attended to in classical theology. For religious believers there are religious authorities; for secular believers there will be philosophic authorities. In this regard, it should be noted that one of the most important functions of a methodology is to keep the evaluative standards connected to the factual elements. Good methodologies help to keep medical ethics away from the danger of false generalization and rooted in real-life situations.

Casuistry and Clinical Ethics

A marvelous example of how a methodology organizes intelligence to arrive at defensible decisions can be seen in casuistry, a methodology that had its origins in Stoicism and Cicero and that flourished in the fifteenth and sixteenth centuries, mainly among Jesuit theologians. Casuistry is defined as "the interpretation of moral issues, using procedures of reasoning based on paradigms and analogies, leading to the formulation of expert opinion about the existence and stringency of certain particular obligations, framed in terms of rules or maxims that are general but not universal or invariable, since they hold good with certainty only in the typical conditions of the agent and circumstances of action."[3] Theoretical assumptions (e.g., natural law theory) certainly were operative in casuistic thinking, as they are in modern medical ethics (e.g., deontology and utilitarianism); but the closer one gets to clinical problem-solving, the farther one gets from explicit and overt theoretical considerations.

A clinical case (from *cadere*, "to happen") is a statement about actions or affairs that makes reference to what classic theology called circumstances: Who? What? When? Where? Why? How? and By what means? In the casuistic method the circumstances (*circum*, "around," *stare*, "to stand") literally stood around the core elements, which were called "maxims" (rules or moral directives that guide moral decision-making). Maxims—in the sense of moral rules of thumb—much more than theory continue to be the major evaluative elements in clinical ethics. Examples of some common maxims include "competent patients have a right to decide"; "doctors should strive for the patient's medical good"; and "doctors should not take the life of a patient."

The usefulness of a maxim, its "cash value," resides in the assistance it can provide in making quick defensible decisions. Most often, however, more than one maxim is embedded in a case, and the clinical ethicist's task is to determine which one really rules. Furthermore, any change in the circumstances will tend to make other maxims emerge, so that careful and continuing attention must always be paid to the particulars of the case. In the past casuistry and now clinical ethics both center around cases, and circumstances are critical for each in deciding what is right or wrong.

In classic casuistry certain cases served as paradigms, illustrating which maxims prevailed in a given set of circumstances. As a case under consideration was shown similar to or different from the paradigm case, a particular decision or rule about right and wrong was thought to be more or less certainly applicable. Everything depended upon the interplay of circumstances and maxims. The same is true of medical clinical ethics. A decision about right and wrong action in a clinical case is based on circumstances and justified by a maxim or a rule. Thus casuistry, which Voltaire and others thought they had killed with cynical criticism, seems alive and well in contemporary medical ethics.

Clinical medical ethics lacks the time, interest, and inclination to be engaged in abstract consideration of theoretical ethics. Besides, ab-

---

[3]A. R. Jonsen and S. E. Toulmin, *The Abuse of Casuistry*, University of California Press, Berkeley, 1988, p. 257. This is a valuable reference for anyone interested in casuistry but particularly for clinical ethicists. The authors make a convincing case for the idea that modern medical ethics is casuistry.

stract theory has no payoff in clinical decision-making. Casuistry, on the other hand, focuses on the circumstances of a case and prefers concrete directives (maxims). In the contemporary clinical context, like the historic situation in which casuistry developed, there is pressure to decide as well as a need to justify the decision. The casuist was faced with a confessional case or a dilemma in spiritual direction; the medical ethicist is faced with options in a medical case that must be assessed and chosen quickly. Certain topics or considerations must always be covered, and these one finds identified in the different methodologies available to guide clinical medical ethics.

Contemporary U.S. Methodologies[4]

Shortly after contemporary medical ethics emerged into public awareness in the late 1960s and 1970s, David Thomasma developed a clinical ethics program at the University of Tennessee in Memphis. Thomasma's program was immersed in the clinical setting, and the methodology he developed for ethical decision-making paralleled the methodology used by doctors to make medical decisions. Briefly, he distilled the moral reasoning process about cases into six steps which clinicians were trained to follow. These steps have been slightly altered by him over the years, but in essence they are as follows:[5]

1. Describe the medical facts of the case.
2. Describe the values (goals, interests) of all parties involved in the case: physicians, patients, house staff, hospital, society.
3. Determine the principal value clash.
4. Determine possible courses of action which could protect as many of the values in the case as possible.

5. Choose a course of action.
6. Defend this course of action.

Thomasma defended his methodology and the need for clinicians to learn ethical reasoning procedures in a book he wrote in 1981 with Edmund Pellegrino.[6]

In 1982 Albert Jonsen, Mark Siegler, and William Winslade published a small volume on medical ethics written specifically for doctors and aimed toward the facilitation of clinical decision-making.[7] They transformed Thomasma's six steps into four areas of concern, into which they packed many complex considerations. Recognizing that doctors are used to making medical decisions that follow a certain methodology but are uncomfortable with ethical decisions, the authors discussed the reasons for physician discomforts and then worked to overcome them through a systematic approach to ethical problems. Their method was designed to provide a checklist for physicians that would ensure all relevant considerations were taken into account: What facts are most relevant to the case? How should the facts be organized to develop critical considerations? and How should the various ethical considerations be weighed? The four areas of concern that they described are as follows:

1. *Medical indications (the physician's domain)*: Diagnosis, prognosis, therapeutic alternatives, clinical strategy based on risks and benefits of various courses of management, and particular characteristics of the patient.
2. *Patient preferences (patient decision-making based on medical indicators)*: How to handle a conflict between medical indicators and patient preferences; competency considerations; overriding a patient's refusal; what to do when a patient is incompetent and dying.

[4]The methodologies presented in this article are shortened versions or outlines of the originals.
[5]D. Thomasma, Training in medical ethics: An ethical workup, *Forum on Medicine* 1(12):36, 1978. The workup cited is an update of the 1978 version that Thomasma uses at Loyola University's Stritch School of Medicine.

[7]A. Jonsen, M. Siegler, and W. Winslade, *Clinical Ethics*, Macmillan, New York, 1982. Mark Siegler later wrote a separate article on methodology (M. Siegler, Decision-making strategy for clinical-ethical problems in medicine, *Arch Intern Med* 142:2,178–2,179, 1982).

3. *Quality of life consideration (when patients cannot decide for themselves):* When a patient is unable to make his or her decisions, a surrogate must decide whether treatment creates more benefit or more burden (Is the surgery, radiation, medical regime, etc. worth it?). A value is placed on features of human experience (consciousness, capacity for relationship, pain, function). Such quality of life evaluations occur only when patients are unable to make judgments, their preferences are unknown, and the medical goals are limited (e.g., in cases involving terminal illness, permanently unconscious patients, handicapped neonates, or an order not to apply cardiopulmonary resuscitation).

4. *External factors (effects of decisions upon others):* Clinical decisions commonly have impacts extending beyond the doctor/patient/surrogate triad; they affect the patient's family, limited resources, limited finances, medical teaching needs, and the safety and well-being of society. These factors are weighed last and are not given great weight in routine decisions.

The decision-maker using this methodology is not only guided in his or her considerations of basic subjects, but is advised when to introduce each consideration and how much weight to assign it. The four general areas of concern are relatively simple, but within each category many different elements and levels of ethical reflection are included.

An ethical workup designed by the author of this article[8] attempts to separate out the different elements and levels of discourse, as well as to show how decision-makers logically proceed from one to the other. Like the former model, it has four main parts:

Expository phase: Guiding the identification of relevant factual material.

1. *Medical factors:* Diagnosis, prognosis, therapeutic options, realistic medical goals, treatment effectiveness, uncertainties associated with scientific understanding in medical practice.

2. *Ethical factors:* Who is the patient and what does he or she want? What are the interests, wishes, feelings, intuitions, and preferences of the patient, physicians, staff, hospital administrators, society?

3. *Socioeconomic factors:* Costs borne by patient, family, hospital, HMO, insurance company, national government, or local community.

Rational phase: Guide to reasoning about the relevant data.

1. *Medical ethical categories:* Terms like informed consent, refusal of treatment, confidentiality, experimentation, and euthanasia create a general taxonomy for organizing data and referral to available literature. The language of medical ethics provides the tools for thinking about cases.

2. *Principles and maxims:* Beneficence, autonomy, respect, truth, fidelity, sanctity of life, and justice are widely accepted guides for reflection. More concrete guides come in the form of specific rules: Do not prolong death; always relieve suffering; respect competent patients' wishes.

3. *Legal decisions and professional codes:* Paradigm legal cases guide reflection about other cases (for example, a Quinlan-type case). Professional codes, updated by proclamations of professional organizations, also guide reflection.

Volitional phase: Moving from facts and reflection to decision-making.

1. *Ordering the goods:* When more than one good value or interest is realizable, all must be listed according to a scale of priorities. For example, competent patient preferences have priority over physician or family preferences; in an epidemic, societal goods take preference over individual goods.

2. *Ordering principles:* When principles come into conflict, they are ordered according to personal beliefs and professional commitments. For physicians, beneficence (caring for a patient, curing, saving life, relieving pain) takes priority. Other principles are respected but are never preferred to beneficence.

3. *Making a decision:* Professional people decide, with as much prudence and sensitivity as their personality development permits. Special care is required whenever a decision will result in a patient's death.

---

[8]J. F. Drane, Ethical workup guides clinical decision-making, *Health Progress* 69(11):64–67, 1988.

Public phase: Preparing for public scrutiny and defense of decisions:

1. Making assumptions explicit, becoming aware of subjective factors and underlying beliefs.
2. Correlating reasons and feelings, striving for consistency in using principles, maxims, and rules.
3. Organizing arguments for public discourse. In a pluralistic society an acceptable ethic is supported by convincing reasons.

The methodologies of Thomasma, Siegler, and Drane all touch the same basic points. They differ in the explicitness with which key elements are reflected in the outline. However, none of the three would disagree about any element included in the others' models. Each model attempts to provide a procedural system that can be used by clinical decision-makers no matter what their theoretical beliefs (utilitarian or deontologist, religious or secular).[9] The methodologies differ, then, in choice of terms, ordering of topics, prominence of themes, and temporal sequences.

A European/Latin American Methodology

Hans-Martin Sass, former Director of the Bochum Center for Medical Ethics in West Germany, is the author of the Bochum Protocol. José A. Mainetti, Director of the Institute of Medical Humanities at the University of La Plata, Argentina, strongly endorses this methodology as an alternative to "made in USA" approaches to bioethics,[10] which Mainetti feels reflect a North American culture, society, and medicine that is technologized, secular, and pluralistic. (Recently, however, Mainetti has seen

North American medical ethics moving toward European and Latin American styles.)

In this view medical traditions in Europe and Latin America are more humanistic, and their medical ethics are not so tied to deontological and utilitarian theories. Because they are less formalistic, theory-driven, and rule-dominated, according to Mainetti and Lebener, they can help renew medical practice.

Because European medical ethics is more sensitive to virtue considerations and less dominated by principles, it needs its own methodology—one that avoids even the appearance of an engineering strategy applied by technical experts—to bring about socially acceptable solutions. Mainetti finds such a method in Hans Martin-Sass' Bochum Protocol, which, like two of the other models we have seen, has four phases, each of which is divided into subsections. This model consists largely of questions:

Identification of scientific/medical findings: What treatment would be best in light of the scientific medical facts?

1. *General reflections:* Diagnosis, prognosis, treatment alternatives, treatment benefits or results, prognosis without treatment?
2. *Special reflections:* How do treatment options with their benefits and burdens apply to this particular patient?
3. *Physician's task:* Are clinical conditions such as to provide adequate treatment? Is the doctor competent? Is medical knowledge clear? Is medical ignorance recognized?

Identification of ethical/medical findings: What treatment would be best in light of ethical/medical factors?

1. *Patient health and well-being:* What burdens (physical or spiritual) are associated with each therapeutic alternative?
2. *Patient self-determination:* What are the patient's values, attitudes, and level of understanding? Can the patient's participation and decision-making be respected, or will it be set aside in favor of a surrogate's decision?
3. *Medical responsibility:* Can conflicts between doctor, patient, staff, and family be mediated

---

[9]H. Brody, *Ethical Decisions in Medicine (second ed.)*, Little Brown, Boston, 1981. In this book the author provides an outline of different methodologies, depending on one's theoretical belief (utilitarian, deontologist, etc.).

[10]H. M. Sass, H. Viefhues, and J. A. Mainetti, *Protocolo de Bochum para la práctica ético-médica (second ed.)*, Zentrum für Medizinische Ethik, Bochum, 1988.

without undermining trust, confidentiality, or truth? How much clarity, certainty, or doubt exists about the appropriateness of ethical categories and their interrelationships?

Case management: What decision is best, in light of all the above considerations?

1. What are the most acceptable options given the medical ethical findings? Is further consultation or patient transfer required?
2. What are the concrete obligations of the physician, patient, staff, and family in light of the treatment chosen?
3. Are there arguments against the decision? Was the decision discussed with the patient? Was the patient's consent received?

Additional questions regarding ethical evaluation:

1. In cases requiring prolonged treatment: Regarding routine review of medical treatment and ethical appraisal, Is the treatment plan flexible? Are palliative measures considered when prognosis is dismal? Is consideration of the patient's expressed and presumed wishes assured?
2. When social factors are present: Regarding family, emotional, professional, and economic complications, Can the complications be borne by the patient, family, and community? Is the patient's social integration, happiness, and personality development being promoted? How are these social factors to be evaluated vis-à-vis the medical/scientific and medical/ethical considerations?
3. In therapeutic and nontherapeutic experimentation: How does the experiment affect the medical/ethical considerations? If disclosure to the patient is incomplete or is not understood, can the experiment be justified? If the patient has not consented, can it be justified? Was patient selection fair? Can the patient withdraw at any time?

Similarities and Differences

Similarities between the European/Latin American and the U.S. methodologies are many, but the former does show several distinguishing characteristics. Although the principles turn out to be the same, less prominence is given to autonomy in the Bochum Protocol. The section on patient self-determination, for example, is written from a physician's perspective. The protocol asks what the doctor knows about the patient's value system, attitudes, and understanding. This approach leads to the question "To what extent can the patient be taken into consideration or to what extent can he (she) be completely set aside?"[11] Such phrasing would be inconceivable in a United States methodology, where the cultural emphasis on patient autonomy is strong. Similarly, the Bochum Protocol makes treatment decisions primarily the doctor's responsibility (the physician is asked to consider discussing issues with patients and then to decide whether or not to follow patient preferences). And a comparable difference regarding patient autonomy is seen in the section on experimentation. (The protocol asks questions about justifying research when the patient is not informed or has not consented to participate. In the United States any such medical behavior would be ethically and legally indefensible.)

In general, the Bochum Protocol is as formalistic and technical as the North American models but displays certain elements not found in the latter. For instance, more explicit reference is made to epistemologic issues ("What important factors is the doctor ignorant of?" "Are the medical concepts sufficiently clear?"). Taking medical ignorance and lack of clarity into consideration is not quite the North American style. Young doctors, in fact, work hard during medical training to develop an impression of certainty and self-confidence (some would say infallibility).

Concluding Remarks

The four methodologies just described move

---

[11]H. M. Sass, H. Viefhues, and J. A. Mainetti, *Protocolo de Bochum para la práctica ético-médica (second ed.)*, Zentrum für Medizinische Ethik, Bochum, 1988.

from the relatively simple to the relatively complex. Thomasma's model provides the simplest outline of critical issues. Siegler lists only four topics but includes many more complex considerations under each. Drane unpacks some of the complex issues and organizes them according to an epistemologically progressive schema. The Bochum Protocol incorporates clinical, ethical, and epistemologic issues and, in addition, covers different clinical settings.

An evaluation of the different models would require a testing of their effectiveness and usefulness to practitioners: How well are the crucial elements kept before the decision-maker? Is the decision-maker sensitized to critical problem areas? Are potentially unrecognized issues signaled? Is the model pragmatic and clinically workable?

Personally, I see advantages and disadvantages in each model and suspect that practitioners will decide for themselves which one works best and how the most workable model can be improved.

The fact that there are different approaches to ethical decision-making in different regions is readily understandable. European medicine is more humanistic, in the sense that medical training continues to include philosophy of medicine, history of medicine, medical anthropology, and now medical ethics. It is easier with such a background to consider a less technical and more philosophically sophisticated decision-making approach. North American doctors and medicine, on the other hand, are more clinically focused and less appreciative of philosophic issues in medical practice. Their strengths lie more along pragmatic lines. Ideally, however, the best methodology would be both clinically practical and philosophically sophisticated. If cooperation between North American, European, and Latin American ethicists moves forward, then both goals might come closer to realization.

Know Well to Do Good

M. Angélica Piwonka de A., Isabel Bustos D.,
Eliana Gaete Q., and Mila Urrutia B.

Today's society is characterized by an emphasis on technology, accelerated change, and dehumanization. This situation makes it especially important that medical attention given to the individual should be strongly predicated upon humanistic training.

This calls for comprehensive instruction, not just accumulating and transmitting a body of information. Furthermore, because it provides the basis for a well-rounded education, humanistic training should be a requirement for all—prospective scientists as well as prospective lawyers—and should underlie the practice of any profession. Any good professional should be, in his or her own way, a humanist. Not in vain has it been said that ours is the time of "humanisms," especially when one recognizes the "greatness and misery of man manifesting, sustaining, and favoring his total dignity."[1]

Conflict-laden situations arise in the exercise of any profession. Besides extensive training and an understanding of mankind's spiritual and transcendent nature, proper handling of such situations demands an empathetic vocation to provide service—a predisposition to help one's fellows—arising from a confluence of knowledge, compassion, and activity that may properly be considered an embodiment of the concept of wisdom.

Wisdom of this sort, of the natural order of things, is identified with philosophy, the discipline of order *par excellence*, precisely because philosophy deals with the highest principles underlying reality and—above all—the goals of human life. If we feel disoriented and confused, it is because we lack a universal and profound understanding capable of integrating more specialized sorts of knowledge, a comprehensive and radical understanding that even in the midst of advancing technology will remind us that human dignity does not reside necessarily in this advance, but rather in man himself.

Thus, given the shared dignity inherent in each individual and all mankind, the study of humanity provides the basis for a complete education and understanding of a well-defined set of standards based on fundamental and universal ethical precepts. Such study must be included in both basic programs for health professionals and programs of continuing education in order to train qualified professionals who can shoulder their career responsibilities and help others in such a way as to preserve and enhance the dignity of those receiving their assistance.

This inherent dignity, a basic human need, calls for us to rethink ends and means—not only in extreme situations but in small daily routine tasks. The service that a nurse provides, at all times and in tending to the smallest details of her work, is simply her response to what our society requires.

On the basis of the foregoing, it appears worthwhile to examine some situations more or less representative of those a nurse encounters daily. These are not limited to extreme situations with obvious ethical connotations, but also include lesser ones that should be assessed the same way—situations that all nurses experience in routine daily contact with their patients.

---

[1]See John Paul II, *Christifideles laici*, Ediciones Paulinas, Bogotá, 1988, p. 16.

Case 1: Nursing Routines

To establish nursing routines, the nurse must consider the following factors:

- ☐ The patient: his needs (psychobiological and social as well as spiritual), his problems, and his family, as well as the number of patients to be tended.
- ☐ The type of care involved: its nature, amount, complexity, frequency, and scheduling.
- ☐ The material resources available.
- ☐ The nursing staff: the type and number of staff members providing care and the scheduling of their work times.
- ☐ The environment: the care facility's structural features, cleanliness and appearance, and the psychosocial ambience.
- ☐ The time-frame: the pace of life in the facility and the customary schedule of daily activities.

Executing a nursing care plan for a group of patients calls for assessment of the above factors using an organized approach that will ensure safe, efficient, and personalized nursing care. The nurse responsible for doing this faces a dilemma implicit in service standards, because these standards are usually geared to the functioning of the service rather than the patients' needs.

Standards are necessary, of course, but they should be flexible; and the nurse should decide what to do from that standpoint, remembering that the subject entrusted to her care is a human being. This is true despite the fact that it is easier to rigidly follow some standard than to assume a commitment and exercise one's own judgment before the patient, the person responsible for authorizing departures from the norm, and one's colleagues.

Some matters involving standards that commonly need modification are as follows:

Hospital Visiting Hours

"Visiting hours" commonly coincide with times when adults are working and children are at school, thus making it difficult for friends and relatives to visit hospitalized patients. Also, the period assigned for visiting hours is often very short, affording the patients little time to spend with their visitors. In such cases the system neglects to recognize that most patients have families, that the patient's presence in the hospital is merely an accidental occurrence in his life, and that the situation through which he is living can be markedly brightened by the support, understanding, and presence of friends and family members.

Schedules

When a patient is in pain, nurses sometimes adhere strictly to the drug administration schedule for giving analgesics, or they delay giving the medication so that the patient "will have a good night." Both practices frequently occur without careful evaluation of the patient's pain and needs. As a result, analgesics are often administered at times indicated on the chart, or at times most convenient for the night staff, rather than when the patient really needs the medication.

Similarly, other schedules, including those for mealtimes and administration of a wide range of medications, are frequently geared to the service's smooth operation and the hospital staff's convenience rather than accommodation of the patients' needs and customary behavior patterns.

Case 2: Research

Nurse 1: "They finally gave me the funds to try this new solution for cleaning eschars. Now I need to select the experimental and control groups."

Nurse 2: "You'll have to make sure the patients in the test group on whom you're going to try the solution are conscious and lucid, so that you can tell them what it's about and obtain their consent."

Nurse 1: "But do you really think that's so important? After all, it's not going to harm them."

To improve the quality of their care, nurses must study and try out new procedures calculated to benefit their patients. However, when a new technique or medication involving the patient is being tested, nurses are prone to commit two errors: neglecting to obtain or heed their patients' opinions and ignoring or bypassing the ethical standard requiring that the patient's informed consent be obtained.

Case 3: Gossip

Nurse 1 (on coffee-break): "I think the patient I've just admitted has AIDS! He's a well-known homosexual. . . . Even uses make-up. You should have seen the person who brought him in!"

Nurse 2: "You don't say. I'm going to take a look. What room is he in?"

Nurse 1: "He's in 2-A, beside the emphysema case, the one that's terminal."

Sometimes health care personnel make light or idle comments about a patient's circumstances that are unimportant to those talking but that could be extremely important to the patient.

Such gossip should be strongly discouraged, for professional confidentiality is one of the principal obligations of the nursing oath. The patient confides in the nursing professional as a result of his condition, and it is implicitly understood that the information provided will not be revealed. This understanding extends to all matters within the purview of the profession when disclosure might in any way harm the patient.

Case 4: Private Nursing

Nurse 1 (at a private nursing bureau): "They're calling to ask for someone to take care of an incontinent old man who can't feed himself. They want someone who is good-natured, patient, and helpful."

Nurse 2: "We don't have anyone available right now. The only possibility would be to send Jane, but we don't know what she's like, she's only been here

a week. . . . Well, let's send her anyway. After all, it's just an old man."

Scientific and technologic advances have brought changes to the nursing profession, especially regarding specialization and new kinds of care. This has had a major impact upon the field of private nursing—which has expanded recently and seems destined to grow more. Nevertheless, the nature of this type of nursing care continues to make it unusually vulnerable to ethical problems. Specifically, there is less opportunity for one professional to consult with another, less external control over the quality of care rendered, and none of the compulsory supervision that exists at health care facilities. These circumstances can significantly increase the risks to which the patient and his family are exposed.

Adding to the difficulty, early discharge of patients has become a common hospital practice. Such early discharge permits better utilization of hospital beds and provides multiple benefits for the patients and their families. But in many cases it also requires that home nursing care be provided by suitable and qualified personnel.

Within this context, the nurse's responsibility for delegating functions is a powerful tool subject to possible misuse. That is, ignorance of the particular status of a patient or of specific staff members' technical and moral qualifications can lead to decisions potentially harmful to the patient and his family. Therefore, in exercising this authority it is essential that the nurse be sensitive and assume an ethical responsibility that extends beyond the scope of her strictly legal obligations.

Case 5: Dying with Dignity

Nurse: "Angelina, move the patient in bed seven to isolation; he is critical and needs to be alone. Alert the doctor and don't admit any visitors. . . ."

Aide: "I've already put the screen around his bed so the other patients in the room won't see him, but if you like I'll move him to isolation."

Dialogues such as this are commonplace in hospitals, especially in the general medical and surgical services. The gravely ill patient who seems about to die tends to be isolated and removed from his roommates, possibly to prevent their confronting the frightening life experience that is the act of dying.

The nurse visits the patient when she has to perform routine control and treatment procedures. Her focus is on the execution of techniques, while interpersonal relations are avoided—perhaps out of fear, or perhaps because she is not prepared to stay with a dying patient, it being an "unlearned role" in our society.

We who typically avoid thinking about death commonly fail to realize that only to the extent that the nurse is capable of facing her own death will she really be able to help the patient undergoing this last and most solitary experience. Paradoxically, however, the patient who is dying asks very little of others: to be left alone with his loved ones and to receive spiritual aid in accord with his religious beliefs. From the nurse he asks specifically for a personal relationship: to listen to him and let him know, even without words, "I'm here beside you at this decisive moment."

As this suggests, care of a dying patient involves ethical responsibilities that the nurse should be aware of and for which she should be prepared—so that up to the last moment of his life the patient can receive the care his human condition merits and can die with dignity.

Bibliography

Arcusa, E. *Responsabilidad médica. Manual de deontología médica: Orientaciones, soluciones, casos prácticos (second ed.).* Ediciones Paulinas, Bogotá, 1968.

Beauchamp, T. L., and L. B. McCullough. *Medical Ethics: The Moral Responsibilities of Physicians.* Prentice Hall, Englewood Cliffs, 1984.

Colegio Médico de Chile. *Etica médica: Normas y documentos.* Editorial Antárctica, Santiago, 1986.

Consejo Pontificio COR UNUM. *Algunas cuestiones de ética relativas a los enfermos graves y a los moribundos.* Vatican City, 1976.

Gaete Q., E. Address at the graduation of the 1986 class of nurse-midwives. Escuela de Enfermería, Pontificia Universidad Católica, Santiago, Chile, 1986.

Rodríguez-Luno, A. *Etica.* EUNSA, Pamplona, 1982.

Sarmiento, A., I. Adeva, and J. Escos. *Etica profesional de la enfermería.* EUNSA, Pamplona, 1977.

Hospital Ethics Committees

Juan Carlos Tealdi and José Alberto Mainetti

Hospital ethics committees (HECs) are interdisciplinary bodies that perform teaching, research, and consultative functions dealing with the ethical problems that arise during the practice of hospital medicine. These bodies emerged in response to problems posed by new medical technologies and a new social awareness oriented toward evaluation of prolonged treatments, decisions not to treat newborns with serious malformations, and other deliberations of an ethical nature.

In 1982, only 1% of the hospitals in the United States had committees of this kind, but in 1988 the percentage had risen to 60% for hospitals with more than 200 beds (1). Today's reality in Latin America, however, continues to show little such development. This article presents a historical analysis of HECs' legal basis, describes their structure and Argentina's experience with them, and makes some recommendations.

The Praxeologic-Ethics Committee

In his decision of 31 March 1976, Judge Richard Hughes of the U.S. State Supreme Court of New Jersey responded to a request to suspend the artificial respiration of a young woman in a deep coma by noting that the ethics committee of the institution where the woman was a patient should be consulted. In his decision, Hughes cited a recent article by the pediatrician Karen Teel (2) in which she proposed having an ethics committee composed of physicians, social workers, lawyers, and theologians serve as an instrument for evaluating different therapeutic options applicable to a given patient.

The Morris View Nursing Home, the institution where the young woman, Karen Quinlan, was in a coma, formed an ethics committee composed of two representatives of the clergy, the institution's director, a social worker, a physician who was not treating Karen Quinlan, and its own legal representative. The committee, which was not the envisaged panel of experts, went beyond the framework of prognostic review proposed by the judge to consider ethical aspects involved in making decisions about the case. In this way, without awareness of the principal actors, Teel's critical article, the unfortunate Karen Quinlan, the informed Judge Hughes, and the determined Morris View Nursing Home gave forward impetus to the most recent chapter in a fascinating human history.

Extensive publicity surrounding the Quinlan case called attention to the ethics committee, an entity almost nonexistent until then (3), and prompted its formal consolidation; but it was the March 1983 report (4) of the President's Commission for the Study of Ethical Problems in Medicine and Biomedical and Behavioral Research that gave a decisive boost to such committees by proposing their organization and use in making decisions about terminal patients. This report provided a model for establishing such committees, a list of already existing ones (only 1% of the hospitals in the United States had them at that time), and a survey of their activities.

When a baby with Down's syndrome and esophageal atresia was born at Bloomington, Indiana, in the spring of 1982, a year before the presidential report, another key event in the history of HECs began. The life of the newborn depended upon an operation that would allow it to be fed. The baby's parents refused treatment; and the infant, abandoned to its fate in a home, died of starvation in six days while the medical team tried without success to get a court to intervene in the case (5). The following year the U.S. Department of Health and Human Services proposed a regulation to evaluate the treatment of disabled children and suggested government intervention in such cases (6). The American Academy of Pediatrics responded to this by proposing the creation of specialized ethics committees, each of which would be specifically designated an "Infant Bioethical Review Committee" (7).

Then, on 11 October 1983, the child who would be known as "Baby Jane Doe" was born at Port Jefferson, New York (8). This infant was born with multiple neurologic deficits, spina bifida, microcephaly, and hydrocephaly. The medical team caring for her to prevent infections but not to treat her malformations indicated the baby might benefit from surgical intervention. Her parents, preferring conservative treatment, rejected the intervention proposal, but a court ruled that the operation should be carried out. The decision was reversed by the New York State Court of Appeals, and Baby Doe was taken home without treatment. Confronted with this situation, in February 1984 the U.S. Department of Health and Human Services ordered an investigation of parental decisions about the treatment of disabled babies and opened a telephone hot line for reporting cases of negligence.

On 23 May of that year, U.S. District Court Judge Charles L. Brieant of the Southern District of New York, Manhattan, summarily vacated the federal "Baby Doe rules" for violating the medical duty of confidentiality and the parents' right to privacy. Brieant thus dealt with the complaints of the American Medical Association, American Hospital Association, and other

societies. The Department of Health and Human Services accepted the decision in part, and although it adhered to Washington's prevailing guidelines and emphasized the possibility of investigating such cases, it offered great freedom of action to hospitals having infant care review committees. Within this context, debate over decision-making revolved about three alternatives: leaving decisions to parents and physicians, establishing direct government intervention and control, or taking cases to court (8). Another strong alternative confronting these three was the option of utilizing HECs, an option that was to undergo major development.

The Legal-Scientific Committee

An earlier chapter of the story began 30 years before the Quinlan case. On 1 October 1946 an international tribunal at Nuremberg, Germany, sentenced 22 members of the Nazi Party for crimes against humanity. The following year, after having uncovered atrocious experiments carried out on prisoners of war, the tribunal proclaimed the Nuremberg Code,[1] which established a set of principles that should be respected in conducting medical experiments on human subjects.

The code's influence was immense: It was discussed at a national conference in Chicago in 1958 (9). It provided the basis for a Draft Code of Ethics on Human Experimentation that was drawn up by the World Medical Association in Geneva in 1961 (10) and developed into the World Medical Assembly's Declaration of Helsinki of 1964 (11). It was also contained in the Twenty-ninth World Medical Assembly's amendment of that declaration in Tokyo in 1975, which expressly recommended that each phase of experimentation with human subjects, after being defined in an experimental protocol,

---

[1] The international codes cited in this chapter are reprinted in full or in part as appendices to this book, pp. 217–229.

be submitted for consideration to an independent committee specially formed to advise and render an opinion on it, so that the basic recommendations of the Nuremberg Code could be more thoroughly applied.

In this way research ethics committees, which have since functioned in various health institutions including hospitals, were consolidated globally under the basic concept of human responsibility. That same year, 1975, saw the publication of the previously noted article by Karen Teel (2).

Six years later, in 1981, the World Health Organization disseminated its "Proposed International Guidelines for Biomedical Research involving Human Subjects." This proposal sought to point up the usefulness of applying the Declaration of Helsinki, revised at Tokyo, to developing countries (12). Particular attention was drawn to Latin America as a region that seemed especially suitable for establishment of ethics review committees.

The Deontologic-Technical Committee

The origins of our story's first chapter are lost in the mists of time. It is believed that toward the end of the fifth century B.C. or the first half of the fourth century B.C., the shortest and most influential of known medical texts took shape in Greece. Its author is unknown.

Physicians found that the text offered a set of standards enabling them to practice their profession morally, and also established the basis for powerful social action through the universality of its language (13). Reproduced through the centuries from times when men worshipped Aesculapius, the Greco-Roman God of Medicine, considered by Erotian a work about *téchne*, prescribed by Pope Clement VII's bull *Quod jusiurandum* in 1531 to all those graduating as physicians, used as their standard by the Asclepiads in K. Deichgräber's view (14), and as the Pythagorean manifesto in L. Edelstein's (15),

the Hippocratic Oath has influenced medical ethics until today. The World Medical Association's General Assembly adapted it for its Declaration of Geneva in 1948 and International Code of Medical Ethics in 1949. Moreover, by invoking professional commitment and a code of ethics, the Oath made itself the major antecedent of the ethics committees serving medical associations, colleges, and schools of medicine, institutions that often extended this model to hospitals.

HEC Organization According to the Three Models Presented

A distinction established between the three models just presented is useful in enabling us to define the concept of the "praxeologic-ethics committee" with greater precision. That is because the praxeologic-ethics committee's worth resides in the fact that it is charged with making ethical decisions involving both facts and values—scientific concepts, technical rules, and philosophic ideas.

The commission or delegation of authority which falls to the committee, though proposed by some person or group, must in any case come from the hospital itself. It should be borne in mind that a legal-scientific or deontologic-technical committee is deferring to one or another sort of outside entity (government, universities, associations, etc.), whereas the HEC serves as the "conscience of the institution" (16). The definition of Cranford and Doudera (17), who describe this committee as "a multidisciplinary group of health professionals at a health institution who carry out the function of managing the ethical dilemmas that occur within the institution," makes this clear.

Our concept seems even clearer if we compare the legal and deontologic options with the ethical one. As Diego Gracia (18) observes, this shows that HECs need to have a methodology for analyzing the moral problems they confront. He suggests that this methodology should include the following phases: initial evaluation of the problem; analysis of the proposed act's correctness; analysis of its goodness; and decision-making. In turn, Kieffer (19) proposes the following phases: presentation of the problem; identification of alternative courses of action; analysis of the results of each course of action; ordering of existing values; and selection of a course of action based on the analysis. Other authors have proposed different approaches (20).

In any case, it seems evident that useful tools for the committee's work are clinical ethics protocols, including that of Bochum (21). For the committee is not merely applying already established moral standards geared fundamentally to maintaining professional decorum or carefully noting the legal consequences of a bold scientific undertaking; instead, its aim is that of providing a truly ethical process.

We can also say that HECs are eminently praxeologic (oriented to human behavior) rather than scientific or technical, because they concentrate primarily upon the multiple implications of particular actions and decisions (22, 23). This is the point, we believe, at which we should ask ourselves, "What is an HEC's ethic?" and at which we will inevitably encounter metaethical issues.

Bearing in mind that everyone involved in the ethical dilemma is represented, Bertomeu (24) believes it possible to employ a communication ethic like that of Apel and Habermas which excludes the strategic negotiating interests of the parties in order to initiate a true moral process. For this to happen it is necessary, irrespective of any objections (25), that philosophers be able to enter hospitals and ensure the probity and rigor of the moral debate among health professionals and laymen at the same time (as Toulmin posits—26) that they establish their own status. In any event, clinical ethics requires special training (27, 28).

In addition, it is necessary to note the multidisciplinary nature of an HEC compared to a committee of experts (a legal-scientific committee) or a committee of notables (a deontologic-technical committee). At the same time, the HEC's functions will be much more varied—since the existence of any conflict in values may convoke it, while the other two types of committees have more limited domains.

The Argentine Experience

In recent years a few ethics committees have been created in Argentina; and because they have arisen during the great resurgence of interest in bioethics, they may be considered immersed in this subject.

More specifically, on 5 December 1984 the Ethics Committee of the University of Buenos Aires' Hospital de Clínicas was created as a result of a few episodes of medical malpractice and certain clinical investigations that had not been evaluated from an ethics standpoint. Among the deeper considerations motivating the hospital's decision was its need for an agency capable of overseeing research and malpractice, channeling complaints by patients and family members, providing ethical education for students and graduates, and defining standards of medical activity. Members were chosen from among physicians of "recognized ethical stature associated with the hospital." This ethics committee, which stopped operating a few years later, was basically of the deontologic-technical type, though it may also have considered dealing with legal-scientific matters.

Elsewhere in Buenos Aires, an HEC was created at the Italian Hospital.

In Tucumán, two ethics committees were created in 1988. One, the Bioethics Society of the Medical College of Tucumán, is devoted to the study of reproductive technologies and contraception. The other, the Ethics Committee of the Faculty of Medicine, is composed of 10 members, three of them physicians; it has been assigned advisory and consultative duties. There are no hospital ethics committees in Tucumán.

In Mendoza, the Central Hospital created a bioethics committee in October 1987. This multidisciplinary body, which has been going through a formative period, holds meetings every 15 days.

Elsewhere, a bioethics committee is being organized at the Lagomayor Hospital. The Psychiatric Hospital of Sauce has appointed a coordinator and plans to organize an HEC. And in Mar del Plata the Deontothanatology Committee of the Community Hospital, created in 1984, may become an HEC.

Within this context, the Ethics Committee of the Oncologic Center of Excellence of Gonnet was created under our direction in 1987 in response to the mounting moral problems being encountered in the health care field. A result of extensive previous work in the field of medical humanities and bioethics, the committee consists of six to 12 professionals from a variety of disciplines and is designed to perform educational, normative, and consultative tasks. In general, its purpose is to make recommendations that are not binding upon the parties involved.

During the first two years of its existence the committee engaged mostly in research and instruction. However, since December 1988 it has come to devote itself increasingly to care-oriented consultative work. Its present membership includes an anthropologist and a priest, though a majority of the members are physicians or philosophers. The committee's weekly meetings are devoted to reading and discussing cases. All hospital personnel participate in the committee's plenary meetings. The greatest shortcoming of this approach encountered to date is difficulty in simultaneously achieving effective group integration and methodologic progress.

The main questions that the committee has dealt with to date fall into the following areas: theoretical and practical aspects of ethical decision-making; understanding and adaptation of clinical ethics protocols; analysis of the professional-patient relationship; health care; new technologies; experimentation involving human subjects; and death and dying. From the standpoint of its composition, functions, and methodology, the committee may be considered a unique example of the praxeologic ethics type.

It has come increasingly to serve as a reference center for hospitals in the area, to which it provides advice and instruction, and its educational role has grown steadily.

Recommendations on HEC Organization

On a daily basis, HECs are the most efficacious tool available for working in the field of biomedical ethics, from three standpoints: theoretically and conceptually in terms of ethics communication; methodologically, for bringing to bear a clinical approach intermediate between casuistry and situation ethics; and administratively, by providing a sound basis for prescriptive action. This suggests that a good share of our ideas for stimulating bioethics in our countries may come to crystallize around HECs, despite the fact that it is not easy to guide their organization.

In its guidelines for ethics committees, the American (U.S.) Academy of Pediatrics asserts that a hospital's management should appoint the HEC's individual members, who should include a staff physician, a hospital administrator, an ethicist or member of the clergy, a legal representative (lawyer or judge), a representative of the disabled, a member of the community, a member of the medical staff, and a nurse. The hospital should provide the necessary resources for operation of the committee, which should meet regularly or upon request.

The guidelines further state that the committee should be charged with developing standards to deal with both general issues and specific cases, should retrospectively review clinical histories considered morally questionable, and should review specific cases by holding meetings open to all the affected parties, said meetings to be called on 24 hours' notice at the request of members of the HEC, hospital administration, or patient's family. The committee should keep a record of all its deliberations and of the specific cases considered, but should also maintain institutional confidentiality, its records being available to outsiders only on court order or at the special request of an accredited organization.

The American Hospital Association's recommendations for hospital biomedical ethics committees hold that their functions should be oriented toward managing biomedical ethics education programs, providing forums for discussion between physicians and other professionals within or outside the hospital community about topics in biomedical ethics, providing consultative services for people involved in biomedical decision-making, and evaluating institutional experiences through review of decisions with biomedical ethics implications. Such committees should not concern themselves with review of professional conduct; their reviews should not substitute for legal or judicial reviews; and they should not make decisions about biomedical ethics problems. (That is, the committees should in no way supplant traditional decision-making authorities in such matters.)

These recommendations also indicate that committee members should be chosen with the committee's foregoing aims in mind and should encompass a broad spectrum of views and experiences. This multidisciplinary membership should be drawn from the ranks of physicians, nurses, administrators, social workers, clerics, trustees, lawyers, ethicists, and patient representatives. A hospital's legal adviser may take part in the meetings and should review the committee's recommendations.

For greater efficiency, the committee should have the hospital's support and should operate as a stable entity meeting regularly and when necessary. As a general rule, no one personally involved in a case the committee is deliberating may participate on the committee while the case is being considered. The recommendations of the committee should be regarded as valid for the entire team intervening in the treatment. The patient's privacy and the confidentiality of patient information must be respected. The circumstances under which the committee's recommendations may appear in clinical histories should be determined by each hospital.

Veatch (29) identifies four general types of HEC: those that review ethical or other values in decisions about an individual patient's care (the kind proposed by Karen Teel); those that deal with ethically more general decisions and policies (distribution of resources, hospital readiness to deal with given problems, etc.); those that consult (their function is to provide advice—especially in cases involving terminal patients); and those dealing with prognoses (as was proposed by Judge Hughes in the Quinlan case).

Spinsanti (30) adds a fifth model, characteristic of institutions with religious sponsorship, wherein the committee takes special account of the need to reconcile activities with religious morals.

John Robertson (31) has suggested four possible HEC models: optional-optional, in which there is no obligation to consult the committee or to follow its recommendations; imperative-imperative, in which consultation and adherence to the committee's recommendations are mandatory; imperative-optional; and optional-imperative.

In any case, we believe it suitable for an HEC to be able to advance progressively (32) from formative development through retrospective review of cases to establishment of general standards to adoption of an active consultative role. It is hard for us to believe that the organization of an HEC should be a perfectly standardized matter. Each hospital, each group, each individual will have its unique experience within very general lines.

But ethics is a philosophic discipline, not a categorial science. Its knowledge is enshrouded, approximate, and based on denial of the "non-ethical." An HEC's first step is therefore Socratic—identification of ethical sensitivity, concern for good, eagerness for instruction. Initially, therefore, the need is to find similarities; and, to facilitate this process, it is our "recommendation" that a course on hospital ethics committees be organized in which these sensitivities and concerns can be developed. This course should be designed to provide the minimal theoretical and practical elements appropriate for such development.

Beyond this, he who views ethical issues through the eyes of the HEC will be able to see the multiform faces of all his past and present patients, the long corridors of life and death, hope and anguish. He will see the respirators and the beds and the eyes, the scalpel that bleeds over open flesh, the agony of Jane Doe and the resigned gesture that Karen Quinlan made when, in a wink, there was no more air. He will also see laws, codes, and the masses of people maltreated in the name of health and the glory of scientific research. He will see the centuries pass by, and, in the timeless bottom of a land worked by men of all nations, on the eroded hill of centuries, the yellowed and indestructible stone of the Temple of Aesculapius.

References

1. Cohen, C. Ethics committees: Birth of a network. *Hastings Cent Rep* 18(1):11, 1988.
2. Teel, K. The physician's dilemma, a doctor's view: What the law should be. *Baylor Law Rev* 27:6–9, 1975.
3. Kosnik, A. Developing a health facility medical-moral committee. *Hosp Prog* 8:40–44, 1974.
4. United States, President's Commission for the Study of Ethical Problems in Medicine and Biomedical and Behavioral Research. Hospital Ethics Committees: Proposed Statute and National Survey. In: *Deciding to Forego Life-Sustaining Treatment.* U.S. Government Printing Office, Washington, D.C., 1983, pp. 439–457.
5. Pless, E. The story of Baby Doe. *New Engl J Med* 309(11):663, 1983.
6. United States, Department of Health and Human Services. Proposed Rule 45 CFR Part 84, Nondiscriminations on the Basis of Handicap Relating to Health Care for Handicapped Infants. *Fed Regist* 48(129):30850, 1983.
7. American Academy of Pediatrics. Comments of the American Academy of Pediatrics on Proposed Rule Regarding Nondiscriminations on the Basis of Handicap Relating to Health Care for Handicapped Infants. Internal document.
8. Fleishman, A. R., and H. Murray. Ethics committees for infants Doe? *Hastings Cent Rep* 13(6):5–9, 1983.
9. National Conference on the Legal Environment of Medical Science. *Clinical Research: Legal and Ethical Aspects, Session III. Report of the National Conference on the Legal Environment of Medical Science.* National Society for Medical Research and Chicago University, 1960.
10. World Medical Association. Draft code of ethics on human experimentation. *Br Med J* 2:1119, 1962.
11. World Medical Association. *Declaration of Helsinki: Recommendations Guiding Physicians in Biomedical Research Involving Human Subjects.* 1964.
12. World Health Organization. Proposed International Guidelines for Biomedical Research involving Human Subjects. 1982.
13. Mainetti, J. A. El Juramento Hipocrático. *Quiron* (La Plata) 11(2):97–101, 1980.
14. Deichgräber, K. Die ärztliche Standesethic des hippokratischen Eides. *Quellen und Studien zur geschichte der Naturwissenschaften und der Medizin* 3:29–49, 1933.
15. Edelstein, L. *The Hippocratic Oath: Text, Translation, and Interpretation.* Johns Hopkins, Baltimore, 1943.
16. Gibson, J. M., and T. K. Kushner. Will the 'conscience of an institution' become society's servant? *Hastings Cent Rep* 16(3):9–11, 1986.
17. Cranford, R., and A. E. Doudera. The Emergence of Institutional Ethics Committees. In: Health Administration Press. *Institutional Ethics Committees and Health Care Decision-Making.* Ann Arbor, Michigan, 1984, pp. 6–7.
18. Gracia, D. Panorama actual de las humanidades médicas y de la bioética. Paper presented at the VI International Bioethics Symposium held at Gonnet, Buenos Aires, Argentina on 30 November 1988.
19. Kieffer, G. H. Toma de decisiones éticas. In: *Bioética.* Alhambra, Madrid, 1983, pp. 47–90.
20. Thomasma, D.C. Training in medical ethics: An ethical work-up. *Forum Med* 1(9):33–36, 1978.
21. Sass, H.-M., H. Viefhues, and J. A. Mainetti. *Protocolo de Bochum para la práctica ético-médica (second edition).* Zentrum für Medizinische Ethik, Bochum, 1988.
22. Hucklenbroich, P. Action theory as a source for philosophy of medicine. *Metamedicine* 2(1):55–73, 1981.
23. Sadegh-Zadeh, K. Foundations of clinical praxeology; Part I: The relativity of medical diagnosis. *Metamedicine* 2(2):183–196, 1981.
24. Bertomeu, M. J. La ética en los comités de ética. *Quiron* (La Plata) 19(1):81–83, 1988.
25. Ruddick, W., and W. Finn. Objections to hospital philosophers. *J Med Ethics* 11(1):42–46, 1985.
26. Toulmin, S. How medicine saved the life of ethics. *Perspect Biol Med* 25(4):737–750, 1982.
27. Erde, E. L. On peeling, slicing, and dicing an onion: The complexity of taxonomies of values and medicine. *Theor Med* 4(1):7–26, 1983.
28. Self, D. J. A study of the foundations of ethical decision making of physicians. *Theor Med* 4:57–69, 1983.
29. Veatch, R. Hospital ethics committees: Is there a role? *Hastings Cent Rep* 7(3):22–25, 1977.
30. Spinsanti, S. I comitati di etica negli ospedali. In: *L'Alleanza Terapeutica: Le dimensione della salute.* Citta Nuova Editrice, Rome, 1988, pp. 99–112.
31. Robertson, J. Ethics committees in hospitals: Alternative structures and responsibilities. *Quality Rev Bull* 10(1):6–10, 1984.
32. Levine, C. Questions and (some very tentative) answers about hospital ethics committees. *Hastings Cent Rep* 14(3):9–12, 1984.

On Informed Consent

María del Carmen Lara and Juan Ramón de la Fuente

In recent years there has been considerable debate about whether patients should influence medical decisions. There are at present no guidelines that may be regarded as valid for all physicians or all countries. Those involved are divided into two main camps on the basis of ethical principles regulating not only the physician's behavior but also that of the society to which he belongs.

If it is held that the paramount value in medical practice is the patient's well-being, his participation in the making of decisions may be secondary. If, contrariwise, respect for the patient is the higher ethical value, then it is possible, in some circumstances, for the patient to make decisions that do not further his well-being.

For the patient to make a decision, it is essential that he be autonomous and competent to do so. There are, of course, circumstances that interfere with the patient's competence to act autonomously. However, neither autonomy nor competence should be regarded as absolute concepts, but rather ones that should be related to each particular case.

There is no general model governing how the patient is to be given the information he needs to provide the basis for his decision. Furthermore, the significance of the patient's informed consent regarding what is done by his physician varies from case to case. Subjecting the patient to normal therapeutic procedures, for example, is not the same thing as including him in a clinical research project, especially one where he is assigned at random to a particular treatment group in a controlled clinical trial.

The Concept of Autonomy

The conduct of the physician as such is governed as much by his personal values as by the basic ethical principles of medical practice. Now, there are two general ethical frameworks in medical practice: In one, interest in the patient's autonomy is subordinated to his well-being, and in the other the reference point is respect for the patient and the exercise of his autonomy (1).

In the former, actions are seen as correct if they are conducive to the patient's well-being. This is an ethic geared to outcome, in which autonomy is marginal and paternalism is wrong only when the benefits desired for the patient are not attained. It is clear that many people prefer to be treated paternalistically and "put themselves in the doctor's hands." For them, the exercise of autonomy is more a source of frustration and anxiety than of satisfaction.

On the other hand, in the ethic oriented toward what is done rather than its outcome, the point of departure is the conditions under which action is taken. Autonomy becomes fundamental as a condition for action. For a person to exercise his autonomy, he must be treated with respect. This means that his consent must be sought for any procedure carried out, and all coercion—including paternalistic coercion—must be avoided.

Some persons, however, lack the thinking capacity and volition needed for autonomous action, and in a medical context their state of health may be such as to reduce these abilities still more.

As this suggests, a consensus is difficult to

reach when the controversy over autonomy is viewed in absolute terms. Ethical rules cannot be framed that apply to all patients under all circumstances. Hence, it must be concluded that autonomy is not all-or-nothing, but rather that differing situations exist wherein autonomy can be exercised to a greater or lesser degree (1).

Incapacity

If respect for autonomy is fundamental, so is the attempt to restore those capacities that make it possible. Survival is necessary but insufficient. Indeed, it is still a matter of controversy whether survival without autonomy is a valid goal of medical practice. On the other hand, it seems clear that a risky treatment can be performed to reestablish some functions of autonomous life even if survival is more assured without it.

Lack of Capacity for Autonomous Action

This circumstance arises most often in cases involving children, the original subjects of paternalism. In addition, within the context of medical practice, prolonged and debilitating physical and mental diseases tend to impose a variety of limitations on autonomous action.

In such cases, ongoing evaluation is essential. It is also true that there are situations in which both parents and physicians should restrain their paternalism and leave some decisions to their children and patients, depending on how they are progressing.

Permanent Loss of Autonomy

In this case physicians and close relatives can apply a hypothetical notion of consent: What decision would the patient make if he could? If an answer can be given, then some (if only vestigial) respect can be preserved for what the patient had been and his erstwhile autonomy.

Total Lack of Autonomy

Here, even if the question "What would he have done?" can be asked, the idea of respect for autonomy is meaningless, and medical practice is inevitably paternalistic to some extent. So the question becomes, Who is going to exercise the paternalism, the patient's relatives or the physician?

Information and Consent

Granting or refusing consent to a medical procedure is a particular manifestation of autonomous action. However, medical advice is accepted or rejected by the patient on the basis of information available to him about his disease, its prognosis, and possible treatment options. Therefore, the question arises as to what the patient should know.

The answer to this question will depend on the ethical framework within which the physician functions. If his conduct is governed by the principle of maximum benefit to the patient, he will withhold information if he feels that revealing it may generate anxiety, depression, or self-destructive behavior. Conversely, if the physician's actions are governed by respect for the patient's autonomy, he will provide all necessary information before taking any decision.

There are at least two settings in which the patient can be given information: the therapeutic setting and the research setting. Though in some cases they overlap, it is useful to consider each setting independently.

Within this context, it should be noted that the relevant information can be provided to the patient either through a frank discussion or on a printed sheet or form requesting his consent. Use of the printed form is very common in some countries, but it seems clear that such forms often fail to accomplish the purpose of informing the patient. Patients read them and sign them, but they often cannot remember afterwards what they read, or even whether they read it (2).

Criticism of such written information is mainly of two kinds. For one thing, it has been noted that there is an increasing tendency to provide such written information mainly in order to comply with legal requirements and avoid possible legal problems, rather than to communicate with the patient (3). Thus, once the patient has signed his "informed consent" form, a lawsuit is less likely to prosper, for it can always be argued that the patient "was aware" of what he would undergo. Of course, it often happens in emergencies that neither the patient (who is sometimes unconscious) nor the close relatives (who are usually distressed) have the cognitive capacity to read and understand the information so provided (4).

The second criticism of this written information, specifically that presented on printed consent forms, relates to its structure and content. Such forms often use a language that only a highly educated patient can grasp and sometimes present information that is incomplete (2), too extensive, or hard to understand (5). There has been much discussion of other ways information might be presented (by videotape, brochure, group discussion, etc.), but no studies have yet been done to determine the relative merits of these methods (5).

It has also been proposed that, in addition to preprinted legal consent forms, other forms should be drafted by professional writers with the advice of physicians, evaluated through presentation to healthy subjects and patients to make sure they can be understood, and put to use. Such prepared material could include detailed information on the nature, risks, and benefits of the intended procedure, and the patient could be given a copy for discussion with his family and friends (6). Though not a bad idea, it is felt that this approach would work only in certain cases.

More generally, it should be noted that there is no need to polarize the alternatives: The patient need not know everything, and the physician need not decide everything. The act of informing is part of the doctor-patient relationship, and within this context the doctor can decide which information may be appropriately given to the patient he is interacting with. Some information can be not just unnecessary but indeed undesirable for the patient to know (2, 3).

Some authors maintain that the patient's capacity to make a decision about his treatment needs to be confirmed only if he and his physician disagree (7). Under these somewhat ill-defined circumstances the patient's competence must be evaluated, and (except where there are legal questions) it is ultimately the physician who determines whether the patient is or is not competent to refuse a course of treatment.

In psychiatry, for example, patients have increasingly been refusing treatment with antipsychotic drugs. Nevertheless, it has still been possible to treat these patients legally, despite their refusal (8), by establishing through medical evaluation that the limitations of their mental functions make a truly autonomous choice impossible.

For consent to be a manifestation of autonomy, the patient must be aware of, understand, and appreciate his disease, the therapeutic alternatives, and the risks involved. In addition to adequate cognitive function, the patient's affective state is critical, for any affective disorder can distort the patient's view.

A model has been proposed for determining the need for the patient's consent and his ability to give it based on the characteristics of the treatment (9). This model is summarized as follows:

☐ If for a given disorder or disease (which may be fatal) there is an effective, risk-free treatment, and there is no therapeutic alternative, tacit consent may be assumed. Conversely, a terminal patient who knows that a treatment will be futile is competent to reject it.

☐ If there is any alternative treatment, or if the treatment proposed involves some risk, the patient must understand the differences between the existing alternatives and/or the risks involved and must be capable of making a decision on the basis of that understanding. Ignorance or inability to understand renders the patient incompetent; in such cases, it is correct for the physician to choose what he considers the best option.

☐ The extent of the patient's competence must be especially carefully evaluated when he makes decisions that appear irrational, dangerous, or at odds with medical judgment. To be deemed competent, the patient needs to appreciate the nature and consequences of the decision he is making. The term "appreciate" in this context signifies understanding at the highest level. To be deemed competent in making an apparently irrational decision, the patient must show that he knows and understands all the relevant details of his disease and the therapeutic options, and must be able to state the reasons for his decision.

The foregoing model briefly summarizes some broad guidelines that can be useful in practice. The greatest problems arise when the patient's decisions, apparently irrational and destructive, are not true expressions of autonomy but are a by-product of his disease, which the physician is obliged to treat (10).

Consent in Clinical Research

Among the problems relating to informed consent controversies, those posed by patient participation in controlled clinical trials stand out. Indeed, sometimes the ethical and methodologic interests in this area seem diametrically opposed, though often the contradictions are more apparent than real.

In general, the best experimental design available for determining the efficacy or efficiency of a given treatment is that of the controlled clinical trial. In such a trial, different groups of patients receive different treatments (or one group serving as a control may receive no treatment), and the ensuing results are compared. The treatment each patient receives is determined by ran-

dom selection, and it is here that the principal ethical questions arise, notably, Is random selection necessary? and Is the patient's consent essential for participation in these trials?

Random selection is a very important methodologic condition, for it permits the investigators to minimize other differences while examining the effects of different treatments. Hence, what is at issue in the debate over clinical trials is not their utility, scientific importance, or methodologic appropriateness, but rather their ethical aspects, to the extent that they may compromise the physician's obligation to his patient as well as the patient's rights and welfare.

To resolve this seeming dilemma between medical progress and the patient's well-being, it is necessary to properly apply the following ethical principles governing research on human beings: First, the prime consideration is protection of the patient's rights and well-being; second, treating the patient takes precedence over research; and finally, in evaluating different treatments the best possible experimental design must be used, useless or harmful procedures must be eliminated, and loss of time and resources must be avoided. In this vein, it should be noted that a new procedure can always be compared with "the best available procedure"; the patient always has the right to refuse to participate in a controlled clinical trial; and the researchers always have an obligation to request the patient's consent.

Where disagreement often arises is over what to tell the patient. Among other things, it has been observed that in some studies consent may influence the studies' outcome (11). However, for a person to participate in a clinical trial it is necessary that his consent be voluntary, that he be competent to give it, and that he base his consent on the information needed to arrive at a sound decision. This information must include a description of the study's nature, purpose, duration, procedures, and probable risks and benefits, plus descriptions of the alternative procedures available, how confidentiality will be protected, the institution's policy on compensation, to whom the patient must turn if he has any questions or if other symptoms emerge, the voluntary nature of his participation, and his right to withdraw from the study at any time.

Unfortunately, situations do arise in which apparently voluntary consent has been secured with a degree of manipulation. This happens when the patient is made an offer that is hard to refuse, when he is made to think that care will be withheld afterwards if he decides not to participate, if he is given wrong or alarmist information about his prognosis, or if he is simply not informed about other treatment options.

On the other hand, there are cases in which the request for consent is couched in excessively rigorous terms, which increases the likelihood that patients will refuse to participate. As a result, the recruitment phase is prolonged, the number of withdrawals increases, random assignment is distorted, and sampling errors occur—all of which impairs the clinical trial's reliability. In these cases care should be taken not to make the request for consent too rigorous, or else the clinical trial should be forgone. After all, there are other research designs (12). All in all, therefore, even in the area of clinical trials, there is no solid argument for supposed incompatibility between scientific medicine and medical ethics.

References

1. O'Neill, O. Paternalism and partial autonomy. *J Med Ethics* 10:173–178, 1984.
2. Riecken, H. W., and R. Ravich. Informed consent to biomedical research in Veterans' Administration hospitals. *JAMA* 248:344–348, 1982.
3. Lewis, P. The drawbacks of research ethics committees. *J Med Ethics* 8:61–64, 1982.
4. Weatherall, D. J. Commentary. *J Med Ethics* 8:63–64, 1982.
5. Meisel, A., and L. Roth. What we do and do not know about informed consent. *JAMA* 246:2473–2477, 1981.
6. Adequately informed consent (editorial). *J Med Ethics* 11:115–116, 1985.
7. Spencer, E. Competency and consent to treatment. *JAMA* 253:778–779, 1985.
8. Applebaum, P. The right to refuse treatment with antipsychotic medications: Retrospect and prospect. *Am J Psychiatry* 145:413–419, 1988.
9. Drane, J. Competency to give an informed consent. *JAMA* 252:925–927, 1984.
10. Drane, J. In reply to Spencer. *JAMA* 253:779, 1985.
11. Dahan, R., C. Caulin, L. Figea, et al. Does informed consent influence therapeutic outcome? A clinical trial of the hypnotic activity of placebo in patients admitted to hospital. *Br Med J* 293:363–364, 1986.
12. Kopelman, L. Consent and randomized clinical trials: Are there moral or design problems? *J Med Philos* 11:317–345, 1986.

APPLICATUM

Organ Transplantation: The Latin American Legislative Response[1]

Hernán L. Fuenzalida-Puelma

In recent years the world has witnessed major advances in the technology of organ transplantation, defined by Norrie as "the medical procedure whereby tissues of a human body are removed from the body and reimplanted . . . in . . . that of another human being, with the intention that the transplanted tissue should perform in its new position the function it previously carried out" (1).

As medical barriers to organ transplantations (both postmortem and inter-vivos) have been overcome, legal and ethical obstacles that severely limit the availability of organs have arisen. As these obstacles require fundamental societal decisions, the prospects for transplantation therapy will depend increasingly upon the regulatory environment established by national governments (2).

In 1987 the World Health Organization recognized the need for development of guidelines on organ transplantation by adopting World Health Assembly Resolution 40.13 calling for the study of the legal and ethical issues associated with this delicate medical procedure. In general, the importance of legal regulations in organ transplantation make it imperative that this procedure be comprehensively addressed by legislation (2), so as to ensure that the rights of both donor and recipient, whom the Declaration on Human Transplantation of 1987 recognizes as patients (3), are respected and that the main ethical concerns regarding transplantation are met. In light of the vast array of legal and ethical problems raised by the technology of organ transplantation, it is particularly important to determine which issues legislation has chosen to consider, and also which issues are not addressed by law.

This study examines the legislation (including laws, decrees, decree-laws, and legal regulations) governing the procurement and transplantation of human organs in 16 Latin American countries[2] on an issue-by-issue basis and reviews policy statements about organ transplantation that have been issued by the World Health Organization.

Postmortem Donations

Concern about postmortem donations tends to focus on (a) the form of consent required of the donor and his or her relatives, (b) recipient selection, (c) determination of death, and (d) conflicts of interest that could arise in the course of the procedure. Another matter, funding, that is of general concern, will be taken up in the section on inter-vivos donations.

[1]Edited version of a presentation to the International Congress on Ethics, Justice, and Commerce in Transplantation held in Ottawa, Canada, on 20–24 August 1989.

[2]Argentina, Bolivia, Brazil, Chile, Colombia, Costa Rica, Cuba, the Dominican Republic, Ecuador, Guatemala, Honduras, Mexico, Panama, Paraguay, Peru, and Venezuela.

Donor Consent

Two main approaches to donor consent are commonly referred to as "affirmative" donor consent and consent based on "required request."

Affirmative Donor Consent

This is the critical concept behind voluntary organ donation. Affirmative consent has contributed to the rapid and relatively noncontroversial adoption of organ transplantation in the countries that use this method. There are essentially three types of organ donation by affirmative consent, these being (1) donation by will, (2) donation by donor card, and (3) donation by presumed consent.

Donation by will. Dickens reports that in former times common law did not allow a person to donate his or her body by will because the body was not considered property in law, and so was not part of the estate governed by the will (4). Today, however, a number of civil law countries such as the Dominican Republic and Costa Rica allow a person to consent to organ donation by will.

Nevertheless, in practical terms this form of donation is highly unreliable, since will provisions are seldom revealed in time for suitable organ donation. The process is further delayed by the obligation to provide the potential recipient with details about the transplant in order for the gift to take effect upon the donor's death (4). Thus, special civil procedures should be enacted to accelerate the opening of such wills when death occurs. This advice is aimed especially at Latin American countries with strong formalistic traditions and those where relatively complex and lengthy procedures required to open a will make organ retrieval well-nigh impossible. Nevertheless, despite these problems, donation by will has an advantage: It is not subject to veto by the donor's relatives (4).

Donation by donor card. This procedure, used in Argentina, Canada, and Cuba, appears to be the best form of voluntary organ donation. Its advantage lies in the fact that the donor carries the card with him or her at all times. Thus, the hospital may search for the card and immediately act upon it, rather than having to ask the donor's relatives if a living will exists, and so the efficiency of organ donation is enhanced.

Paradoxically, however, adoption of donation by donor card has contributed to the current organ shortage. To begin with, the procedure tends to be lengthy and impractical. As Cotton and Sandler state, ". . . first, healthy individuals must contemplate their mortality and make a conscious decision to have their organs surgically removed after their death. Second, these individuals must carry with them at all times a signed card noting this decision. Third, public safety or hospital personnel must locate the document and notify the recovery team in sufficient time for recovery to be organized and accomplished."[3]

Beyond that, Latin American countries are generally reluctant to address the issue of death in this way, which is culturally regarded as simplistic. And a recent survey in the United States studying the efficiency of this type of system led to the discovery that no state had a procedure to be followed by law enforcement or medical personnel for the routine identification of card-carrying donors.[4]

More generally, a number of Latin American countries with affirmative donor consent legislation establish a hierarchy of consent (usually by the donor's relatives) for donation of the cadaver. Relatives are generally given the power to veto consent from a relative of the same or lower affinity to the decedent. In certain countries, the relatives may not consent to cadaver use if they are aware that the decedent objected to donation.

Such legal sensitivity to the nearest relatives' preferences regarding donation influences medical practice.[5] Hospitals and physicians are hesi-

---

[3]R. D. Cotton and A. L. Sandler (2), p. 64.
[4]R. D. Cotton and A. L. Sandler (2), p. 64.
[5]B. Dickens (4), p. 6.

tant to remove organs from donors without family consent, even if the deceased possessed a signed donor card. This reluctance has three basic causes. It stems primarily from a fear of future legal action by the donor's family members, who could, for instance, allege that consent to organ donation was subsequently revoked by the donor. Physicians also say that this reluctance arises from a moral obligation to comply with the wishes of the family regarding the deceased person. Finally, the organ donation community is sensitive to the possibility of bad press arising from a situation where an organ is removed despite family objections, which could jeopardize the voluntary donation system.[6]

Therefore, even when a signed donor card is found on a potential donor, physicians often verify that close relatives have no objection to the donation. As Dickens states, "keeping faith with the recently deceased represents an important social value."[7]

Presumed consent. The third form of affirmative donation, donation by presumed consent, calls for removing cadaver organs routinely unless objections are raised before removal (e.g., by the donor prior to death or by a relative, provided the deceased did not specifically authorize donation). Presumed consent laws relieve the grieving family from having to deliberate on the physician's request for organs. This form of donation ensures a larger supply of organs than other forms of affirmative donor consent (5).

Obviously, however, physicians hesitate to remove organs without family consent. Therefore, the number of organs available has not increased significantly. Also, there is concern that presumed consent circumscribes the individual's right to determine what happens to his or her body, since he or she must take affirmative action to prevent organ removal (6). Furthermore, for presumed consent to be valid, the potential donor must understand what is involved, including the provision that failure to dissent will

be construed as consent. This requires widespread education efforts in order to meet minimal legal and ethical standards.

Since 1976 the Council of Europe has been advising European countries to gradually develop their consent laws in the direction of presumed consent for the removal of donor organs.[8] However, this method is not presently utilized in Latin America.

A variation of the presumed consent approach is to acquire organs through the presumed consent/required notification rule. This rule requires that a reasonable effort be made to contact next of kin, so that the latter has the option to refuse donation. Then, if the deceased person did not object to the donation, and if no next of kin or guardian is available after an exhaustive search, the hospital is allowed to remove any needed organ.[9]

Required Request

According to Cohen, who uses this term the way it is employed by Arthur Caplan (7), "the primary hindrance to organ donation is not clinical ignorance, financial obstacles, or even legal concerns . . . It is simply a failure to ask" (5). Required request would abolish this failure by obliging hospitals to discuss the possibility of organ recovery with a potential donor's next of kin upon the donor's death. This relieves physicians of the need to decide whether to question a potential donor's relatives about this matter. Thus, as Cotton and Sandler state, "required request preserves the voluntary nature of the system, but forces a decision to be made" regarding donation.[10] In this way, it is hoped, the boost in organ requests will bring about an increase in the number of available organs.

However, this procedure may be less effective than expected if it becomes perfunctory (4). Prottas feels that required request "flows from a sense that organ procurement more closely re-

---

[6] R. D. Cotton and A. L. Sandler (2), pp. 64–65.
[7] B. Dickens (4), p. 7.

[8] B. Cohen (5), p. 78.
[9] R. D. Cotton and A. L. Sandler (2), p. 65.
[10] R. D. Cotton and A. L. Sandler (2), p.67.

sembles a positive obligation rather than a spontaneous act of generosity."[11]

Moreover, physicians may fail to emphasize the need for charitable donations, and so refusal to donate may tend to become automatic.

Recipient Selection

Living donors may designate the recipients of their gifts, and in most cases the donation is made to a relative. But by what standards should postmortem donations, which are generally made without the recipient being specified, be distributed?

It can be argued that morally, donated organs belong to the community. Therefore, they must be allocated equitably among transplant centers and among patients. Following this approach, McDonald suggests "a system of priorities for which several factors can be used to determine which patients on a local list of waiting patients should have the highest priority in receiving an available organ" (8). This is a difficult task, for if the public perceives the distribution policy as unfair or contrary to important social values, it will be reluctant to donate organs (9).

There is general agreement that the primary criteria should be medical, and that the two main criteria should be medical need and probability of success. Yet judgments about the probability of an organ transplant's success are debatable. And as Prottas notes, while some contraindications such as mismatched immunologic characteristics have been established, others such as the ability of parents to provide postoperative care are more controversial (10).

In the United States, for instance, an infant known as Baby Jesse was initially refused a heart transplant because doctors felt that "Jesse's young, unwed parents . . . were incapable of providing him with the exhaustive care he would require after surgery" (11). Yet although family support may be extremely important in post-

operative care, the absence of family as defined in traditional terms should not serve as a reason to consider a patient unfit for a transplant.

Also, a conflict sometimes exists between urgency of need and probability of success. In that case, Annas feels, the most crucial thing is to define "clinical suitability" for transplantation in a manner that concentrates upon benefit to the patient in terms of lifestyle and rehabilitation rather than upon simple survival (9).

Besides applying medical criteria, some argue that it is also appropriate to consider the age and social utility of the prospective recipient, i.e., the likely pattern of future services to be rendered by the patient upon recovery. Such standards would be difficult to formulate and adopt; furthermore, they could lead to value judgments about the relative worth of people's jobs and lifestyles. In this connection, one should note Annas' view that "arbitrary patient selection excluders . . . such as income, age, and personal habits" should be shunned altogether (9).

In addition, unlike social utility, lifestyle is already taken into consideration in selecting patients, under the category of medical utility. That is, it is not deemed unjust to assign priority to transplant candidates whose lifestyles contributed significantly to their end-stage organ failure. Knowledge of a patient's lifestyle may also be useful in predicting the probability of success of the transplant. For example, continued heavy use of alcohol would greatly reduce the likelihood of a successful liver transplant. Yet it may be difficult to effectively apply such criteria, because the connection between a recipient's disease and his or her lifestyle can seldom be proved irrefutably.

To counter these various problems, medical criteria must be adopted that are objective and independent of social worth categories. Annas suggests the adoption of uniform medical screening criteria to be reviewed and approved by an ethics committee with significant public representation (9).

Most Latin American countries do not specify recipient criteria in their legislation on organ transplantation—beyond general requirements

---

[11] J. M. Prottas (6), p.191.

of medical need, compatibility, and relationship to the donor. However, despite the fact that ongoing development of medical technology makes defining workable criteria difficult, countries should consider enacting provisions indicating criteria that would be considered inappropriate.

Determination of Death

Until fairly recently, death was traditionally defined as cessation of cardiorespiratory function (12). However, as medical technology developed, artificial respirators began being used to maintain individuals after severe injury. It soon became apparent that there was another use for the respirator beyond sustaining a person's life; namely, in a case of severe neurologic injury from which recovery was impossible, the patient's organs could best be preserved for transplantation by keeping them in the body where they grew and maintaining them through artificial support systems (6). Therefore, it became necessary to define death in terms of brain function.

Legislation currently employs three general approaches in defining death: (1) No criteria are defined, and death is determined by ordinary or accepted medical practice; this approach is used in Costa Rica, Cuba, Mexico, Venezuela, and most provinces of Canada. (2) Death is defined as brain death; this is done in Chile and Colombia, and also under the terms of a 1987 law in Bolivia. (3) Sequential definitions are used that include brain death; this is done in Ecuador, Panama, and Peru (13).

Approach (1) is adequate where a common law system is followed (i.e., within this hemisphere in Canada, the United States, and the English-speaking Caribbean). In such countries there is less need for legislation on organ transplantation, thus facilitating organ recovery (2).

Approaches (2) and (3) are more characteristic of countries using a civil law system—among them all the countries of Latin America. Dickens considers definition (2), which depends on purely neurologic criteria, to be limiting in that it requires repetition of tests at least 24 hours after the initial determination of irreversible coma. He finds that "this may be desirable where coma originates . . . in drug overdose or when a patient is in shock, but less so in more obvious cases, such as severe trauma." Delay in determination of death may unnecessarily prejudice the suitability of tissues for organ transplant without affording benefit to dying patients. "Furthermore," Dickens continues,". . . this may be a demanding test to satisfy . . . by physicians in small towns [who often lack] convenient access to complex machinery . . . necessary to . . . conduct such tests." (13)

Approach (3) permits application of a brain test only to patients who are receiving artificial life supports. The test has the advantage of reducing physicians' discretion when patients have lost brain function but have retained other systemic functions (13).

Conflict of Interest

"Medical ethics," Dickens feels, "require that physicians involved with death of persons who may be suitable organ donors after death should not be, nor appear to be, caught in a conflict of interest. . . . Their practice should not be tainted by the suspicion that their concern for patients is distracted by thoughts of the benefit death may represent to potential recipients of organs," a suspicion that could cause voluntary organ donations to substantially decrease.[12]

Accordingly, in most Latin American countries legislation ensures that physicians responsible for determining death do not belong to a transplant team. Only two countries, Ecuador and Paraguay, are silent on this subject. According to Dickens, this measure also spares a dying patient the indignity and discomfort of being taken to die in a facility where organ retrieval can be undertaken conveniently. However, "it has the effect," Dickens continues, "of relieving

_____
[12] B. Dickens (4), p.5.

the physician dealing with the family at death of the patient from any responsibility to address the question of organ donation."[13] This is a disadvantage, in that it requires hospitals to assign this responsibility to another person, although it is the aforementioned physician who must notify the authorities that a donor is available once death has occurred.

Inter-vivos Donations

Concerns about inter-vivos donations tend to focus on four key points: (a) donor consent, (b) funding and donor compensation, (c) commercialization, and (d) international sharing of organs.

Donor Consent

The removal of healthy organs from living patients presents a number of unique legal questions, because it is a surgical procedure generally performed "for the therapeutic benefit not of the donor but of another person." In Norrie's view, the main concern in the case of competent adult donors is ensuring that informed consent is voluntarily given.[14] When the donor is a minor, or is mentally or legally incompetent, difficult issues arise.

According to Cotton and Sandler, "the doctrine of informed consent derives from a tradition of patient self-determination within the context of the physician-patient relationship. . . . Informed consent is achieved when a physician meets the duty to adequately disclose to the patient the nature of the proposed treatment or procedure, the risks involved therein, available alternatives, if any, and the reasonable benefits to be expected" (2). Most Latin American countries require that the potential donor give written consent to the procedure. However, he or she may withdraw this consent up to the time of

the operation without incurring any legal consequences. This allows the donor to consider his or her decision carefully; it also protects the physician and the hospital by providing a legal record of consent, should the donor regret his or her decision after the operation.

Most countries only permit written consent to organ donation by sound-minded donors over the age of majority. Primarily, this decision arises from concern that minors and mentally (or in some cases legally) incompetent individuals will not fully appreciate the consequences of the operation and could be easily swayed or taken advantage of in order to benefit a potential recipient. Thus a number of countries, notably Bolivia and Mexico, prohibit minors, mental incompetents, prisoners, and pregnant women from donating organs. Certain other countries, including Argentina, allow some forms of donation by such persons, but also attempt to provide safeguards for the individuals at risk.

Total prohibition, according to Sharpe, may be too severe in this situation, in view of the current, and probably ongoing, scarcity of organs (14). Therefore, donor requirements should be rendered more flexible in order to meet the need for organs, especially in the case of children, who require organs that closely approximate the size of the diseased organ. Hence minors, and for similar reasons mental incompetents, should be allowed to donate, provided controls are imposed to prevent abuse. Likewise, it seems paternalistic of certain countries to classify pregnant women as incapable of donation. However, prohibition of organ donation by prisoners to people outside their families may be justified by the concern that they might be induced to donate organs for early parole, a situation that has reportedly occurred in the Philippines.

Funding and Donor Compensation

Something that must be considered in both postmortem and inter-vivos transplantation is the simple fact that an organ transplant is a very

---

[13] B. Dickens, (4), p.5.
[14] K. M. Norrie (1), p.453.

expensive proposition. In 1985 the one-year cost of a heart transplant in the United States ranged from US$170,000 to $200,000, a liver transplant in the same country cost between $230,000 and $340,000, and immunosuppressive therapy, which must be continued for life, cost approximately $6,000 per year (9). These prices put transplant operations beyond the reach of most people unless they are privately insured. Therefore, McDonald supports government funding of organ transplantation, so that "all recipients would have equal access to available organs and would be equitably treated" (8). It should be noted, however, that in providing organ transplantation services, the government may be forced to displace other, higher priority health care services (9). This type of dilemma would tend to be especially acute in poorer, less developed countries.

Also, while the foregoing procedure is egalitarian in principle, Dickens feels that "the presumption . . . that government may properly deny wanted services to persons with the means to acquire them . . . is open to ethical challenge" (15). Denial of the use of organ transplantation services must thus be based on more profound objections than mere inequality of opportunity for others.

Regarding compensation to donors, it is generally felt that donors should not incur any kind of expenses related to the removal of the donated organ. This principle is different from that which supports the donation of organs itself, which is gratuitous. A number of countries, notably Canada and Panama, provide public funding of the recipient costs associated with organ transplantation. In other countries (including Argentina) the law ordains that the recipients' social security shall cover the donor's expenses. Yet, interestingly, none of the legislation reviewed provides a definition of the term "expenses."

Cotton and Sandler suggest that donor compensation should include both lost earnings and expenses incurred by the donor in connection with the organ donation (2). The former covers wages, salaries, and associated benefits accorded

by specific labor legislation. The latter covers expenses for six sorts of items: examinations preceding the donation, logistical costs (for transportation, housing, and meals), surgical removal of the organ or organs, patient recovery, insurance coverage for immediate and future risks, and insurance coverage for damage that may result from the organ's removal.

Commercialization

Demand for organs currently exceeds supply and will likely continue to do so, especially with the further development of medical technology. Given this circumstance, the sale of human organs is likely to flourish unless strongly deterred by legal or ethical controls.

Such a market could alleviate the shortage of organs and tissues, thus saving and improving the quality of more lives. It would also respect the freedom of individuals to do as they wish so long as they do not harm others.

Yet Professor Dickens finds "the prospect of a free commercial market in organs . . . morally intolerable . . . it would favor well-insured or rich recipients over poor, and induce the poor . . . to sell their body tissues," a situation reported to occur in Bombay (15). Furthermore, there is concern that the existence of such a market would eliminate all current voluntary organ donations and reduce the "altruistic" nature of our society regarding human health (14).

Commerce in organs, i.e., both for-profit transactions and international trade of human organs (especially live kidneys from developing countries), for transplant purposes has been widely condemned, in both international fora and most of the national legislation involved. The most relevant international declarations are the Statement on Live Organ Trade by the 37th World Medical Assembly (Brussels, October 1985—16) and World Health Assembly Resolution 42.5 of 1989 (17). A number of Latin American countries have specific legislation that prohibits the sale of organs. Certain other countries—notably Brazil, the Dominican Republic, Paraguay, and Peru—do not expressly prohibit it, and so the practice is not barred by law.

International Sharing of Organs

The matching of available organs to the best possible recipients based on immunologic criteria has been an important factor in increasing graft survival in recent years. This situation encourages measures calling for international sharing of organs, a development that would increase the likelihood of a perfect match between donor and recipient. In that event, human organs would no longer be viewed as a scarce national resource, but rather as a scarce international resource.

In a voluntary system of organ donation, it seems appropriate to assign priority to citizens of the country in which the organ was donated, but it may be commendable to share organs with nonimmigrant aliens. (Only one country, Colombia, expressly prohibits the international sharing of organs, while Canada and the United States already appear to have an informal reciprocity agreement that allows citizens of either country to be recipients of organs donated in the other country.) Overall, there appear to be strong moral arguments for sharing organs with other countries and participating in a system marked by reciprocity. Eventually, as the technology of organ transplantation advances and the rate of organ donation increases in other countries, an exchange program may become feasible on an international scale.

Concluding Remarks

The study upon which this article is based has explored the current legal regulation of organ transplantation in many Latin American countries. It is immediately apparent that very few of the countries involved have comprehensive legislation in this area. And while certain countries have made provision in their legisla-

tion for passage of regulations, as of 1989 they had failed to draft such regulations. Also, some Latin American countries (including Costa Rica) still follow the cumbersome procedure of donation by will, which incurs excessive delays making organ retrieval almost impossible. In addition, Latin American legislation needs to consider the donation potential represented by minors and certain incompetents, despite the ethical debate that surrounds the right of these individuals to become donors.

Regarding commerce in human organs, it is true that society has a duty to encourage the availability of sufficient organs and also that considerable legal advances are needed in the organ transplant field. Nevertheless, the solution to the organ shortage does not lie in commercialization. Among other things, such commerce would discriminate against those who do not possess adequate financial means for acquiring the needed organ.

On the other hand, a lack of distinction between commerce in organs and compensation of donors for related costs has created a legislative and regulatory vacuum of considerable importance. The resulting absence of a legal base for donor compensation, besides failing to encourage donations, makes it very difficult to conduct adequate information and education campaigns pertaining to organ donation and donor rights (1). Regrettably, this vacuum makes the matter of compensation subject to private understandings between donors and recipients.

As the foregoing indicates, organ transplant technology has raised a number of important ethical and legal issues. In seeking to ensure that the principal issues among these are addressed, the World Health Organization has recommended that guidelines be promulgated to help countries develop more comprehensive government legislation on organ procurement and transplantation (2). Such comprehensive legislation is clearly needed, for as Gerson points out, "ultimately, the potential for organ transplantation will depend not only on advanced medical technology, but also on progress in the legal technology of organ donation" (18). This observation is relevant for the nations of Latin America.

Acknowledgments. I would like to express my deepest gratitude to Ms. Leslie Creeper of Canada, Ms. Maud Calegari of France, and Ms. Ana María Linares of Colombia for their collaboration on this study.

References

1. Norrie, K. M. Human tissue transplants: Legal liability in different jurisdictions. *International and Comparative Law Quarterly* 34(3):442, 1985.
2. Cotton, R. D., and A. L. Sandler. The regulation of organ procurement and transplantation in the United States. *J Leg Med* 7(1):55–56, 1986.
3. 39th World Medical Assembly. The Declaration on Human Transplantation. World Medical Association, Madrid, October 1987.
4. Dickens, B. Legal issues pertaining to the role of the family in organ retrieval. *Transplantation Today* 2:4, 1987.
5. Cohen, B. Organ donor shortage: European situation and possible solutions. *Scand J Urol Nephrol Suppl* 19(3):79, 1985.
6. Prottas, J. M. The rules for asking and answering: The role of law in organ donation. *University of Detroit Law Review* 63(145):186–187, 1985.
7. Caplan, A. L. Ethical and policy issues in the procurement of cadaver organs for transplantation. *N Engl J Med* 311(15): 981–983, 1984.
8. McDonald, J. C. The national procurement and transplantation network. *JAMA* 259(5):725–726, 1988.
9. Annas, G. J. Report on the Massachusetts Task Force on Organ Transplantation in regulating heart and liver transplants in Massachusetts: An overview of the Report of the Task Force on Organ Transplantation. *Law, Medicine, and Health Care* 13(1):8–39, 1985.
10. Prottas, J. M. The structure and effectiveness of the U.S. Organ Procurement System. *Inquiry* 22(4):365–376, 1985.
11. Wallis, C. Of television and transplants. *Time* 127(25):68, 1986.
12. Rosenberg, J. C., and M. P. Kaplan. Evolving legal and ethical attitudes toward organ transplantation from cadaver donors. *Dialysis and Transplantation* 8(9):907, 1979.
13. Dickens, B. Legal evolution of the concept of brain death. *Transplantation Today* 2:62–63, 1985.
14. Sharpe, G. Commerce in tissue and organs. *Health Law in Canada* 2:27–44, 1985.
15. Dickens, B. Legal and ethical issues in buying and selling organs. *Transplantation Today* 4:5–21, 1987.
16. 37th World Medical Assembly. Statement on Live Organ Trade. World Medical Association, Brussels, October 1985.
17. World Health Organization. World Health Assembly Resolution 42.5. Geneva, 1989.
18. Gerson, W. N. Refining the law of organ donation: Lessons from the French law of presumed consent. *Journal of International Law and Politics* (New York University) 19(4):1013–1032, 1987.

Annex 1. Legal sources.

Country	Reference	Date	Abbreviation used
Argentina	Law 21,541	21 March 1977	L77
Argentina	Law 23,464 (amendment to Law 21,541 of 21 March 1977)	23 March 1987	L87
Argentina	Decree 397/89	28 March 1989	D89
Bolivia	Decree Law 15,629	18 July 1978 (summary)	DL78
Bolivia	Regulations	March 1982 (summary)	R82
Brazil	Law 4,280	6 November 1963	L63
Chile	Law 18,173	15 November 1982	L82
Chile	Regulations	3 December 1983	R83
Colombia	Law 9	January 1979 (summary)	L79
Colombia	Decree 2,363 (superseded Law 73 of 20 December 1988; no new provisions have been adopted)	25 July 1986	D86
Costa Rica	Law 5,560	20 August 1974	L74
Cuba	Law 41	13 July 1983	L83
Dominican Republic	Law 391	1 December 1981	L81
Ecuador	Law 64	15 June 1987	L87
Guatemala	Decree 45–79	9 August 1979 (summary)	D79
Guatemala	Regulations	7 October 1986	R86
Honduras	Decree 131	7 June 1983	D83
Mexico	Sanitary Code	26 February 1973	HC73
Mexico	Regulations	16 August 1976	R76
Panama	Law 10	11 July 1983	L83
Paraguay	Law 836/80	12 December 1980 (summary)	L80
Peru	Law 23,415	4 June 1982	L82
Peru	Regulations	6 May 1983	R83
Venezuela	Law 72	28 August 1972	L72

Annex 2. Organ donations between living persons.

Legal reference by country	Consent of the donor			Recipients
	Regenerating organs	Nonregenerating organs	Incompetence	
Argentina:				
L77	Excluded	Over 18 years of age. Consent of a legally compentent donor	If the donor is mentally incompetent, relatives can give the required consent	Depends on relationship to the donor: parents, children, and siblings; on an exceptional basis, spouse and adoptive children
L87	Over 18 years of age. Consent of a legally competent donor	Over 18 years of age. Consent of a legally compentent donor	...[b]	Depends on relationship to the donor: parents, blood-related siblings; on an exceptional basis, spouse, adoptive children, relatives to the second degree of consanguinity, and collateral relatives to the fourth degree of consanguinity
D89	Written informed consent of donor and recipient. Donor must specify the organs that he/she wishes to donate	Written informed consent of donor and recipient. Donor must specify the organs that he/she wishes to donate	...	...
Bolivia:				
DL78[a]	Consent of a mentally and legally competent donor	Donor consent	Minors and mentally incompentent persons. Prisoners can only donate to relatives	...
R82[a]	Consent of the donor in the presence of a notary public	Consent of the donor in the presence of a notary public	Minors and mentally incompentent persons. Prisoners can only donate to relatives	...
Brazil:				
L63	...	...	...	...
Chile:				
L82	Over 18 years of age. Written informed consent by a legally competent donor or a married female donor	Over 18 years of age. Written informed consent by a legally competent donor or a married female donor	...	...

77

Annex 2. (Continued)

Legal reference by country	Consent of the donor			Recipients
	Regenerating organs	Nonregenerating organs	Incompetence	
Chile: R83	Written consent of a legally competent donor or a married female donor	Written consent of a legally competent donor or a married female donor	…	…
Colombia: L79	Donor consent	Donor consent	…	…
D86[a]	Over 18 years of age Written consent of the donor	Over 18 years of age Written consent of the donor	Minors and prisoners	…
Costa Rica: L74	Of legal age Written consent of the donor in the presence of two witnesses	…	…	Depends on relationship to the donor: relatives to the fourth degree of consanguinity or third degree of kinship, and spouse
Cuba: L83	Pursuant to regulations of the Ministry of Public Health			
Dominican Republic: L81	…	…	…	…
Ecuador: L87	Consent of a legally competent donor	Consent of a legally competent donor	Mentally incompetent persons	Depends on medical necessity and compatibility
Guatemala: D79	…	…	…	…
R86[a]	Over 18 years of age Written consent of the donor and recipient	Written consent of the donor and recipient	Minors, mentally incompetent persons, prisoners, and unconcious persons	Depends on medical necessity, compatibility, and age (preferably under 55 years of age)

Country: Law				
Honduras: D83[a]	Over 21 years of age / Voluntary consent of a donor in full possession of his/her mental faculties	Over 21 years of age / Voluntary consent of a donor in full possession of his/her mental faculties	Unconcious persons	Depends on relationship to the donor: siblings
Mexico: HC73[a]	Excluded	Written consent of the donor	Minors, mentally incompetent persons, and prisoners	Depends on Ministry of Health procedures
R76[a]	Written consent of the donor signed in the presence of two witnesses over 18 and under 60 years of age		Minors, mentally incompetent persons, and prisoners	Depends on relationship to donor (preferably first-degree relative), medical necessity, and age (under 60 years)
Panama: L83	Written consent of the donor	...	Minors, mentally incompetent persons, and prisoners	Depends on medical necessity
Paraguay: L80[a]	Written consent of the donor	...	Detainees and mentally incompetent persons	...
Peru: L82	Written consent of the donor	...	...	Depends on medical necessity
L83	...	...	...	...
Venezuela: L72	Written consent of a donor in full possession of his/her mental faculties Only parents, children, and siblings of the recipient can donate	...	...	Depends on relationship to the donor: parents, adult children, and adult siblings

a Pregnant women cannot donate.
b ...The law does not address this matter specifically.

79

Annex 3. Commerce.

Legal reference by country	Prohibition of commerce	Penalty		Comments
		Fine	Jail	
Argentina:				
L77	Yes	...[a]	Yes	...
L87	Yes	...	Yes	...
D89	...	...	...	...
Bolivia:				
L78	Yes	...	...	Commerce prohibited except when authorized for charitable purposes
DL78	...	...	...	...
Brazil:				
L63	...	...	...	...
Chile:				
L82	Yes	...	...	Acts or contracts for profit are null and void
R83	Yes	...	...	...
Colombia:				
L79	Yes	...	...	...
D86	Yes	Yes	...	Commerce is prohibited except for reasons of grave public disaster or human solidarity
Costa Rica:				
L74	Yes	Yes	...	Commerce is regarded as profaning the deceased and is punishable under the criminal code
Cuba:				
L83				Pursuant to regulations of the Ministry of Public Health
Dominican Republic:				
L81	...	...	...	...
Ecuador:				
L87	Yes	Yes	...	Acts or contracts for profit are null and void
Guatemala:				
D79	...	...	...	...
R86	Yes	...	...	...
Honduras:				
D83	Yes	Yes	Yes	...
Mexico:				
HC73	...	...	...	...
R76	Yes	...	...	...
Panama:				
L83	Yes	...	...	...
Paraguay:				
L80	...	...	...	...
Peru:				
L82	...	...	...	...
R83	...	...	...	...
Venezuela:				
L72	Yes	Yes	...	...

[a] ... = The law does not address this matter specifically.

Annex 4. Donor compensation.

Legal reference by country	Compensation for:		Payment made by:		Comment
	Lost income	Expenses	Social Security	Recipient	
Argentina:					
L77	...[a]	Yes	Yes	Yes	The donor is exempt from all payment or reimbursement of costs relating to surgery
L87	...	...	...	...	...
D89	...	...	Yes	...	...
Bolivia:					
DL78	...	...	...	...	...
R82	...	...	...	...	...
Brazil:					
L63	Yes	...	The Ministry of Health pays for indigents	Yes	...
Chile:					
L82	...	...	...	...	...
R83	...	...	...	...	...
Colombia:					
L79	Yes	...	Yes	...	...
D86	...	...	Recipient or persons responsible for recipient	...	...
Costa Rica:					
L74	...	...	...	...	...
Cuba:					
L83	Pursuant to regulations of the Ministry of Public Health				
Dominican Republic:					
L81	...	...	...	...	...
Ecuador:					
L87	...	...	...	...	...
Guatemala:					
D79	...	...	...	...	...
D86	...	...	...	...	...
Honduras:					
D83	...	...	...	...	...
Mexico:					
HC73	...	...	...	...	...
R76	...	...	...	...	...
Panama:					
L83	Yes	Yes	...	...	Donor and recipient are entitled to free medical treatment
Paraguay:					
L80	...	...	...	...	...
Peru:					
L82	...	...	...	...	...
R83	...	...	...	...	...
Venezuela:					
L72	...	...	...	...	...

[a] ... = The law does not address this matter specifically.

Annex 5. Determination of death.

Legal reference by country	Definition of death	Physicians responsible for determining death	Hospital situation
Argentina:			
L77	Cessation of brain function	A clinician, a neurologist or neurosurgeon, and a cardiologist[a]	Qualified
L87	To be established in a regulation (not yet adopted)	...	...
D89	Cessation of brain function	A clinician and a neurologist or neurosurgeon;[a] the death certificate must be signed by the second, as well as by members of the family present at the time of death	Qualified
Bolivia:			
DL78	Current diagnostic methods	Two physicians[a]	Qualified
R82	Cessation of brain function	Three physicians[a]	Qualified
Brazil:			
L63	...	The director of the hospital or his legal representative	...
Chile:			
L82	...	...	...
R83	Absence of brain function	Two surgeons, at least one of whom must be a neurologist or neurosurgeon	...
Colombia:			
L79	...	Two physicians[a]	Qualified
D86	Cessation of brain function	Two physicians[a] and one of the physicians who is to perform the transplant	Qualified
Costa Rica:			
L74	Confirmed by appropriate procedures	Two physicians[a]	Authorized
Cuba:			
L83	Pursuant to regulations of the Ministry of Public Health		
Dominican Republic:			
L81	...	Three physicians	Specialized in organ transplants

Legal reference by country	Definition of death	Physicians responsible for determining death	Hospital situation
Ecuador:			
L87	Absence of cardiac, respiratory, and brain function	...	Authorized
Guatemala:			
D79	...	...	Public or private, but must comply with the regulations
R86	...	Three physicians (surgeons)	...
Honduras:			
D83	...	A neurologist or neurosurgeon and a cardiologist or internist	Authorized
Mexico:			
HC73	Certified by methods established by the Ministry of Health and Welfare	Two physicians[a]	Authorized institutions
R76	...	...	Qualified
Panama:			
L83	Spontaneous cessation of respiratory and circulatory or brain function, if artificial support measures are used	Three physicians[a]	Authorized
Paraguay:			
L80	...	...	Qualified
Peru:			
L82	Cessation of brain activity or cardiorespiratory function	Three physicians	...
LR83	Cessation of brain or cardiovascular activity	Medical board: the director of the hospital, a neurologist, and the chief physician	
Venezuela:			
L72	Appropriate procedures	Three physicians[a]	Authorized

[a] The physicians indicated cannot be members of the transplant team.
[b] ... = The law does not address this matter specifically.

Annex 6. Postmortem organ donation.

Legal reference by country	Donation requirements	Order of consent for donation of the cadaver[a]	Use of cadaver in medico-legal cases
Argentina:			
L77	Over 18 years of age Written consent of a legally competent donor	Spouse, adult children, parents, siblings (adults), grandparents and grandchildren, relatives to the fourth degree of consanguinity, or relatives to the second degree of kinship	...[b]
L87	Over 18 years of age Consent by a donor in full possession of his/her mental faculties	Spouse, adult children, parents, siblings (adults), grandparents and grandchildren, relatives to the fourth degree of consanguinity, or relatives to the second degree of kinship	...
D89	Written consent of the donor and recipient	If no relatives are present at the time of death and if the Sole Coordinating Center for Organ Removal and Implants agrees, the cadaver may be used	...
Bolivia:			
DL78	Donor consent	Legally authorized relative The cadaver may be used if it has been abandoned	...
R82	Written consent If the cadaver is to be embalmed or cremated, it may be used automatically	Legally authorized relative If the cadaver has been abandoned, the hospital director may authorize its use	With the authorization of the health authorities
Brazil:			
L63	Written consent of the donor	The donor's spouse, relatives to the second degree of consanguinity, religious institutions, or persons legally responsible for the donor	...
Chile:			
L82	Written consent of the donor	The cadaver may be used if is abandoned, or with the consent of relatives to the first degree of consanguinity or the donor's spouse	...

R83	Written consent of a legally competent donor or of a married female donor	The cadaver may be used if it is not claimed within two hours of death, or with the consent of the donor's spouse or legitimate parents	...
Colombia: L79	Donor consent	A legally authorized relative may give consent / The cadaver may be used if it has been abandoned	...
D86	Donor consent	Spouse, relatives to the fourth degree of consanguinity, relatives to the second degree of kinship, or adopted parents or children	...
Costa Rica: L74	Written consent of the donor	Spouse, adult children, parents, adult siblings, or the hospital director	With the authorization of the coroner
Cuba: L83		Pursuant to regulations of the Ministry of Public Health	
Dominican Republic: L81	Written consent of the donor in his/her will	...	...
Ecuador: L87	Consent of a legally competent donor or a married female donor	Spouse, children, parents, or siblings	...
Guatemala: D79	...	The cadaver may be used if the relatives agree, or if it has been abandoned	...
R86	Written consent of the donor	If the donor consents while alive, upon death the cadaver may be used without need of relatives' consent	...
Honduras: D83	Written consent of a legally competent donor	Spouse, adult children, parents, adult siblings, or grandparents	...

Annex 6. (Continued)

Legal reference by country	Donation requirements	Order of consent for donation of the cadaver[a]	Use of cadaver in medico-legal cases
Mexico: HC73	Written consent of the donor	...	...
R76	Written consent of the donor	Relatives If the cadaver has been abandoned, it may be used without consent	...
Panama: L83	Donor must be of legal age Written consent by a donor in full possession of his/her mental faculties If the donor is a minor, the minor's guardian must consent	Spouse, adult child, parents, the person who determines the disposition of the cadaver If the cadaver has been abandoned, it may be used without consent	Corneas only
Paraguay: L80	Written consent of the donor	...	
Peru: L82	Written consent of the donor If death occurs in a health center, organs may be removed without consent unless the donor has recorded his/her objection in the Register	Parents, children, or spouse	...
R83	Voluntary written informed consent of the donor	Whether consent has been given [by the donor] or not, it can be given by parents, spouse, or children	...
Venezuela: L72	Written consent of the donor	Spouse, adult children, parents, or siblings	If the cause of death is definitely known, organs may be removed

a Persons who may give consent in the absence of consent or objection.
b ... = The law does not address this matter specifically.

Human Dying Has Changed

Alfonso Llano Escobar

Man's passage from life on earth has a dual dimension: the existential process of dying and the transcendent, mysterious dimension of the beyond. This article examines the first dimension, the existential process of man's death, without forgetting the unfathomable mystery of spiritual transcendence. More specifically, it describes the characteristics of the new form of human dying as an effect of modern science, technology, and life; examines the serious problem created for the patient by the change in the form of dying; and attempts to describe the solution to this problem that has begun to emerge around the world in recent decades.

The Altered Form of Dying

Let us start with an easily verifiable fact: Modern medical science and technology, the philosophers of the last century, the writers of the present century, our communication and entertainment media, and the consumer society of the present century have changed the dying process from what was traditional in almost all countries, at least in the Western world. It is not necessary to point out the specific scientific and technologic factors involved to observe that ". . . health care in hospitals, with their highly developed technology, has changed the form of dying" (1).

In past times, most people died at home, knowing they were going to die, surrounded by their loved ones, with religious care, and in possession of all the facilities required for making both minor and major decisions with regard to their situation. At present, to the contrary,

". . . statistics from the United States of America reveal that more than 80% of natural deaths take place in clinics and hospitals where the means for prolonging life are increasing every day and are provided to practically all patients. Very frequently these patients end their days in isolation and solitude with tubes inserted into all their orifices and with needles in their veins, waiting to breathe their last breath" (2).

Death is becoming "hospitalized"; that is, it is being taken out of homes and social life and being hidden in clinics and hospitals. Anesthesia, drugs, and tranquilizers diminish the patient's consciousness, and with it the patient's freedom.

Frequently, the truth is kept from patients with regard to the seriousness of their situation. "Somehow," a physician notes, "many of us have come to believe that we have a right to lie to patients under the assumption that we are protecting them from the cruelties and realities of life and death. This is the first step in the destruction of an honest relationship with the patient" (3).

Recently, in the United States at least, the pendulum has been swinging back. In the 1960s the practice of nearly all U.S. physicians was to hide the truth from their patients. In the 1980s, however, more than 80% apparently believed in telling them the entire truth. Nevertheless, this change has not taken place in other countries of the Americas, most notably those of Latin America, where patients and their families tend to leave nearly all the initiative regarding information and treatment up to the physician.

Together with these data of scientific origin regarding death, it would be well to provide some social information. Not many years ago, N. Versluis (1) presented a good analysis on this subject in which he made the following observations:

> Our times fail to recognize death in the full measure of its gravity. There is no place in modern life for thinking of death. It is feared, and perhaps because of this, contemporary man prefers ignoring it and playing with it (which is another form of avoiding it) rather than facing it by attempting to understand it and accept it as part of real existence. We are so familiar with death through the communications media that we have made ourselves insensitive to the possibility of dying and prefer to consider it as something alien to us. Motion pictures, television, novels, and soap operas are abusing the phenomenon of death, which they circulate as an easily acquired commodity for consumption. The public demands it in great quantities, accompanied by violence, which it accepts and even enjoys with lamentable debasement (1).

The American sociologist G. Gorer has a name for this phenomenon of the consumer society, the manipulation and enjoyment of violent death. He calls it "the pornography of death" (4).

What a strange contradiction the twentieth century manifests with regard to death. On the one hand it wishes to ignore real death, and at the same time it abuses death's image in the form of play and violence through the communications and entertainment media. The increasingly common attempt in various countries of the world to conceal death as much as possible by making up corpses in order to give viewers a lifelike impression may be considered symbolic of the social concealment of death. On the other hand, children are taught "to kill" in play, and adults are sold the article of death in motion pictures and television programs.

Another important change in the form of dying involves prolongation of human existence on two levels: First, most people today die in middle or advanced age; and second, the act of dying itself has been prolonged.

In most countries life expectancy at birth has practically doubled. In past centuries, as a result of wars and plagues, life expectancy at birth was roughly 30 years for men and 35 for women (5). Today, life expectancy in the developed countries is more than 70 years. It is true that middle age has been extended, but it is also true that the infirmities of old age have increased and become generalized. The number of elderly people is increasing disproportionately around the world, accompanied by the well-known problems of this stage of life and even some new ones.

Science and technology are also contributing to prolonging the process of dying. The scientific and technical progress achieved in the health sciences in this century are of such magnitude that one might say with pardonable exaggeration that physicians are no longer allowing death to happen. If in past centuries a cancer of the pancreas or myocardial infarction typically left the afflicted with little time to live, those who suffer them today may survive for months or even years enduring a slow death; there are even those who make full recoveries and return to normal life.

If, in addition to this prolongation of life, it is considered that many physicians say little if anything to their patients regarding their true situation, and at most provide only family members with information about the patient's status, it can be seen that more and more frequently the patient is no longer master of his own death, since he does not know when he is going to die, nor can he make appropriate decisions based on pertinent information.

In summarizing the new form of dying in the twentieth century, it can be said that death has been largely postponed until old age, since life expectancy in many countries is now more than 70 years. Furthermore, the act of dying has been prolonged, since it may go on for months and even years; it has become "scientific," since nowadays people die in hospitals, surrounded by health personnel and ministered to by technical equipment that tries the dying person's patience; it has become passive, since in many places physicians, in agreement with family members, make decisions regarding hospitalization, surgery, operations, and the like without even consulting the patient; it has become profane, since religious services in accordance with the beliefs of the patient are tending to diminish and even to disappear in some health centers; and it has become isolated, since the patient dies alone and abandoned, even while surrounded by the most varied and attentive health personnel.

Real death has thus been "hospitalized," in contrast to the social image of death disseminated and manipulated by the communications media; and so real death is often deprived of its significance and transcendent relationship to the beyond. It has become superficial and trivial.

The Problem with the New Form of Dying

Clearly, all this creates a serious and delicate problem for the patient. Therefore, rather than enumerating a series of problems, as if each were independent one from the other, it appears more worthwhile to bring the difficulties involved together and consider them as one central problem for the purpose of exploring their ramifications and consequences.

The one fact which appears to underlie almost all the characteristics of modern dying just described is precisely that science, technology, and society have wrested death from the patient, since he now behaves in a passive manner with regard to the dying process.

In general, physicians and health personnel devote themselves to treating the patient with all kinds of technologic advances, guided by the supreme criterion of prolonging his life, if only his purely biological life. The hospital, and to some extent family members, take charge of the death of the patient, who is no longer allowed to die his own death. He suffers it but is not master of it, for they have taken it away from him. This may be done with his complicity. His desire to live forces him to deliver himself into the hands of health professionals, who from the surgeon to the stretcher carrier are in charge of all matters, great and small, regarding the patient and his physical and personal surroundings.

In this way hospital centers have taken over the patient's process of dying. They advance or delay the moment of his death. They send him to an intensive care unit or to the operating room when they wish, and also remove him at will, usually in accordance with the demands of science and technology.

This is perhaps what most characterizes present-day dying. People die "scientifically" in hospitals and clinics, surrounded by strange men and women dressed in white and supplied with all kinds of apparatuses. They are removed from their families and religious settings and interned in a white jungle where physicians are in charge and science and technology prevail—all this with a view to distancing death and prolonging life to the utmost extent that the scientific and technologic capabilities of the institution will allow.

The key people making decisions here are not the patients but rather their closest family members and the health professionals involved. We use the plural here advisedly, since it is more in keeping with the fact that relatives are typically numerous and health professionals legion.

It is worth repeating that the inevitable result of this kind of medical treatment, which is becoming known as "aggressive" or "invasive" medicine, is to take death away from the patient. The individual does not make either major or minor decisions, largely because he is ignorant of the diagnosis of his illness and of its prognosis. Treatments are concealed from him, and neither his collaboration nor his active opinion with regard to his illness is requested of him. He is isolated as a precautionary measure, and visits from family members and friends are restricted. Such isolation is accentuated to a maximum degree when he is transferred to an intensive care unit.

This process of physical internment and isolation can be regarded as "deprivation of death."

From the traditional act of dying at home, surrounded by loved ones and provided with religious support, a solitary death has been created in which there is an increasingly limited encounter between a blurred and poorly informed consciousness on the one hand, and an increasingly silenced and silent transcendence (God) on the other. If this circumstance is combined with reduction and practical absence of the patient's freedom, it is neither unreasonable nor exaggerated to say that science and technology have deprived the patient of his death.

What problem is created for the patient by this cutting off of the personality, this isolation from others, this passivity, this ending of existence without consciousness of the end or the beyond? To begin with, the absence of the self and lack of consciousness and freedom signify a regrettable diminution of the patient's personality. Man is truly measured by his personal dimension, not by his physical size, weight, or build; neither is he measured by his biological life or the number of years it endures, without due regard for its quality or the participation of the individual in healing processes.

Illness and, above all, the dying process place man, even if he does not believe in God, before the most important decisions of his life; and what the healthy man does not understand if he has never suffered severe illness, is that as the body becomes ill, the lucidity of the personal self is not spared. The mind, the spirit, and the total man also fall ill, and in this circumstance he must confront the meaning of his last days.

Today, more than ever before, the physician needs initiation in a sound anthropology that will teach him to approach each patient and treat him as the human being he is, one whose interior world is being put to the test, whose anxieties and fears cannot be ignored; a human being with his own transcendence and his own overture to God. To deprive the patient of his mental lucidity and the degree of consciousness required to dispose of his goods, to keep him from saying goodbye to his loved ones, speaking to his lawyer and to the chaplain about his problems of conscience and his desire to put himself

at peace with God and mankind, is to create a problem for him, the problem of having to make decisions with regard to God and his fellow creatures and not being able to do so for lack of information and freedom.

This is precisely what is known as dying an undignified death, dying like a plant or animal.

We must defend the rights of the patient, and we must find again the most essentially human way of dying—that of dying in full awareness and in freedom.

Modern-day medicine, which deserves great praise and gratitude for its enormous conquests, must recover the human values of the physician and the patient as a means of making health professionals see the need to restore the patient's awareness and freedom, together with his right to assume his place regarding God precisely at the moment when he is terminating his earthly life.

The patient tends to benefit from such a cooperative attitude, since treatment typically promotes a cure when it replaces a passive attitude with active participation (6).

The need to recover death is great. What can be done, then, to retrieve it?

Toward Possible Solutions

Let us attempt to generalize about what has been done in recent decades throughout most of the world, since the new form of dying has been appearing everywhere, and everywhere has been evoking a similar response.

The response has been somewhat delayed. The modern world has become insensitive to traditional moral values, and perhaps for this reason the effects of the involuntary dehumanization of medicine were not immediately felt, either in the area of research or in that of treatment provided at hospitals and clinics.

However, the response, when it came, assumed a name: bioethics. From it and with it we are going to see the world's response in favor of maintaining contact not only with the fact of death but also with the health of human life in general, with research into human life from conception until death, and with the applications of research. Bioethics is not a discipline that is cold, calculating, abstract, defined, and precise in its methods and content. It is rather a movement, an interdisciplinary effort, a growing process of searching out moral values; and as such it must be given time to assume form, meaning, method, and organization. It is not an already-existing standard brought in from the outside with mandatory legal power over the medical world or hospital personnel—as if it were intended to punish a criminal, reprimand him, or deprive him of his life or liberty.

Let us make this point very clear: The health professional is above all a benefactor of mankind. What he is doing for humanity cannot yet be evaluated to its full extent and depth. As the physician since ancient times has been compared to the priest, and has recently been practically transformed into the lord and master of life and death, it is not surprising that he is ironically compared to God himself. Physicians are "playing God," the magazine *Newsweek* noted a few years ago on its cover and in a feature article (7).

Let us not forget the historical-social premise stating that science provides power (8) and technology provides progress and change. Rather than committing a sin, the modern-day physician is making a discernible and regrettable error; he believes in good faith that science and technology have made him the master of human birth and death.

Such, however, is not the case. God must continue to be God; and man, whether a technician or a scholar, must be aware of his limitations and become a tool in the hands of God for the good of humanity.

Let us return to the universal response in favor of the patient's recovery of death and mastery over his dying. Let us recall some of the events that have given rise to this international response in favor of the humanization of medicine and defense of patient rights that is called bioethics.

The greatest violations of human freedom that have taken place in this century—especially those systematically perpetrated more by dictators than by physicians, violations that have regrettably employed the practices of aggressive medicine, in places such as concentration camps and in human experiments carried out on prisoners—have induced the highest authorities to defend the right of all human beings to informed consent prior to any experimentation, hospitalization, or medical treatment.

Nuremberg, Helsinki, Rome, the United Nations, the World Health Organization, the Pan American Health Organization, Geneva, and the Holy See (9) are names that will long be associated with human welfare. They are the names of sites or of international organizations linked to pronouncements made at the highest level in defense of human freedom, especially of those suffering from conditions found in prisons and concentration camps and those with physical or mental disability.

To cite another example, the World Medical Association, meeting in Lisbon in 1981, approved a Declaration on the Rights of the Patient, which, *inter alia*, provides that after having been properly informed of the treatment proposed, the patient has the right to accept or reject it and to die a dignified death.

The intervention of governments through their legislative and judicial organs has played an important role in emphasizing the ethical nature of medical acts, and the communications media have seen fit to publicize such interventions nationally and internationally. This has had a great influence on the emergence of bioethics, particularly in the United States (10).

As the popular saying goes, "for great ills great remedies." Such a broad and offensive abuse of human freedom required a commensurate solution. It was this state of affairs that gave rise to the world response in support of twentieth century man.

It is patently evident that the highly developed research of this century has placed more emphasis on science than on ethics. And, on the whole, the situation in which modern medicine and hospital technologies have placed the patient is one where his freedom is restricted and even abused, since he usually dies without realizing what is happening.

Given these circumstances, it is not surprising that a response favoring patients' rights has emerged and that the influence of the Foundation for the Right to Die with Dignity is spreading throughout the world. This worldwide movement has set itself the goal of helping all human beings become aware of their right to die as people and recover and exercise their right to make the most important decisions with regard to the process of dying.

The Birth and Nature of Bioethics

The worldwide response of international organizations; local governments; legislative, judiciary, scientific, and religious authorities; and individual researchers and scientists was given the name of "bioethics" less than 20 years ago by a United States oncologist (11). This author sought to create a new field of study and a movement among scientists around the world, and to initiate interdisciplinary research that would serve as a bridge between ethics and the biomedical sciences.

What are the goals of this new discipline? Bioethics seeks to link ethics with biomedicine, to humanize medicine, and among other things to help all patients (and we will all be patients someday) become aware of the right that will help them to die with dignity.

Bioethics is characterized by the following features:

☐ It has evolved in a scientific setting as a need perceived by health professionals themselves in the broadest sense to protect human life and the environment.

☐ It arises from an interdisciplinary effort by many health professionals. It is a search of various fields of biomedical and professional knowledge in which sociologists, psychologists, ethicists, philosophers, and theologians, among others, are participating, joining together to explore the human values that inspire their work.

☐ It is not a ready-made science with "prefabricated" ethical formulas. As many biomedical

problems are new ones, it is not surprising that a need has arisen to seek new perspectives capable of guiding investigative work in this area. So although bioethics' point of departure is traditional principles and values, it seeks to use these to find new solutions to the new problems posed by biology, genetics, and many other sciences.

☐ It is founded more on reason and the good moral judgment of its practitioners than on any school of philosophy or religious authority. Consequently, its principles and orientation are of an autonomous and universal nature.

☐ It does not seek so much to involve itself with elaborate theories as with practice, so as to provide ethical guidance for researchers, technicians, scientists, lawmakers, and political leaders that will help them correctly assess the human repercussions of their work and will enable them to respond with appropriate measures.

☐ It especially seeks to humanize the environment in clinics and hospitals, and to promote the patient's rights to exercise a healthy liberty and to end his days with a dignified death.

☐ It does not seek to regulate medical practice with regard to the doctor-patient relationship (which remains a concern of medical ethics). Rather, it seeks to make all biomedical professionals aware of the international codes on human experimentation and of legal requirements with regard to health practices in their respective countries.

☐ It seeks to integrate ethics with the biomedical sciences for the purpose of persuading health professionals everywhere of the need to take account of the patient's humanity and to include the ethical dimension of health problems in all medical decisions.

☐ Because bioethics is not yet a clearly defined field, it is not surprising that a certain vagueness and imprecision blur its concepts, scope, and operating methods.

☐ The presence of bioethics is most evident at bioethical centers and institutes where interdisciplinary teams are engaged full-time in exploring, teaching, and disseminating moral values capable of serving as a basis for biomedical research. Its influence is also clearly felt at national and international conferences, on committees and commissions, in libraries and specialized journals, and in all kinds of publications.

☐ Bioethics is more concerned with seeking the ethical dimensions of new problems created by the biomedical sciences than it is with traditional treatment of medical subjects. This is evident from the content of any publication that deals with bioethics. When it studies traditional themes—for example, abortion or euthanasia—it does so in its own way with new perspectives.

☐ While bioethics is being taught to future physicians at medical schools, its principal aims at present are outside the classroom. That is, it seeks to make itself a presence in scientific research circles and hospitals in order to offer humanizing and moral values and to see patients' rights prevail.

References

1. Versluis, N. Desconocimiento social de la muerte. *Concilium: Revista Internacional de Teología (Madrid)* 65:291–299, 1971.

2. Häring, B. *Moral y medicina: Etica médica y sus problemas actuales.* Editorial PS (Perpetuo Socorro), Madrid, 1972, p. 137.

3. Baltzell, W. H. The dying patient: When the focus must be changed. *Arch Intern Med* 127:108, 1971.

4. Gorer, G. *Death, Grief, and Mourning.* New York, 1967. (Cited by N. Versluis, op. cit., p. 292.)

5. Calderan Beltrão, P. *Analisi della popolazione mondiale.* Libreria Editrice dell'Università Gregoriana, Rome, 1967, Chapter 9, p. 70.

6. Bedell, S. E., P. L. Cleary, and T. L. Delbanco. The peaceful stress of hospitalization. *Am J Med* 592–596, 1984.

7. Clark, M., M. Gosnell, and D. Shapiro. When doctors play God: The ethics of life-and-death decisions. *Newsweek*, 31 August 1981.

8. Gracia, D. El poder médico. In: A. Dou (ed.). *Ciencia y poder: Actas de las reuniones de la Asociación Interdisciplinar José de Acosta (vol. 13).* Universidad Pontificia Comillas, Madrid, 1987, p. 141.

9. Faden, R. R., T. L. Beauchamp, and N. M. P. King. *History and Theory of Informed Consent.* Oxford University Press, New York, 1986, p. 91.

10. Castillo Valery, A. *Etica ante el enfermo grave.* Disinlimed, Caracas, 1986, p. 127.

11. Potter, V. R. *Bioethics: Bridge to the Future.* Prentice-Hall, Englewood Cliffs, New Jersey, 1971.

Legal and Ethical Issues Relating to AIDS

Ronald Bayer and Larry Gostin

Acquired immunodeficiency syndrome (AIDS), the first epidemic disease to strike advanced industrial nations in more than a generation, has posed an extraordinary array of ethical and legal challenges. As a lethal illness, spread in the context of the most intimate relationships, it has forced examination of difficult questions about the appropriate public health role of the State. As a disease of the socially vulnerable (those who have been additionally subject to irrational reactions stemming from fears associated with HIV infection) AIDS has compelled modern societies to face issues involving the need to employ the power of the State to protect the weak at moments of social stress.

Both roles of government—that of advancing the public health and that of defending the weak—have been called upon in the first years of the AIDS epidemic. And although these roles have at times been in conflict, more often (and in ways that have reversed conventional assumptions) it has been clear that the protection of the public health and of the weak and vulnerable have been interdependent. Moreover, a common theme has emerged: that aggressive protection of the public health requires the State's coercive powers to be exercised with the greatest restraint, and that creation of a social climate of trust is central to the efforts to foster mass behavioral change.

Both ethical considerations and pragmatic concerns have contributed to the adoption of public health strategies that can be broadly defined as voluntaristic—stressing mass education, counseling, respect for privacy. Yet within the broad voluntaristic strategy there have been tensions, sometimes unresolved. Differences among Western liberal societies have been reflected in the salience given to some matters, the extent to which proposed interventions have been deemed problematic or of no particular moment, the compromises that have been struck. The contrast with authoritarian societies has been more stark.

In this essay we will survey three issues at the juncture of ethics, law, and public policy: discrimination against those with HIV infection, confidentiality and its limits, and the exercise of compulsory State powers to limit the spread of HIV infection.

Much of our detailed discussion will be drawn from the experience of the United States. It is the epicenter of the epidemic in the developed world. It is also the nation where an extraordinary range of AIDS-related legal activity has occurred and where the most vigorous debate about the ethical issues posed by the threat of HIV has taken place. A close examination of the course of events in the United States provides an opportunity to point out options that other societies might well consider. It will also reveal in a sobering way certain paths to be avoided. We have thus made a virtue of necessity, the United States' experience being the case that we know best.

Discrimination

Times of epidemic are also times of social tension. Fears exacerbate already-extant divisions, revealing deepening social fault lines. So it is not surprising that discrimination against persons with HIV infection has become a worldwide phenomenon. The AIDS virus has divided individuals, nations, and ethnic, cultural, and sexual groups; and the potential for greater division is ever-present.

On an international plane, some Americans have blamed Haitians and Africans for the epidemic; some Africans have blamed Europeans; in Japan, foreigners have been blamed; and the French "Right" has blamed Arab immigrants (1). This dreary process is not new, as William McNeill has shown in his social history of epidemics, *Plagues and People* (2).

A natural corollary, and an echo of the international quarantines dating from the fifteenth century, has been the creation of travel barriers. Much of the Far East and Middle East, for example, have placed impediments in the way of travel by returning nationals, foreign students, and foreign businessmen infected with HIV (3). And an ever-growing list of nations demands proof of long-term visitors that they are free of HIV infection.

HIV infection has also been used as a rationale for excluding people from a range of critical social activities. America has read all too frequently about children with HIV being turned away from schools, of employees dismissed from their jobs and losing their life or health insurance, and of AIDS patients being denied appropriate treatment or being forced by circumstances to stay in hospitals because they no longer have a home. Hundreds of cases have been brought before courts and human rights commissions in the United States by people with HIV claiming discrimination. Examples of discrimination have also been reported in many other nations.

Discrimination based upon an infectious condition can be as inequitable as discrimination based on other morally irrelevant grounds such as race, gender, or handicap. The U.S. Supreme Court has recognized that "society's accumulated myths and fears about disability and disease are just as handicapping as are the physical limitations that flow from actual impairment. Few aspects of handicap give rise to the same level of public fear and misapprehension as contagiousness."[1]

But there is a critical difference between discrimination based upon race or gender and discrimination based upon disease status. An infection is potentially transmissible and can affect a person's abilities to perform work-related tasks. A decision to exclude an HIV-infected person from certain activities because of a real risk of transmission or relevant performance criteria would be understandable and would not breach antidiscrimination principles. However, denying such persons rights, benefits, or privileges where health risks are only theoretical or very rare, and when performance is adequate, is morally unacceptable. Since the risk of transmission of HIV in most settings is remote (4), and since persons with HIV infection may function normally when not experiencing serious symptoms, there are no morally acceptable grounds for discrimination.

Irrational fears of AIDS are typically at the root of HIV-related discrimination. Public opinion surveys reveal that a consistent minority harbors anxieties about and antipathies toward those with HIV infection. In the United States some one-fourth of the public believes people with HIV should be excluded from schools, workplaces, and other public settings. Twenty-five percent also assert that individuals suffering from HIV-related disorders should not be treated with compassion. Such findings have been replicated in many regions of the world (5). Fueling both anxieties and antipathies is often a visceral hostility to those groups popularly linked to AIDS—gay men, drug users, and prostitutes.

Not only is discrimination against the HIV-infected morally wrong, it can also be counterproductive from the standpoint of public health. The Institute of Medicine (6), the American

---

[1]School Board of Nassau County v. Arline, 107 s.Ct. 1123 (1987).

Medical Association (7), the Presidential Commission on the HIV Epidemic (8), and federal and state health officials in the United States, as well as public health officials in many other nations and at the World Health Organization (9, 10) have all termed HIV-based discrimination unjustifiable and inimical to the struggle against AIDS.

Fears of a breach of confidentiality and subsequent discrimination discourage individuals from cooperating with vital public health programs and receiving treatment for sexually transmitted diseases and drug dependency. These fears also mobilize opposition to routine voluntary testing and counseling among people with high-risk behaviors. Such resistance to testing might well melt away if individuals believed they were strongly protected by the law.

In the United States the Federal Rehabilitation Act of 1973, section 504, prohibits discrimination against "otherwise qualified" handicapped individuals. There is little doubt among legal scholars that the 1973 Act applies to AIDS, and probably to HIV infection (11, 12). A recent amendment to the Rehabilitation Act states that a person with a contagious disease or infection is protected if he or she does not "constitute a direct threat to health or safety" and is able "to perform the duties of the job" (13). Lower courts, moreover, have consistently held that HIV-related diseases, including asymptomatic HIV infection, are covered under the 1973 Act.[2-4] The major limitation of the 1973 Act is that it is applicable only to programs receiving federal financial assistance and does not extend in any significant way into the private sector.

The 50 states and the District of Columbia have handicap statutes similar to the Federal Rehabilitation Act. In all jurisdictions except five, handicap statutes prohibit discrimination against employees in both the private and public sectors. In 34 states the courts,[5,6] human rights commissions, or attorneys general have formally or informally declared that handicap laws apply to AIDS or HIV infection (14).

A recent global survey of AIDS legislation for the World Health Organization found that only five of the 77 nations surveyed had express provisions for the protection of people with AIDS (3). Whether other nations take the path of legislative enactment, create human rights commissions with the authority to investigate cases of discrimination and enforce norms of equity, or rely on other forms of government intervention, what is critical is that as a matter of public policy those vulnerable because of HIV infection be protected. The most elemental notions of human dignity as well as the public health require no less.

Confidentiality and its Limits

The threat of discrimination has had a profound impact on the extent to which the most articulate among those at risk for HIV infection have demanded ironclad protection of confidentiality.

Both ethical and pragmatic factors contributed to the remarkable emergence of a strong public health interest in articulating and fostering a regime of confidentiality early in the AIDS epidemic. In the face of a serious challenge to communal well-being, the lesson was clear: Privacy and confidentiality are critical to the public health.

---

[2]Chalk v. Orange County Department of Education, 832 F.2d 1158 (9th Cir.) (1987).

[3]Doe v. Ceninela Hospital, 57 u.s.l.w. 2034 (U.S.D.C.D.C. Cal.) (1988).

[4]Ray v. School District of DeSoto County, 666 F. Supp 1524 (M.D. Fla.) (1987).

[5]Shuttlesworth v. Broward Cty., 639 F. Supp 654 (S.D. Fla.) (1986).

[6]Cronan v. New England Tel. Co. (Mass. Sup. Ct. No. 80332) (Aug. 15, 1986). Goaded by their patients and their research subjects, physicians and scientists have amplified the call for protection of clinical records and research files. Even before discovery of the virus etiologically linked to the profound collapse of the immune systems of those who were infected, and before the development and mass production of the test designed to detect antibody to that virus, researchers, public health officials, and clinicians were thus compelled to address the concerns of the populations most at risk for the new disease (15).

When HIV antibody testing began in mid-1985, the importance of protecting confidentiality was already well-understood. Because the test provided the occasion for identifying infected but asymptomatic individuals who would then be subject to employment, housing, and insurance discrimination, public health officials responded by underscoring the critical importance of confidentiality. Indeed, as the United States Centers for Disease Control (CDC) moved toward recommendations for large-scale voluntary testing to accompany an aggressive counseling campaign, they embraced a posture on confidentiality and the need for state and federal legislation to protect HIV records that was striking (16). For those who could not be reassured, for those who believed that no system of confidentiality protection could protect infected persons from the threat of irrational social reactions, health officials responded by providing for testing under conditions of anonymity (17).

In time, the defense of confidentiality endorsed by the Surgeon General, the Association of State and Territorial Health Officials, the American Medical Association, the Institute of Medicine, the National Academy of Sciences, and the Presidential Commission on the HIV Epidemic was to become a centerpiece of the political culture of the national AIDS epidemic. Even before AIDS, all 50 states had enacted generally strong legislative and administrative protection against breaches of medical confidentiality. Since the HIV epidemic's advent a majority of the states have gone further—spurred on by public health officials and advocates of the interests of those most at risk—enacting specific statutes to safeguard the confidentiality and privacy of individuals infected or perceived to be infected with HIV (18). (Internationally, 26 of the 77 countries surveyed for the World Health Organization were found to have legislation regulating confidentiality—3.)

Despite such institutional support, and despite the forceful resistance to political pressures for weakening the commitment to protect confidentiality, there were tensions within the broad medico-political alliance forged in the epidemic's first years. Within the United States, these were most obvious in debates over reporting positive HIV test findings by name to public health departments and in disputes over the extent to which confidentiality might be breached in order to warn unsuspecting sexual partners.

Confidential Reporting of HIV Infection

Soon after the recognition of AIDS by the CDC, state and local health departments had moved to require that physicians and hospitals report, by name, those diagnosed with the new syndrome, thus extending to AIDS the policy that governed venereal and other infectious diseases. The aforementioned global survey of AIDS legislation for WHO found that 51 of the 77 responding nations had enacted legislation for compulsory reporting (notification) of AIDS cases. The United Kingdom Advisory Group has taken a contrasting view, recommending that AIDS not be reportable by law (3).

U.S. officials believed that only such named reporting would permit those responsible for the public health to have an accurate epidemiologic picture of the disease with which they were confronted. Only such reporting would permit application of other appropriate public health measures to the sick. It was widely assumed that the public health required this abrogation of the principle of confidentiality, as had always been the case not only when epidemic threats were involved, but when other infectious diseases posed a challenge.

Many believed that such reporting did not entail any significant breach of confidentiality as long as the public health records thus created were insulated from further disclosure (or subpoena in court cases)—the Supreme Court had given its imprimatur to public health reporting requirements (Whalen *versus* Roe)—but others were dubious. A deep suspicion of government and a strong cultural tradition of individualism led many physicians—at their patients' behests—to ignore reporting requirements, especially where stigmatized illnesses such as sexually transmitted diseases were involved.

It is thus remarkable, given the salience of concerns about the privacy of individuals with AIDS, that there was little resistance to efforts to mandate case reporting by name. However, the relative ease with which AIDS was incorporated under state and local health requirements governing the reporting of communicable and infectious diseases—in the United States such public health regulations are governed by state rather than national law—did not extend to efforts to make results of the antibody tests reportable (19).

The first successful attempts to mandate public health reporting of HIV antibody test results in the United States came in Colorado, a state with relatively few AIDS cases. Proponents of reporting argued that it could alert responsible health agencies to the presence of people likely to be infected with a dangerous virus; allow such agencies to ensure that such people were properly counseled about the significance of their laboratory tests and about what they needed to do to prevent further transmission of the virus; permit those charged with monitoring the prevalence of AIDS virus infection to better accomplish their tasks; and create the possibility of expeditiously notifying the infected when effective antiviral therapeutic agents became available.

On these grounds it was asserted that failure to undertake the logical step from reporting AIDS to reporting asymptomatic infection with the AIDS virus would represent a dereliction of professional public health responsibility in the face of a new deadly disease. Responding to concerns about potential breaches in the confidentiality of health department records that could result in social ostracism, loss of insurability, and loss of employment, state health officials asserted that the system for protecting such public health records had been effective for decades. There was no reason to believe that in the case of infection with the AIDS virus the record would be tarnished.

However, those whose lives had led them to fear the intrusions of the State—whatever the putative benign purpose—were intent on thwarting the move toward reporting. Regardless of the historic and prevailing standards of confidentiality that governed public health records, argued opponents, a repressive turn caused by the hysteria associated with AIDS could well result in social policies that even proponents of reporting would consider anathema. Ironically, gay leaders and civil liberties groups argued, reporting by name would subvert the public health by driving high-risk individuals away from testing. To these objections the advocates of reporting responded, "The issue before us is the reality of a tragic epidemic of AIDS, not the theoretical risk [that] our confidentiality system will be breached" (20).

It was a setback for those who feared the impact of reporting that the final report of the President's Commission on the HIV Epidemic, issued in June 1988 (8), which so forcefully defended the centrality of confidentiality to the public health, recommended that all states follow the course first taken by Colorado—and subsequently followed by an increasing number of states (18 as of this writing). Ultimately more significant, there now appear to be fissures in the broad alliance that had opposed named public health reporting in states where the level of infection is relatively high. In New York State, for example, the Health Commissioner was challenged in court by major constituents of the medical profession in a suit demanding that the state's steadfast refusal to mandate reporting be reversed.[7] Though the court rejected the claims of the plaintiffs, the suit indicated that the shared perspective of the first years of the epidemic was no longer a matter to be taken for granted.

The debate over reporting reveals the ambivalence, or even deep tension, that exists in the United States between respect for personal privacy and the social welfare perspective of public health. In other countries, reporting of HIV infection has been initiated without fanfare. In

---

[7]New York State Society of Surgeons et al. v. Axelrod.

such settings the very concept of privacy does not preclude such reporting. In Scandinavia, for example, under an ethos that gives priority to social welfare, reporting of HIV using numerical identifiers has been undertaken without controversy (3).

What is critical for policy-makers to consider as they contemplate the prospect of HIV reporting is the impact such measures might have on the goal of limiting the spread of AIDS. That is the public health standard against which all interventions must be judged. It is also the preeminent ethical and legal standard against which proposed actions must be measured. In nations where public health records are fully shielded from disclosure, the conditions for reporting exist. Such conditions are necessary but not sufficient. Most critically, a clear and rational public health justification for named reporting exists. It is not adequate to propose such a course simply because the "public health tradition" appears to dictate it. If the legacy of the historic experience of those most at risk for HIV infection would lead them to avoid testing because of reporting, to move in such a direction would be a grave error. The resolution of such conflicts will not be found in the articulation of abstract principles, but rather in the complex political process of building the foundations of confidence.

Warning Third Parties

Despite the well-established role of public health departments in identifying and notifying the sexual contacts of those reported to have venereal diseases, this strategy of intervention—designed to break the chain of disease transmission—played no role in the early response to AIDS. Not until 1985, with development of the antibody test, was it possible to consider contact tracing, since only the test made it possible to detect the asymptomatic carriers of the AIDS virus. But even after the test became available and it was realized that antibody-positive individuals were also carriers of HIV, contact notification was almost never

undertaken by public health departments in the United States. Matters of practicality as well as concern about privacy were involved (19).

Fueling the opposition was deep suspicion about how notification would broaden the extent to which the State would have in its possession the names of the infected, or those whose behavior placed them at increased risk of infection. Contact tracing also raised the specter of the State seeking information about intimate affairs and creating lists of sexual partners. Thus, although contact notification programs were predicated upon the voluntary cooperation of the "index case" in providing the names of those who might have been infected, and upon a promise to preserve the anonymity of the individual providing the names, such programs were viewed as dangerous. Notifying the potentially infected, even for purposes of warning them about the risk they might pose to others, would represent one more step in a threatening course. In the calculus that thus prevailed, the right to privacy took precedence over the right to know information critical to the shaping of sexual and procreative decisions.

Because of such anxieties, concerns about the costs of such a labor-intensive preventive intervention, and uncertainty about how the absence of therapeutic intervention affected the applicability of the traditional rationale for notification, public health officials were notably reluctant to undertake such programs. When they did so, it was typically in relatively low-prevalence areas. It was not until late 1987 that New York City, the epicenter of the U.S. epidemic, overcame its initial opposition to contact notification and made plans to offer the assistance of public health aides to those who could not, because of fear or shame, personally notify past partners who might have been unknowingly infected with HIV.

By mid-1988 little was left of the fractious controversy. The Association of State and Territorial Health Officials (21), the National Academy of Sciences and the Institute of Medicine (6), and the Presidential Commission on the HIV Epidemic (8) had all given their endorsements to such efforts. The fierce opposition by gay leaders had all but vanished. And so, the ideologic battle having been resolved, what remained were the difficult questions centering on the epidemiologic circumstances that could provide an appropriate context for so individualized and so costly an approach to warning those placed at risk of HIV infection through sexual behavior or drug use.

Interest in the possible role of contact tracing as part of an overall strategy to control the spread of HIV is reflected in a 1989 consultation by the WHO Global Program on AIDS. Also, 12 of the 77 countries included in the previously cited international survey reported the use of contact tracing to identify new cases as a way of preventing the further spread of HIV (3).

There is no question that partner notification will be most appropriate in low-prevalence areas, where general education and warnings about the risk of infection may be less effective. So too is it clear that partner notification has a special role to play in alerting unsuspecting individuals, even in high-prevalence areas, that they may have been infected—the paradigmatic case being the female partners of bisexual men. Especially where deep suspicions and fears about coercion and unwarranted disclosure exist, however, public health officials will have to develop programs that display respect for both index cases and contacts, and will have to demonstrate a capacity to understand the fears of those with whom they are working. In particular, the traditional standards of voluntarism and protection of the anonymity of the index case must be preserved—a critical issue now that some legislatures have begun to consider mandatory measures.

Finally, it would be a tragic parody of public health policy were the "retail" efforts to reach individuals at risk to divert energy and resources from the wholesale requirements of mass education. In the end, both programs of mass education and individual warnings must serve the overriding goal of slowing the spread of HIV infection.

A much broader question—debated for many years—is when, if ever, a physician's duties extend beyond a patient to endangered third parties. The importance of confidentiality in the clinical encounter derives from two quite distinct sources. On moral grounds, respect for the patient's dignity and autonomy is held to require that communications made with an expectation that they will be shielded from others be treated as inviolable. And, from a pragmatic perspective, confidentiality is held critical to candor on the part of the patient; for without assurances of confidentiality, patients might be inhibited from revealing clinically relevant information. Without confidentiality the very possibility of establishing a therapeutic relationship might thus be subverted.

But despite the importance of confidentiality to the practice of medicine, physicians on their own, under pressure from colleagues, and most frequently as a result of state requirements, have at times revealed their patients' secrets when some threat to the safety or well-being of others was involved. The moral and pragmatic underpinnings of confidentiality have thus yielded to supervening moral and societal claims.

Many courts in the United States have acknowledged the moral imperative of protecting third parties in immediate danger. The course of judicial opinion, however, has been fraught with controversy. In the most celebrated case, Tarasoff v. Regents of the State of California,[8] the Supreme Court of California held that if a psychotherapist reasonably believes a patient poses a direct physical threat to a third party, the psychotherapist must warn the endangered person.

The Tarasoff decision produced an avalanche of concern about the extent to which patients would be discouraged from confiding their dangerous thoughts to their therapists. Nevertheless, most state supreme courts that have confronted the issue have adopted the Tarasoff reasoning (22). A few have not established a *duty* to warn but only an authority to do so. Under

---

[8]Tarasoff v. Regents of the State of California, 17 Cal. 3d 425, 551 p. 2d 334, 131 Cal. Rptr. 14 (Cal. 1976).

such a standard, the determination of whether to warn would remain a matter of professional discretion.

In virtually all cases, however, the courts have limited their protective concern to *identifiable* third parties at risk of real and probable harm. For example, one court dealing with the threat of hepatitis B recognized that the duty to warn might exist but would require disclosure only to named sexual or needle-sharing partners, not to the community at large.[9]

Those who have considered the ethical, as contrasted with the legal, dimensions of the conflict between the claims of confidentiality and the duty to warn have generally asserted that there are circumstances under which the sanctity of the clinical encounter may be breached. When a physician is uniquely positioned to warn an identifiable individual about an intended grave harm, the principles of medical ethics cannot, according to most interpretations, be held to prevent the physician from warning the potential victim in a timely and effective manner. There is less agreement, however, on the extent to which breaches of confidentiality under such circumstances should be morally obligatory or left to the physician's discretion.

It is against this backdrop that clinicians, public health officials, and politicians have struggled with the question of how to act when an HIV-infected patient refuses to inform identifiable, unsuspecting past or current partners about the dangers of infection. In the case of past partners, concern has centered on the possibility that an unknowingly infected individual might act as the unwitting agent of transmission to yet others. In the case of current partners, the focus has been on the possibility of preventing the transmission of HIV to an as yet uninfected individual.

As these issues were considered, it became clear that the process of warning past sexual partners did not require identification of the

source of potential infection. No public health goal would be served by breaching the cloak of anonymity of the index case. Where an infected individual refused to warn a current partner, however, the situation posed graver difficulties. Without revealing the identity of the source of potential infection, it was possible that no effective protective warning could be done.

At the end of 1987 the American Medical Association issued a broad set of statements on the ethical issues posed by the AIDS epidemic (7). In that document the AMA addressed the issue of warning in a forthright manner. Physicians were to try to convince patients of their obligation to warn the unsuspecting. If they failed in that task they were to seek the intervention of public health officials. Only if public health officials refused or were unwilling to take on the responsibility of warning was it the obligation of the physician to act directly.

When the Presidential Commission on the HIV Epidemic addressed this issue in mid-1988, it too endorsed the notion that physicians should have the right to breach confidentiality in order to warn the unsuspecting, despite the centrality of confidentiality to its overall strategy (8). Reflecting a commitment to professional autonomy, however, the Commission held that the decision about whether to breach confidentiality was to remain with the physician and was not to be imposed as a matter of law.

That too was the stance of a wide spectrum of public health officials and the Association of State and Territorial Health Officials (21), which chose to speak of a "privilege to disclose" rather than a duty to warn. Concerned about the potential public health impact of such efforts, the association's mid-1988 publication, *Guide to Public Health Practice: HIV Partner Notification*, urged that the identity of the index case only be revealed in the "rare case" of ongoing exposure by an individual who would under no conditions be suspected as a potential source of harm. Under such circumstances, the guide indicated, public health officials rather than clinicians should be responsible for making the critical determinations and interventions.

[9]Gammill v. United States, 727 F. 2d 950 (1984).

In some states the legislatures have sought to clarify professional responsibilities. Most states have given professionals the authority to warn specified groups at risk for HIV but have not made it their duty to warn them. The groups involved have included spouses, emergency workers (e.g., ambulance attendants, law enforcement officials), health care workers, funeral workers, etc.

In general, these laws have created more problems than they have solved. A spouse may be at risk for HIV, but what of equally vulnerable sexual or needle-sharing partners who are not married? At the same time, these statutes appear to sanction breaches of confidentiality in order to warn a person whose level of risk is exceedingly low. (A health care worker's level of risk from mucous membrane exposure is considerably less than 0.01%.) It was just such a slippery slope that worried those who have insisted on the absolute inviolability of the principle of confidentiality.

A rational line needs to be drawn, an equitable and prudent standard established. The starting point must be the firm and explicit protection of confidentiality in law. Only then will it be possible to consider exceptions dictated by the need to protect. The authority to breach confidentiality under exceptional circumstances must be formally acknowledged. But because of the complex balancing of risks and benefits, it would be a great error to impose a duty to warn on professional health care workers.

Coercion and its Limits

Despite the progress that has been made in reducing the incidence of HIV infection—an unprecedented success for health education—widespread publicity given the potential for continued spread of the epidemic has charged the ongoing political debate. In an atmosphere of public health crisis, with little early prospect for effective prophylaxis, impatience with the repertoire of voluntary measures has been growing

(23). The fact that the behaviors linked to the spread of HIV infection are volitional and involve acts—sex between men, prostitution, and intravenous drug use—widely regarded as immoral or even criminal has also contributed to the allure of coercion. Some have argued that intentional behaviors posing a threat to the public health should be subject to legal sanctions. Strident calls for "tougher" measures, more specifically for isolation and criminalization, must be understood in this light.

Recourse to the threat of coercion, to the imposition of legal controls as a way of facing the threat of AIDS, has been infrequent in the West. However, 17 nations have enacted legislation placing restrictions on AIDS patients or upon environments conducive to the spread of AIDS. Twelve of these have reserved the right to require isolation, quarantine, or restricted movement of infected individuals. Nine countries have also made exposing another person to transmission of the AIDS virus a criminal offense.

Czechoslovakia's policies are typical of these. That country punishes intentional transmission of the AIDS virus by three years' imprisonment and negligent exposure of others by one year's imprisonment or a fine. The Soviet Union is particularly restrictive, punishing knowing exposure of another person to the AIDS virus by five years' "deprivation of liberty" and knowing transmission of the AIDS virus by eight years' "deprivation of liberty." Several states or territories of Australia punish the falsifying of health certificates for donated blood or other biological material by a fine and/or up to three years' imprisonment (3).

By far the most coercive approach to AIDS has been adopted in Cuba. There a decision has been made to screen the entire population (a third of the nation has already been tested). Such screening is mandatory. The first groups to be tested have been those traveling outside Cuba since 1975, those having regular contact with foreigners traveling in Cuba, all students coming to study in Cuba, all pregnant women, all prisoners, all patients being treated for sexually transmitted diseases, and the sexual contacts of those found to be infected. Some geographically based mass mandatory testing has also been undertaken.

All those testing positive for antibody to HIV are placed in a quarantine center located in a Havana suburb. Thus far, some 250 have been incarcerated. Parents who are infected are separated from their uninfected children, who may not live at the quarantine camp. Married couples in which one partner is infected are separated. Those who are isolated may visit family members and friends every several weeks, but only under the supervision of a chaperon. Married individuals may visit their uninfected partners, and after full warnings to each about the risks of transmission may have sexual relations. Unmarried residents of the quarantine center are prohibited from having sexual relations.

Though isolation of people with HIV infection has rarely occurred in the United States, an increasing number of state legislatures have enacted statutes that permit such control. These statutes authorize confinement of infected people who engage in dangerous behavior, rather than confinement on the basis of disease status alone.

The distinction between antiquated disease-based isolation (the standard in Cuba) and more modern behavior-based isolation is pivotal. The former is concerned with an immutable health status and *assumes* that the infected pose a threat to the community. Such assumptions derive from the infectious nature of the diseases prevalent at an earlier time (24). Behavior-based isolation is more directly targeted to the prevention of dangerous acts and is linked to diseases that are transmitted as a result of volitional behavior.

Isolation under public health law, whether status-based or behavior-based, represents a challenge to fundamental conceptions of liberty, because it can be imposed upon a competent and unwilling person without the procedural protection typically afforded those confronted with the threat of criminal conviction (25). As in the case of criminal sanctions, the State seeks to restrict the liberty of those it isolates under public health law because of a concern for the welfare of others. But unlike the criminal sanction, which is typically time-limited, isolation measures tend to be open-ended. From the public health perspective, the primary concern is not what the individual has done in the past but rather what this individual will do in the future. Prevention rather than retribution and deterrence is the goal.

Of course, isolation based on past behavior and limited by a willingness to assume that after some period of control a change in behavior might be expected would be less repressive than imposition of control based on serologic status alone. But grave problems would remain. After how much time would release be contemplated? And after what degree of certainty about the course of future behavior had been attained? At stake here are the most fundamental matters defining the authority of the State in a liberal society.

In the context of AIDS, any suggestion that isolation measures should be widely applied to individuals who fail to adopt acceptable behaviors must address not only such theoretical matters but a crucial practical question as well: Would the widespread adoption and vigorous enforcement of public health isolation measures affect the course of the AIDS epidemic? There is considerable doubt that the public health would be secured by such measures. Individuals would be controlled, but the goal of mass behavioral change could be adversely affected. Fears generated by the threat of isolation could discourage members of high-risk groups from seeking testing or speaking candidly to counselors about past behavior or behavioral intentions.

Policy-makers and public health officials ought to consider all the potential ramifications of isolation before they embrace such control measures. Appearances may be deceiving and may have counterproductive consequences. Certainly, as the role of such control measures is considered, it will be important to focus on the potential for affecting conditions that give rise to threatening behaviors. The provision of drug abuse treatment programs and the provision of social support services would be crucial in this regard.

As an alternative to the use of isolation, many public prosecutors and state legislators in the United States have turned to criminal law. Such action is politically appealing. The criminal law typically sanctions blameworthy individuals for their dangerous acts. Explicit penalties have been justified on grounds of retribution, incapacitation, and deterrence. Certainly the transmission of a potentially lethal infection with forethought or recklessness falls within the scope of behaviors the criminal law already proscribes.

From the perspective of those concerned with protecting freedom, the criminal law has many advantages over behavior-based isolation. While statutes permitting isolation typically employ terms such as "incorrigibility" and "recalcitrance," criminal statutes must specify the behavior being prohibited. The language of criminal statutes, if it is to survive judicial scrutiny in the United States, must avoid vagueness, always an invitation to unfair enforcement. Isolation statutes require predictions about future behavior—difficult at best (26)—while criminal statutes focus on behavior that has already occurred. In a similar vein, the standards of proof typically required under criminal law before a deprivation of liberty can occur are far more demanding than those required under public health law. And finally, unlike the indeterminate incarceration characteristic of isolation, criminal sanctions are generally finite and proportionate to the gravity of the offense.

Given these circumstances, would it be unreasonable for society to establish clear guidelines concerning the behaviors it will not tolerate in the context of the AIDS epidemic? Would not criminal laws to punish dangerous acts that risk transmission of HIV be desirable? As we shall see, the overreaching need to foster mass behavioral change and the difficulties involved in meeting the standards of the general criminal law might make benefits resulting from frequent recourse to the crude instrument of the criminal law problematic.

In the United States there have been over 50 criminal prosecutions of HIV-infected individuals because of their behavior. Many of these cases have been brought against individuals who knew they were infected with HIV and had sexual intercourse without informing their partners. Others involved biting, spitting, kicking, splattering of blood, or donation of blood by an HIV-infected person. Several of the cases involved military personnel (23). (The Department of Defense orders HIV-infected personnel to refrain from unprotected sex and to inform their partners of their condition. Violation of such "safe sex orders" can result in charges ranging from disobeying a military order to assault with a dangerous weapon and attempted murder.)

The outcomes of these cases point up the great difficulties involved in applying the general criminal law to an infectious disease. For one thing, in the nonmilitary cases involving sexual relations it has been very difficult to prove beyond a reasonable doubt (as required by U.S. criminal law) that the accused intended to transmit HIV or acted with reckless disregard for his or her partner's life. For another, in many cases (especially those not involving sexual relations) the risks of transmission posed by the acts cited have ranged from low to exceedingly remote. (None of the defendants prosecuted to date actually transmitted HIV). For these and other reasons, though there have been convictions, in the overwhelming majority of cases the prosecutions have been dropped or the accused individuals have been acquitted.

Partly in frustration at the difficulty of obtaining convictions under the general criminal law, policy-makers have sought other ways to criminalize behaviors that threaten to transmit AIDS. They have sought to do this primarily by establishing AIDS-specific public health offenses. In this general arena, about half the states already possess public health laws that define engaging in sexual intercourse while knowingly infected with a sexually transmitted disease as a public health offense (27). However, these public health statutes were created to control the spread of syphilis and gonorrhea; most of them do not apply to HIV, because AIDS is not usually classified as a sexually transmitted disease (28). In response to this perceived legal "gap," some state legislators are now seeking to have AIDS reclassified as a sexually transmitted disease.

Also, several states have enacted AIDS-specific statutes. Modeled after older statutes designed to curb public health offenses, they apply solely to HIV transmission. These AIDS-specific statutes differ in scope, but all make it an offense for a person to knowingly engage in some type of behavior that poses a risk of HIV transmission—sexual intercourse, needle-sharing, blood donation, or, more broadly, attempting to transfer any "body fluid." From the prosecutor's perspective, these statutes have a distinct advantage: There is no need to prove any specific intent. The elements of the crime are usually straightforward. The person knew he was infected with HIV, engaged in well-defined risky behavior, and failed to inform his partner of the risk.

Using this general approach, a statute would make the specified behavior a criminal offense only if all the following elements were present: (1) the person knew he was HIV-positive and had been counseled by a health care professional or public health official not to engage in unsafe sexual or needle-sharing behavior; (2) the person did not notify his partner of his HIV status or did not use barrier protection against an exchange of body fluids; and (3) the person engaged in sexual intercourse or needle-sharing. To establish the offense, it would not be necessary to prove either an intent to harm or actual transmission of HIV.

States may also seek to deter HIV-infected individuals from intentionally donating blood or tissue by enacting public health sanctions.

Overall, however, a morbid preoccupation by policy-makers with coercive measures, no matter how carefully crafted, might entail a diversion from the far more difficult task of fostering mass behavioral changes and reinforcing those changes already made. The application of state coercion will make only the most limited contribution toward that goal. More important by far will be programs of focused education, voluntary testing and counseling, and treatment for drug dependence; and it will be through the success or failure of those efforts that the struggle against the further spread of HIV infection will be won or lost. To be sure, such public health measures will be less dramatic than invocation of the states' coercive powers; but such measures are the only ones that may prove effective in the face of AIDS.

Conclusion

At the conclusion to his history of the impact of epidemics upon humanity, William McNeill urges us to recognize that our vulnerability to infectious agents is an inherent feature of our existence (2). Therefore, our culture, politics, and social organization will at critical moments be subjected to strains imposed by the threat of disease. For a brief time—due to historical accident and the discovery of antibiotics—we came to believe that infectious diseases and especially the threat of epidemics was no longer a problem for advanced industrial societies. AIDS has provided a sobering antidote to that hubris.

Now, as efforts are made to slow the spread of HIV infection and care for those already sick, the fundamental values of liberal society are being challenged. The task before us is to define a vigorous course of action that at once protects the public health and the rights of the vulnerable. That is the standard against which we will be judged, and against which history will judge the vitality of liberal societies at a time of crisis.

References

1. Sabatier, R. *Blaming Others: Prejudice, Race and Worldwide AIDS.* Panos Institute and New Society Publishers, Philadelphia, 1988.

2. McNeill, W. *Plagues and People*. Anchor Press, Garden City, 1976.

3. Curran, W. J., and L. Gostin. *International Survey of Legislation Relating to the AIDS Epidemic*. World Health Organization, Geneva, 1988.

4. Friedland, G. H., and R. S. Klein. Transmission of the human immunodeficiency virus. *N Engl J Med* 317:1125–1135, 1987.

5. Blendon, R. J., and K. Donelan. Discrimination against people with AIDS: The public perspective. *N Engl J Med* 319:1022–1026, 1988.

6. Institute of Medicine, National Academy of Sciences. *Confronting AIDS: Directions for Public Health, Health Care, and Research*. National Academy Press, Washington, D.C.,1988.

7. American Medical Association. Prevention and control of AIDS: An interim report. *JAMA* 258:2097–2103, 1987.

8. United States Government Printing Office. *Report of the Presidential Commission on the Human Immunodeficiency Virus Epidemic*. Washington, D.C., 1988.

9. World Summit of Ministers of Health on Programs for AIDS Prevention. *London Declaration on AIDS Prevention*. London, 28 January 1988.

10. World Health Organization. World Health Assembly Resolution 41.24, Avoidance of Discrimination in Relation to HIV Infected People and People with AIDS. WHO document A/41/VR/15. Geneva, 1988.

11. Annas, G. J. Not saints but healers: The legal duties of health care professionals in the AIDS epidemic. *Am J Public Health* 8(7):844–849, 1988.

12. Kmiec, D. W. Memorandum for Counsel to the President: Application of Section 504 of the Rehabilitation Act to HIV-infected Individuals. U.S. Department of Justice, Washington, D.C., 27 September 1988.

13. Civil Rights Restoration Act of 1987, P L 100–259 (S. 557), 22 March 1988.

14. National Gay Rights Advocates. AIDS and Handicap Discrimination: A Survey of the 50 States and the District of Columbia. Washington, D.C., 1986; updated as of Jan. 1988 by the American Dental Association: APHA Annual Meeting: Section on AIDS and Dentistry: Legal and Ethical Issues, Nov. 14, 1988. Unpublished data.

15. Bayer, R., C. Levine, and T. Murray. Guidelines for Confidentiality in Research on AIDS. *IRB: A Review of Human Subjects Research*, 6(6), 1984.

16. United States Centers for Disease Control. Recommended Additional Guidelines for HIV Antibody Counseling and Testing in the Prevention of HIV Infection and AIDS. Mimeographed document. Atlanta, 30 April 1987.

17. Association of State and Territorial Health Officials. *ASTHO Guide to Public Health Practice: HTLV III Antibody Testing and Community Approaches*. Public Health Foundation, Washington, D.C., 1985.

18. Gostin, L. Public health strategies for confronting AIDS. *JAMA* 261:1621–1630, 1989.

19. Bayer, R. *Private Acts, Social Consequences: AIDS and the Politics of Public Health*. The Free Press, New York, 1989.

20. *Rocky Mountain News* (Colorado), 13 October 1985, p. 55.

21. Association of State and Territorial Health Officials. *ASTHO Guide to Public Health Practice: HIV Partner Notification Strategies*. Public Health Foundation, Washington, D.C., 1988.

22. Gostin, L., W. Curran, and M. Clark. The case against compulsory case-finding in controlling AIDS testing, screening, and reporting. *Am J Law Med* 12(1):7–53, 1986.

23. Gostin, L. The politics of AIDS: Compulsory state powers, public health and civil liberties. *Ohio State Law J* 49(4):1,017–1,058, 1989.

24. Gostin, L. Traditional Public Health Strategies. In: H. Dalton and S. Burris (eds.). *AIDS and the Law: A Guide for the Public*. Yale University Press, New Haven, 1987.

25. Merrit, D. Communicable disease control and constitutional law: Controlling AIDS. *N Y U Law Rev* 759, 1986.

26. Monahan, E. *Predicting Violent Behavior: An Assessment of Clinical Techniques*. Sage Publications, Newbury Park, California, 1981.

27. Gostin, L. The future of public health law. *Am J Law Med* 12:461, 1986.

28. Curran, W. J., L. Gostin, and M. Clark. *Acquired Immunodeficiency Syndrome: Legal and Regulatory Policy Analysis*. U.S. Department of Commerce, Washington, D.C., 1988.

Ethical Principles of Biomedical Research on Human Subjects: Their Application and Limitations in Latin America and the Caribbean

Diana Serrano LaVertu and Ana María Linares

Interest in biomedical research on human subjects is based on the legitimate desire to cure or effectively combat disease. And while it is true that most medical advances depend on existing knowledge of physiopathologic processes, it is also important for some of these advances to be tested on human subjects—who will be the ultimate beneficiaries (1).

In the past, most medical research on human subjects was conducted in developed countries, since they were the ones with the necessary economic and technological resources. Over time, however, this situation has been changing, to a point where this type of work is becoming increasingly common in developing countries— much of it being carried out by specialists from developed nations.

There are several explanations for this trend. First, some health problems are peculiar to certain regions; in order for researchers to understand them, the conditions prevailing where they occur must be analyzed. Second, conducting biomedical research in developing countries makes it possible to reduce costs. And third, it sometimes permits avoidance of rules and requirements that are overly complex in the researchers' countries of origin. In many Third World countries, legal provisions providing for ethical surveillance of biomedical research on human subjects have not yet been prepared, while in others these rules exist, but the individuals who, because of their professions, should assume a vigilant role have not been properly identified or are inadequately trained.

From a multicultural perspective, the increasing volume of biomedical research on human subjects conducted in developing countries by investigators from developed nations gives rise to sensitive ethical problems. In principle, ethical considerations applying to human subjects are the same anywhere in the world. One must admit that uniform application of these considerations in different areas is extremely difficult. Nevertheless, is it justifiable for an investigator from a developed country to apply different ethical standards when conducting research in a developing country? And conversely, if one recognizes that in principle he should respect the same ethical principles that he would respect in his own country, what obstacles would he face in conducting research in countries with different levels of economic, industrial, and social development? This work seeks answers to these questions.

Basic Ethical Principles

Many efforts have been made to draw up guidelines for medical research on human subjects. In the international arena, concrete examples can be found in the Nuremberg Code dating back to 1947, the Declaration of Helsinki issued in 1964 and amended in 1975, and the International Guidelines for Biomedical Research Involving Human Subjects proposed in 1982 by the Council for International Organizations of Medical Sciences (CIOMS) and the World Health Organization (WHO). These documents have assisted in charting the ethical principles that are most relevant to biomedical research on human subjects.

Among the more widely discussed ethical principles in the West, three are especially relevant to the subject of research on human subjects, these being (a) the principle of respect for persons, (b) the principle of beneficence, and (c) the principle of justice. However, neither these nor any other principles discussed on these pages offer specific rules for resolving concrete problems relating to research on human subjects. Rather, they provide a frame of reference for obtaining coherent and well-reasoned solutions to specific ethical problems (2).

The Principle of Respect for Persons

The modern basis for this principle lies in the Western concept of the individual as an autonomous being capable of giving shape and meaning to his life. (An autonomous person is someone who follows a specific course of action, in accordance with his own plans and objectives—3.) Excluding the exceptions set forth in law, in principle there is no ethical justification for denying an individual the option of choosing what he will do with his own self.

As it relates to biomedical research on human subjects, this principle has two main aspects: on the one hand, respect for the rights of the person submitting to the research as well as for the actual person; and, on the other, respect for the general well-being of those participating in the research. The first implies a need to provide potential research subjects with the information they need in order to decide if they are willing to participate in the project (4). The second relates to the principle of beneficence, which is discussed later.

Beauchamp and Childress[1] have grouped the elements involved in this principle into two categories: (a) elements pertaining to information, and (b) elements pertaining to consent. The first category relates to communication and understanding of the relevant information. The second focuses on voluntary consent and the ability to provide consent. Overall, the principle of respect seeks to ensure that each individual participating as a research subject does so with full knowledge and understanding of what is to be done, of the possible consequences, and of his right to choose not to participate in the research or even to withdraw from it after it has started.

However, it is clear that being autonomous as a person and having that autonomy respected are two different things. Indeed, many of the ethical problems that arise in practice stem from lack of respect for this autonomy—as illustrated by instances of failure to obtain voluntary informed consent, undue interference in the subject's life, and violation of the confidentiality of medical information pertaining to the subject.

Respect for an individual's autonomy implies recognition of his capabilities and views, including his right to have specific ideas and make specific decisions. Furthermore, it implies that his actions and decisions must not be stymied, except when it is clear that they would adversely affect other people.

In medical research involving human subjects, as CIOMS and WHO assert (1), the ideal would be for every person asked to participate as a research subject to have sufficient intellectual capacity, give sufficient thought to the matter, and know enough about the risks, benefits, and options available to provide effective consent. At the same time, this individual must be sufficiently independent to decide whether or not to participate in the research without fear of later reprisals.

The Principle of Beneficence

Ethical treatment of people not only implies respect for their decisions but also promotion of

[1]T. Beauchamp and J. Childress (3), p. 70.

their well-being. The principle of beneficence is held sacred by the Hippocratic Oath, in the part that states: "I will apply dietetic measures for the benefit of the sick according to my ability and judgment; I will keep them from harm and injustice."[2]

Following the categories of Beauchamp and Childress,[3] on the one hand this implies beneficial action (a) preventing pain or injury, (b) counteracting injury, or (c) otherwise doing or promoting good. On the other, it implies avoiding acts that could be harmful or prejudicial.

This duality of the principle of beneficence can lead to conflict in complex situations where, for example, a beneficial action conflicts with noncommission of an act that could prove prejudicial. In such cases, the doctor must decide between avoiding harm and providing assistance to the patient. In situations like this, as Albert Jonsen says, the doctor gravitates towards the maxim "of doing no harm, unless such harm is intrinsically related to the benefit to be derived" (5).

Among the possible benefits that the doctor tries to obtain for his patient is the curing of a wound or illness. Among the injuries that he wants to avoid are pain, suffering, incapacitation, and illness. In therapeutic research projects, the possible gains and losses—benefits and injuries—are similar to those just mentioned. However, in nontherapeutic research projects the researcher places the focus upon acquisition of scientific knowledge. Therefore, therapeutic research tends to differ from nontherapeutic research in terms of the desired objectives. Nevertheless, the imperative of not harming the research subject is still very important and should be applied effectively in both cases. Within this context, it might be said that therapeutic research can have a wider margin of risk, provided this risk is compensated by potential benefits received by the subject (6).

The difficulty of establishing a clear criterion or procedure to weigh possible risks and poten-

tial benefits is evident. Furthermore, in biomedical research it is recognized that in order to prevent injury, it must first be known what actions have the potential to cause harm. In the process of determining this, some people may be exposed to the risk of harm or even suffer harm.

To guide us in how and where to draw the line between what is justifiable despite the risks involved and what is not because of the magnitude of the risks that must be taken, different international instruments have attempted to establish concrete guidelines. The Nuremberg Code, for example, states that "the degree of risk to be taken should never exceed that determined by the humanitarian importance of the problem to be solved by the experiment" (7). The Declaration of Helsinki clearly states that in biomedical research involving humans, "concern for the interests of the subject must always prevail over the interests of science and society" (8). Similarly, it is generally understood that as a rule the doctor must help the patient, and if he cannot help him must at least be careful not to harm him: *Primum non nocere*," as the Latin sentence ascribed to hippocratic writings states.[4]

The Principle of Justice

This principle, which is hard to define, deals chiefly with the question of who should receive the benefits of research and suffer its damages. The principle of justice has been applied to a person if he is offered treatment that is fair, due, or deserved. Any refusal to offer some benefit, service, or body of information to a person entitled to receive it would be unjust. Similarly, it would be unjust to impose an undue burden or obligation on a person or to demand more of him than is required by law.[5]

Underlying this principle is the idea that irrespective of the criterion adopted, equal people should receive equal treatment. However, this does not tell us how to determine the level of

---

[2]T. Beauchamp and J. Childress (3), p. 106.
[3]T. Beauchamp and J. Childress (3), p. 108.

[4]A. Jonsen (5), p. 200.
[5]T. Beauchamp and L. Walters (6), p. 32.

equality among people. In this sense, the principle leaves the field open to different interpretations of its content. Given the fact that in every group of people there will be many features that stand out as similar and many others that seem different, equality should be understood as "equality in terms of specific features."[6]

Many theories have been put forward to help answer the question of who should bear the burden of research and who should enjoy its benefits. The criteria for measuring fair distribution in either sense can range from the merits of each person to the needs of each. The first part of the question relates to the selection or recruitment of research subjects and the second part deals with distribution of research-derived benefits, or distributive justice.

The process of selecting human subjects for research necessarily entails classifying people. For example: Is it a research requirement to choose a specific type of person? If so, can such people be included in the study without violating ethical principles or the laws of the country in question? And if they can, should the selection process employ some pattern or criterion based on the prospective subjects' personal characteristics?

These distinctions are important insofar as they can encourage the establishment of national policies that deal with the topic more consistently.[7] In many developing countries, the answer to the foregoing questions is fundamental (even though it is often not provided in formal terms), because it provides a means of ensuring adherence to the principles of respect and beneficence and establishes guidelines for local and foreign investigators. In the final analysis, the objective should be to determine whether the real reason for selecting one group of people over another is linked to the type of research itself or to elements that are purely arbitrary or convenient for the investigators.

With regard to the enjoyment of research benefits, although it seems obvious that people

paying the costs of research should receive its benefits, the reality is sometimes different. To begin with, it is generally difficult to come up with an exact estimate of the potential research benefits.[8] It is possible that positive results may not be obtained, or that they may take years to materialize. Beyond that, the benefits of international research conducted in developing countries are not always available to the people of those countries or may not reach them quickly, perhaps on account of those benefits' high cost.

Limitations

Up to this point, we have looked at the theoretical dimension of ethical principles that have critical implications for biomedical research on human subjects. It should be noted, however, that application of these principles in real life poses problems, particularly in the case of international research conducted under diverse conditions.

In the case of Latin America and the Caribbean, each country can be said to have its own characteristics. However, there are certain common features that distinguish the subregion as a unit, among the most notable being marginality, poverty, and inequity. It thus comes as no surprise to observe that what constitutes a basic unmet need in our countries is often a concrete achievement in developed countries.

To cite just one example, most of a developed country's population takes access to basic health services for granted. In contrast, most people in Latin America do not have access to these services. Therefore, the stark contrast between conditions prevailing in a Rio de Janeiro slum and in any U.S. suburb underscores a need to reconsider whether ethical principles really should be applied uniformly in the manner discussed in the first part of this chapter.

We have used the term "limitations" to describe the features analyzed on these pages, since

---

[6]T. Beauchamp and L. Walters (6), p. 33.
[7]T. Beauchamp and J. Childress (3), p. 196.

[8]A. M. Capron (4), p. 143.

failure to heed them can turn them into obstacles for those wishing to conduct research on human subjects in Latin America and the Caribbean. It should also be noted that the particular features covered are only some of the most striking found in this subregion, where extremes of wealth and poverty exist side by side. Our purpose in examining them here is to help foreign investigators understand the context within which they will be working, and, insofar as possible, to facilitate their application of the ethical principles that should guide their work.

Conceptual Limitations

Based on the foregoing, it would be appropriate to ask if the three ethical principles discussed are universally known, and whether they are recognized in Latin America and the Caribbean as the best source for solutions to ethical problems encountered in the course of biomedical research on human subjects.

To help answer this question, we will consider applying the principle of respect for persons. As we have seen, this principle calls for obtaining the voluntary informed consent of anyone asked to be a research subject.

The concept of voluntary informed consent is based on the idea that a conflict of interests exists between society and the individual. In view of the desire to protect all individuals, steps must be taken to ensure that the interests and well-being of each person take priority over those of the society (9). In some parts of Latin America and the Caribbean, however, the relationship of the subject with society is not viewed the same way. Rather, some communities in this area think of each person as a participant in the common efforts of a collective whole. Hence, the life of each person assumes meaning in relation to his role in the community. Accordingly, he is expected to participate in projects that are of interest to the community, putting forward his best effort.

In this type of society it is difficult to imagine how the interests of the subject can conflict with those of his community. Since the needs of this community are generally pressing and affect all its members, the rights of the research subject and the ethics of the project must be viewed in the context of the goals that this society has set for itself.[9] In particular, it is important to note that in many instances the most successful projects are those supported by the official or traditional authorities, who obtain the collaboration of almost everyone. It should be stressed that this is especially apt to be true in remote or isolated places where national authorities have little or no involvement—places such as many of the indigenous communities in various countries of Latin America and the Caribbean, where people tend to live under very difficult conditions, particularly with regard to health.

Insofar as the second aspect of the principle of respect for persons is concerned, it is worth examining the validity of the right to refuse to participate in research. International guidelines call for someone who is a research subject to be aware that he is free to refrain from participating or to withdraw whenever he so desires. But in the small social groups characteristic of rural communities, very strong social pressure is brought to bear on each community member. This has a powerful influence on the decisions that he makes with regard to his personal life. In such a case, the investigator can inform the potential subject that he has the right to withdraw whenever he wishes. However, if the community views his participation as important, the individual's freedom to decide will at the very least be reduced.

Another aspect of the principle of respect for persons that is useful to examine here is the relationship between the investigator and the research subject. If a doctor or investigator is to adhere to the principle of respect for persons and their autonomy, he must be especially careful about the doctor-patient relationship that will inevitably be established. Often, despite the efforts of the doctor or investigator, relation-

---

[9] R. J. Levine (9), p. 20.

ships based on power are established between him and possible research subjects, ones expressed in terms of dependency and submission (10). This is practically inevitable in places where anything foreign is considered "the best" or "the solution." Such a bias is sometimes reinforced by the authorities, without consideration for the well-being of the people where the study is being conducted. It should also be remembered that in places with many needs, the doctor usually plays a key role, to the extent that after the local authorities, he may be the most prominent figure in the community.

Given these special dynamics of the doctor-patient relationship, it typically becomes extremely difficult for the doctor to explain the requirements of the principle of respect for persons and, in addition, for members of the communities involved to even consider the possibility of not participating in research suggested or recommended by the health authorities or local doctor.

Another relevant aspect of the principle of respect for persons relates to the method generally used for obtaining voluntary informed consent, a method that tends to encounter numerous obstacles in isolated rural communities.

Robert Levine[10] makes a distinction between the purpose served by informed consent and the document used to obtain it. The purpose of this consent is to protect the person participating as a research subject. On the other hand, the document seeks to protect the investigator and the institution sponsoring him. Based on this, we can consider the concrete expression of this consent contained in a signed document as almost completely valid among populations with a very low level of illiteracy. Under these circumstances, it can be assumed that the potential research subject will not only be able to read the document he is asked to sign, but will also be able to understand its content and, on the basis of this, make a decision.

However, in many parts of Latin America and the Caribbean this assumption would be totally erroneous. It should be pointed out that although the illiteracy rate has fallen in recent years, the situation has not improved in many sectors, particularly among women. Added to this illiteracy problem is the feeling of mistrust that exists in many communities toward anyone who asks for the signature of a person as a commitment. In countries like those of Latin America, where great importance is attached to legal formalities, and where the person who signs a document may end up with all kinds of unexpected obligations, the fact that an investigator asks for a signature on a document drawn up in language that is hard to understand can give rise to reactions of rejection and mistrust.

It seems evident, therefore, that in certain circumstances rigid application of the informed consent requirement may not be suitable. This is so, for example, when the people who are potential research subjects are part of a culture where the concepts of individuality and freedom to choose do not correspond to typically Western concepts. As WHO and CIOMS have recognized (1), such a situation would call for intervention by the community leader for the purpose of obtaining informed consent. A similar situation arises when individuals do not have the minimum level of scientific knowledge necessary to understand the explanations of the doctor or investigator.

Just as we have discussed some of the aspects of the principle of respect for persons, we could equally well discuss some of the aspects relating to the principles of beneficence and justice that would create problems for any simplistic application of these principles in Latin America and the Caribbean. In sum, it is reasonable to assert that these three ethical principles are not universally known and therefore cannot be rigidly applied to a wide range of diverse situations.[11]

As William Curran (11) points out, the principles called for in the Nuremberg Code and declarations of the World Health Assembly were essentially directed toward implementation in developed countries or very urbanized areas of

---

[10] R. J. Levine (9), p. 26.

[11] R. J. Levine (9), pp. 16, 26.

developing countries. They are principles that reflect a specific concept of the nature of people and their relationship with society. Therefore, cold and merely explanatory imposition of the ethical principles we have described will not satisfy the purpose of guiding doctors or investigators in research projects, since these principles do not properly reflect the specific views of the culture involved or the specific relationships between the individual and society.[12]

Undoubtedly, it would be more appropriate to apply these principles in a way that recognizes the validity of prevailing cultural patterns. There is thus a clear need to understand ethical principles within a framework of cultural relevance, so as to be able to apply them in accordance with local reality. Without renouncing the idea that basic ethical principles are universally valid, one needs to recognize that different contexts require different applications. This does not mean that the principles themselves should be called into question, but rather that the best method of applying them to the specific situation should be sought in order to achieve the best results.

Institutional Limitations

Given the developmental characteristics of most Latin American and Caribbean countries, countless serious problems are caused by an institutional structure that is multiple, crude, overly bureaucratic, and chronically short of technological, human, material, and legal resources. In light of this reality, it is important to underscore the fact that laws, rules, or ordinances regarding the ethical aspects of research on human subjects may not exist. It is clear that in countries where all or almost all basic social needs merit priority, it is impossible to work effectively on all fronts at once.

With regard to the health sector, its role in the economic, industrial, and social develop-

ment of each country is clear. Most Latin American and Caribbean governments are preoccupied with trying to provide their entire populations with basic health services. Coverage in this area is still incomplete. Despite this, there is a growing awareness among people in these countries of the possible benefits to be derived from research projects conducted on their territory.

However, the preparation of rules regulating biomedical research on human subjects is a long and painful process. And even in countries where the first steps have been taken, another major problem is emerging—the problem of how to establish coercive mechanisms to ensure observance of the rules. In many cases such mechanisms do not exist, or else they are too weak, or worse still are not respected. This is a serious general problem for many Latin American and Caribbean justice systems—one that tends to deprive them of both institutional credibility and the opportunity to truly protect their people.

Nor do ministries of health escape widespread difficulties associated with poor resource allocation, a weak political position within the national institutional structure, serious administrative and management problems, and problems relating to excessive bureaucracy. It is undeniable that the health sector receives high priority in every country, but it must also compete with other sectors that may have even more pressing demands. For example, armed conflicts in several countries have forced governments to devote tremendous resources to military matters and relegate other needs to second place.

Then there is the perpetual problem of bureaucracy arising from the government's excessive size. The employees of public entities have responsibilities that cover a host of different areas. This makes it particularly difficult to find those who effectively intervene in the process of studying the matters of interest to us. So decision-making proceeds from desk to desk in a process that is slow and not always based on careful study. In general, the problems of bureaucracy are found with little variation in all of the countries. With regard to our specific field of

---

[12]R. J. Levine (9), p. 26.

interest, the worst problems are the typical slowness and resulting loss of time, since a proposed piece of research must often be done in a specific place and at a specific time.

Furthermore, the ministries of health have not demonstrated the capacity to provide linkages with other social entities—such as social security institutes, universities, and various nongovernmental institutions—that are in a position to contribute to specific research projects. The resulting need to find an entity capable of coordinating the activities of the different health sectors involved in research is thus extremely important, if one wishes to find viable and effective solutions to basic problems confronting both the health field and research within that field.

Also, the Latin American and Caribbean countries have been slow to form ethics committees for monitoring health research projects. Here an important role is being played by research projects sponsored by developed countries. Given the fact that most developed countries require approval of these projects by a local ethics body, committees of this sort have started to emerge for the sole purpose of overseeing such projects. This is a positive development; for once created, regardless of the initial motive, these committees seem destined to continue working and fulfilling the task of monitoring the ethical development of research.

Unfortunately, the institutional problems that plague the Latin American and Caribbean countries are not limited to those specific problems described here. To enumerate all of them would be tedious and out of place. What should be considered, however, is that such problems may be found elsewhere, and that they exist to one degree or another in virtually all countries, irrespective of levels of economic, industrial, or social development.

Conclusion

The current upsurge in international biomedical research projects being conducted in Latin America and the Caribbean has great potential for both the sponsoring and host countries. If the research is carried out properly, the results can be of immense benefit to the host countries—in terms of possible transfer of appropriate technology, access to advances of medical science, and possible discovery of cures or treatments for some of the endemic diseases affecting the subregion.

Even so, the growth of research conducted by foreign investigators in developing countries has understandably roused growing controversy. The foregoing discussion has centered on efforts to apply ethical principles when conducting research on human subjects. Even in this limited area, myriad difficulties can arise when one attempts to put theoretical principles into practice, since those principles reflect a particular view of the world that is not necessarily shared by other peoples.

We have stressed two essential elements. The first is recognition of the universal validity of ethical principles, although this does not mean that the principles involved are necessarily known and accepted equally in all countries. Understanding this discrepancy requires recognition of the cultural differences that exist in different countries and regions. The second element is recognition that knowledge of these differences can provide a useful starting point for adapting principles to circumstances prevailing where they will be applied. We repeat that we are not attempting to encourage research without ethical principles, but rather to familiarize investigators with cultural differences, so that these differences can be taken into account when studies on human subjects are being conducted. In this context, particular differences that seem especially apt to impose limitations on research utilizing human subjects in Latin America and the Caribbean have been underscored.

It should be added that at the moment one of the most effective tools for narrowing the gap between cultural patterns prevailing in Latin American and Caribbean countries and research guidelines issued by developed countries is joint research (*12*). Such joint efforts tend to secure the cooperation of foreign investigators and their local counterparts in each and every phase of the project. Hence, this involves not only sharing responsibility from a scientific and ethical viewpoint, but also working toward a common objective. The closer this co-operation and the more effective the communication between foreign and national investigators, the greater the chance that the research will be carried out with due respect for the host country, its citizens, its laws, and its authorities. Moreover, the associated exchange of ideas helps to remove many obstacles linked to misunderstanding, thereby increasing the likelihood of successfully concluding research that is mutually beneficial and that respects ethical principles within the contexts of different cultures.

References

1. Council for International Organizations of Medical Sciences and World Health Organization (CIOMS/WHO). *Proposed International Guidelines for Biomedical Research Involving Human Subjects.* Geneva, 1982.
2. Veatch, R. (ed.). *Cross Cultural Perspectives in Medical Ethics: Readings.* Jones and Bartlett, Boston, 1989, pp. 196–198.
3. Beauchamp, T., and J. Childress. *Principles of Biomedical Ethics (second ed.).* Oxford University Press, New York, 1983, p. 59.
4. Capron, A. M. Human Experimentation in Medical Ethics. In: R. Veatch (ed.). *Cross Cultural Perspectives in Medical Ethics: Readings.* Jones and Bartlett, Boston, 1989, p. 137.
5. Jonsen, A. Do No Harm. In: R. Veatch (ed.). *Cross Cultural Perspectives in Medical Ethics: Readings.* Jones and Bartlett, Boston, 1989, p. 206.
6. Beauchamp, T., and L. Walters. *Contemporary Issues in Bioethics (third ed.).* Wadsworth, Belmont (California), 1989, p. 31.
7. United States, U.S. Government Printing Office. *Trials of War Criminals before the Nuremberg Military Tribunals under Control Council Law No. 10 (vol. 2).* Washington, D.C., 1949, pp. 181–182.
8. World Medical Association. *The Declaration of Helsinki: Recommendations Guiding Physicians in Biomedical Research Involving Human Subjects.* As adopted by the 18th World Medical Assembly, Helsinki, Finland, 1964, and as revised by the 29th World Medical Assembly, Tokyo, 1975.
9. Levine, R. J. Validity of Consent Procedures in Technologically Developing Countries. In: Z. Bankowski and N. Howard-Jones (eds.). *Human Experimentation and Medical Ethics: XV CIOMS Round Table Conference.* CIOMS Round Table Conferences, No. 15. Council for International Organizations of the Medical Sciences, Geneva, 1982, p. 19.
10. Shannon, T., and J. DiGiacomo. *An Introduction to Bioethics.* Paulist Press, New York, 1979, pp. 105–110.
11. Curran, W. J. Subject Consent Requirements in Clinical Research: An International Perspective for Industrial and Developing Countries. In: Z. Bankowski and N. Howard-Jones (eds.). *Human Experimentation and Medical Ethics: XV CIOMS Round Table Conference.* Council for International Organizations of Medical Sciences, Geneva, 1982, p. 57.
12. Ofosu-Amaah, O. Ethical Aspects of Externally Sponsored Research in Developing Countries: An African Viewpoint. In: Z. Bankowski and N. Howard-Jones (eds.). *Human Experimentation and Medical Ethics: XV CIOMS Round Table Conference.* Council for International Organizations of Medical Sciences, Geneva, 1982, p. 274.

REGIONAL PANORAMA

Present Status and Prospects of Bioethics in Argentina

Justo Zanier, Pedro Hooft, Cristina Di Domenico,
Orlanda Señoriño, Cristina Gurrea, Teresa Asnariz, Jorge Manzini,
Natalia Biló, Emilia Pepa, Héctor Brunamontini, Orlando Calo,
Ana María Petriella, María I. Pacenza, and Laura Golpe

Creation of Argentina's Institute of Medical Humanities in 1972 represented a milestone in the history of Argentine bioethics and led subsequently to establishment of the Chair of Medical Humanities at the La Plata University Medical School in 1980. This concern for research, teaching, and public reporting of health matters related to the humanities and bioethics is attributed in great measure to Dr. José Alberto Mainetti, who has devoted himself to the teaching and development of this area of study. In addition, in recent years a Bioethics Center created at the Institute of Medical Humanities has promoted the formation of similar centers in Buenos Aires, Tucumán, Mendoza, and Mar del Plata.

It should be noted, however, that most of the interest in bioethics does not extend outside these centers, some hospitals, and certain other private health care institutions. Articles about the subject do appear sporadically in the press, and one does hear comments about it on the radio. In general, the Catholic Church is the institution that has contributed most to publicizing bioethics, but its concern has generally been limited to *in vitro* fertilization, embryo implantation, and other aspects of reproductive technology.

The technologic and scientific advances of our time have made it possible for people to intervene in the affairs of others and their environment, and this has produced basic, profound, unprecedented changes in the field of science. Even today, in a time of major technologic expansion, we cannot foretell what the limits of such changes will ultimately be.

As Tyrrel (see bibliography) has noted, there is no proof that present-day man has evolved mentally and morally at the same pace as this technologic explosion has occurred. This absence of proof raises certain questions about man's ability to administer with restraint, equity, and humanitarianism the dizzying advances occurring in every scientific field. The emerging discipline that we today call bioethics, and which some authors pursuing a wider meaning call "scientific ethics" or "technoethics," tries to find answers to such questions.

Although in Argentina the main concerns of this nature that have arisen have related to specific aspects of medical practice (abortion, euthanasia, etc.), it has also become necessary to extend bioethics to the basic sciences, which are the foundation of medical practice and health care, in order to broaden the sphere of interests involved and to adopt interdisciplinary criteria capable of encompassing the problems found.

Many people view present-day scientific and technical advances with a mixture of concern and hope deriving from the broad avenues these advances have opened up. They feel concern because of these advances' unforeseeable consequences, the lack of legal standards limiting their application to both man and his environment, and the great responsibility borne by the present generation in making decisions affecting future generations.

With this in mind, the National University of Mar del Plata has brought together a group of representatives specializing in different disciplines who are interested in these matters. This team includes anthropologists, biologists, educators, jurists, philosophers, physicians, psychologists, and sociologists belonging to the university's teaching and technical teams and other professional and scientific bodies of the community.

The team considers bioethics as a discipline reflecting the ethical problems derived from current scientific and technologic expansion, one that adopts an interdisciplinary approach to those problems with a view to having them considered in the course of actual scientific and professional activities as well as in legislation and public decision-making. The product of a year and a half of work by this group has crystallized into two quite important undertakings: design of a postgraduate bioethics course and the organization of the First Mar del Plata Workshop on Bioethics as part of the VI International Symposium on Bioethics.

Philosophic Foundation and Frame of Reference

The sciences dealing with humanity enable us to know with increasing precision what a human being is, but they do not explain to us that being's essence and the meaning of its existence. In contrast to the situation prevailing in antiquity, expansion of such knowledge and the rapidity with which it has been changing make it impossible for a single person to comprehend it all. Therefore, specialization in different areas of knowledge and even in proliferating subareas is necessary. While recognizing this need, however, it should be noted that such specialization places us in danger of losing sight of the whole.

Moreover, to understand even a part of the whole, and to avoid losing sight of our origins,

we must have some reasonable guiding ideas about the nature of that whole. Hence, we believe there is an urgent need for clear answers to the following questions: What sort of human development is desired? What sort of society? and What sort of science do we need?

Regarding the first question, a human being may be seen as a unique and unreplicable person who requires sufficient freedom to develop individually and socially in a responsible way. As a person, this being does not deal with the world indifferently but makes value judgments through which he or she discerns and judges what things mean.

Regarding the second question, a person's social life constitutes an essential dimension of that person. Indeed, a person's intimate, personal, and social relations are inseparable, together comprising that person's life in the community. Freedom for human beings will therefore be achieved fully and authentically in a society that ensures recognition and realization of equal freedom for all in an environment of necessary interdependence between individuals and society. Within this context, bioethical training of educators, professionals, and scientists is essential in order that they can identify problems needing axiologic study and devote appropriate attention to those matters.

Regarding the type of science that we need, it is important that science not be autonomous or sterile, since the knowledge that it generates should be at the service of human beings conceived as ends and never merely as means to others' ends. However, the more we know the more power we accumulate, and this presents us with the risk of using human beings as tools for our own purposes.

It is unquestionable that science has provided positive benefits for humanity and will be able to provide more in the future. Despite this, it must also be borne in mind that science is neither the only nor the ultimate criterion of truth. And the man or woman of science must be aware of personal dignity (both his or her own and that of others), always regarding the human being as the end. Otherwise we run the risk that technoscience values will be deemed worth more than human values, and that all done in the name of technoscience will be justified, even when it leads to increasing dehumanization.

It must be noted that not everything that is technically possible is ethically justifiable. Science and philosophy, then, are not separate things, but instead are disciplines that must be practiced together, complementing each other in the eternal search for knowledge.

In the field of the life sciences, the scientific and technologic revolution is of such a magnitude that today it presents physicians, biologists, lawyers, and other professionals with problems that cannot be solved with technical information alone. It is also necessary to take philosophic questions into consideration if we do not want a cold and technified world dominated by a science without conscience—a world that might very well be headed toward its own destruction.

Graduate Bioethics Course

This course was proposed to the University of Mar del Plata's Governing Council and approved in August 1988. Its structure conforms to existing regulations governing university graduate programs, being of two years' duration and demanding successful completion of appropriate evaluative requisites for promotion. The course is directed at professionals in all disciplines whose work affects the individual and social lives of people or which takes this as a general subject of study.

The course's aims are as follows: to motivate and train professionals and investigators to identify and resolve bioethical problems in their own areas of work; to train "multiplier" agents in bioethics who can act in government and within the scientific community at large; and to create the first group of teachers and investigators in this field, looking toward its future organization as an independent discipline.

The course has been designed by subject so as to focus upon certain problem nuclei—these be-

ing relationships between society and bioethics, institutions and bioethics, professions and bioethics, and humanity and bioethics (Annex 1). These relationships embrace aspects of the reality to be analyzed, and on this basis the content of the course has been established.

As the Annex shows, six central themes appropriate to the problem nuclei have been selected. These are health and illness, genetics and health, euthanasia, work and society, behavior manipulation, and delinquency and society. The first three of these have their roots in ecologic biology, while the last three have their origins in psychology.

These themes relate to one another in an interdisciplinary manner so that they can be arranged in an articulate and ordered sequence, and so that within the ground encompassed by each theme relevant material pertaining to the four problem nuclei and each of various areas within these nuclei are available for study.

Keeping in mind the course's design features, a multimedia teaching strategy was chosen—a strategy in which information is transmitted not only through the instructor's words in a personal encounter, as in a theoretical class, but is also conveyed through printed matter, audiovisual materials, case analyses, and other methods.

A Bioethics Workshop

The second part of the VI International Symposium on Bioethics and the First Mar del Plata Workshop on Bioethics were held at Mar del Plata on 2 and 3 December 1988. As part of this event, three round table discussions were held. These dealt with "The Major Themes of Bioethics," "A Multidisciplinary Approach to Genetic Counseling," and "Presentation of the Postgraduate Course in Bioethics." Four lectures were also given.

The First Iberoamerican Studies in Bioethics Group was organized at the symposium. This group's objectives are to develop links among its members; promote the organization of a scientific society for research in this area; sponsor and organize research in related disciplines through courses, seminars, conferences, workshops, and congresses; participate in international congresses and workshops in the country and abroad; and maintain permanent contact with universities, research centers, specialists, and allied institutions.

Bibliography

Bunge, M. *Etica y ciencia*. Siglo XX, Buenos Aires, 1986.

Kieffer, G. H. *Bioética*. Alhambra, Madrid, 1983.

Tyrrel, G. N. *La personalidad del hombre*. Paidós, Buenos Aires, 1976.

Annex 1. Design of the Graduate Bioethics Course, Mar del Plata National University, Argentina. Each central theme is intended to develop comprehension, analysis, thought, and decision-making for application to specific problems of an ethical nature.

A. Central Theme: Health and Disease

Area	Problem nuclei			
	Society and bioethics	Institutions and bioethics	Professions and bioethics	Humanity and bioethics
Biologic-ecologic	Health: Naturalistic and individualistic concepts Historic evolution of the concept of health Health as a social asset Standards of living and health indicators Psychosociosomatic illnesses Social implications of the health diagnosis Research on health needs Research on health systems Scheduling and planning (resource use and allocation)	Institutions and health Education and health, education and ecology Psychosociosomatic diseases Professional ethics and institutions Control of environmental management	Importance and participation of the different professions in public health Disease as a subjectively lived reality Psychosociosomatic diseases Application of the medical-social approach to clinical patient management Criteria for reasoning about health status Epidemiology as an interdisciplinary science Preparation of the health professional Professional ethics Professional confidentiality and medical-social information	Health as value; health as equilibrium Vulnerability to disease: A defective attribute of human beings Disease as a subjectively lived reality Psychosociosomatic illnesses Diagnosis of health status Medical technology and man
Psychologic	Health, disease, and normality Historic evolution of mental health Health criteria in relation to society and culture Psychopathologic epidemiology Health education	Public and private institutions The family and its influence on health and disease Education and prevention	The psychologist, the psychoanalyst, and the psychiatrist Psychology and medicine Psychopathology The professional-patient relationship Psychologic and psychiatric epidemiology Preparation of the health professional	Life and death: Eros and Thanatos Health promotion
Philosophic	Health as reward and punishment The dignity of the individual Philosophic concepts and their projection in life systems Philosophic views of the individual Humanism Values and their hierarchy	Normative ethics: Standards throughout history Educational systems as projections of values	Responsibility of the scientist and technologist Critical analysis of the various deontologies The concepts of "person" and "liberty" Axiology	The individual: Human acts and moral acts Will and free choice
Anthropologic	Anthropology and health Medical anthropology: Epistemologic formulations Psychiatric anthropology: The intercultural perspective and the notion of health Culture and subculture Community and global culture The emergence of bioethics as a social need: Implications Society and biotechnologic advances Endoculturation of social patterns	Institutions as generators of new sociocultural patterns at the level of public health medicine	Sociocultural contributions and the medical and behavioral sciences The anthropologist's role in the health field: Anthropology and public health Myths and beliefs in disease therapeutics The doctor-patient relationship: Incorporation of the anthropologic perspective in medicine and psychology	The human being as a biopsychosocial entity belonging to a cultural universe Man as a sick animal

123

Annex 1. (Continued)

A. Central Theme: Health and Disease

Area	Problem nuclei			
	Society and bioethics	Institutions and bioethics	Professions and bioethics	Humanity and bioethics
	Implementation of health programs in society Sociogenesis of disease Cultural factors in disease diagnosis and treatment Transculturation and disease: The case of immigrant families The healer seen through the intercultural stereoptican The therapeutic role of magic Socioanthropologic categories in health situation diagnosis The doctor-patient relationship Lactation and health: Bioethical considerations Health and sexuality Society, health, and marginality Prevention in groups at risk Incorporation of new sociocultural patterns into the community		Epidemiology: Anthropologic contributions about marginality	Human rights vis-à-vis scientific and technical development
Legal	Health as a fundamental human right Health as a protected legal asset Mental health and the law Mental health and legal responsibility Health policies Legal projection of health Ecology and law Conditions of habitability and theories of justice Legal aspects of the doctor-patient relationship Diagnosis: Responsibility Public health policies	Legal regulation of health Rights to privacy, education, and health Ecology and the police power	Professional legal responsibility Codes of professional ethics The legal nature of the doctor-patient relationship Responsibility in the face of diagnostic errors Legislation on these matters	
Sociologic	Sociologic concept of health Historical-social transformations: Their implications for health models Production and health Man-machine analogy Concept of health and disease Level of development and social stratification Research and prevention and their relationship to social integration	Different types of medical institutions The family: Different forms of health promotion The school as transmitter of general public health patterns The role, development, and production of disease	The sociologist in epidemiologic work: Research and prevention Social discrimination regarding disease and disability Social forms of health recognition in different cultures Sociologic contributions to epidemiologic knowledge Maladjustment between social needs and individual choices of profession Level of specialization: Loss of the holistic concept of health	

B. Central Theme: Genetics and Health

Area	Problem nuclei			
	Society and bioethics	Institutions and bioethics	Professions and bioethics	Humanity and bioethics
Biologic-ecologic	Genetics and health: Society-based selective criterion Standards tending to meet this objective Reproductive techniques Future genetic technologies Limits of genetic research: The degree of control that society has in this area Ecology and genetic research	Genetics and health: Centralized or decentralized planning Birth control Limits of genetic research: Institutional norms and prescriptions in this area Ecology and genetic research	Genetics as a branch of medicine: Its scope and objectives Limits of genetic research from a professional standpoint (deontologic criteria) Extension to all living things	Consideration of man as an end or a means
Psychologic	Psychosocial effects derived from genetic research and genetic engineering Psychologic counseling Consideration of the psychosocial effects that can be foreseen from use of future genetic technologies	Incentives and limitations on clinical research and internment institutions	Directed or undirected counseling Incentives and limitations on clinical research Artificial intelligence and psychologic identity	Consideration of man as an end or a means
Philo-sophic	Concept of the individual Humanism and the hierarchy of values Concept of the individual in political ideologies and projects Need for an ethics of the future Different contemporary ethics (lifeboat morality) Liberty, will, and free choice	Institutional customs Implementation of projects through institutions	Deontologies	Values: Concept of the individual; self-ness
Anthropologic	Genetic anthropology Control of birth and marginality Reproductive technology from the anthropologic viewpoint Bioethical considerations regarding sterilization Social construction of the bioethical paradigm Social limits on biotechnologic advances Respect for the human species	Institutions and genetic advances Institutions and the various bioethics positions on birth control and reproductive techniques	Anthropologic genetics: The professional and marginal groups Professional limitations and sociocultural patterns	Human identity Genetic manipulation
Legal	Inviolability of the individual as a fundamental human right Protection of the genetic heritage Comparative law Need for regulation Genetic manipulation and its limits Genetics, artificial fertility, and the law	Population policy Institutions, autonomy of the individual, and birth control Limits of genetic manipulation	Professional responsibility Constitutional and legal limits on genetic research	The individual as an object or subject of the law The personal rights of the individual
Sociologic	Development of biotechnology: Social consequences Social Darwinism: The humanistic reaction Biologic assignment of social roles	Family planning: Social institutions Family planning: The family and consumption	The role of science in contemporary society	Man as a means or an end The human ideal

125

Annex 1. (Continued)

C. Central Theme: Euthanasia

Area	Problem nuclei			
	Society and bioethics	Institutions and bioethics	Professions and bioethics	Humanity and bioethics
Biologic-ecologic	Sustaining life by artificial means Consequences of the diagnosis of death Euthanasia: Social criteria regarding euthanasia Terminal illness The Baby Doe problem	Sustaining life by artificial means Consequences of determination of death Euthanasia: Medical-legal aspects (regulation by law) The Baby Doe problem	Problem of determination of death (technical aspects) Euthanasia: Technical aspects, active and passive euthanasia Terminal illness The Baby Doe problem	Consequences of determination of death Terminal illness The Baby Doe problem
Psychologic	Man and death Psychologic representation of death Denial of death	Need for institutions to provide psychologic assistance for the patient, family, and staff Need for reflection on possible intervention in terminal situations	Need for reflection on possible intervention in terminal situations Interdisciplinary contributions to the problem of determination of death	The individual and death Psychologic representation of death Denial of death
Philosophic	The meaning of death	Concept of the individual	Concept of the individual	The meaning of death
Anthropologic	Nature and culture: The terminal patient's sociocultural universe Organ donation, the social problem Human suffering The anthropology of death: Implications The sacred and the profane Euthanasia: Social and cultural aspects and considerations relating to the manipulation of life	Institutions and transplants: The institution and human suffering Death and institutions	The anthropologist and euthanasia The anthropology of suffering The anthropology of death The terminal patient	The sacred and profane of death Human suffering The individual, marginality, and subculture Human dignity and codes of ethics
Legal	Organ transplants Life as a legally protected asset Legal criteria for determination of death	Conflict between humanistic values via-à-vis technologic and practical values and their projection in the law Comparative law Euthanasia and the law	Codes of professional ethics Legal regulation of the medical professions Euthanasia and the law	The right to die with dignity
Sociologic	The social being and the biologic individual Scientific efficiency, its reflection in society Science as a manipulator of social values	Conflict between the system of values of the medical institution and the family		

D. Central Theme: Society and Delinquency

Area	Problem nuclei			
	Society and bioethics	Institutions and bioethics	Professions and bioethics	Humanity and bioethics
Biologic-ecologic	Biological basis of aggression			
Psychologic	Society and delinquency	Administration of justice Internment institutions: Penitentiaries and institutions for minors	Psychologic assistance and counseling on crime prevention, resocialization, and skill development Experimentation with behavior	Crime and responsibility Disease and responsibility Liberty and responsibility Liberty and the common good
Philo-sophic	Hierarchy of values Education systems	Hierarchy of values Education systems	Hierarchy of values Education systems	The concept of self-ness The individual and liberty
Anthropologic	The delinquency subculture	The delinquency subculture	Subculture and delinquency	Subculture and delinquency
Legal	Criminology and criminal law	Preventive systems Penal systems: Education and treatment Auxiliary sciences	Need for legal assistance Legal regulation of the auxiliary legal professions Dignity of the individual as a limit on human experimentation	Concepts of fraud and culpability The limits of imputability
Sociologic	Anomie and social disintegration	Established (institutionalized) concepts	Sociology and criminality Development of sociologic skills The problem of social insertion	Crime and its causes from the perspective of society

Annex 1. (Continued)

E. Central Theme: Behavior Modification

Area	Problem nuclei			
	Society and bioethics	Institutions and bioethics	Professions and bioethics	Humanity and bioethics
Biologic-ecologic	Production-consumption equilibrium Ecology and rational use of natural resources		Behavior modification using surgical methods and medications	The therapeutic value of talk The relationship between man and the freedom of others
Psychologic	Production-consumption in contemporary society Advertising and behavior modification	Public relations agencies and communications media Legal regulation of programming and publicity	Psychology and communication The psychologist as public relations adviser Psychologic techniques in behavior modification	Communication as a characteristic of man Communication and liberty Free versus induced choice
Philo-sophic	Inversion of the scale of values Regarding the individual as a means to an end	Inversion of the scale of values Regarding the individual as a means to an end	Inversion of the scale of values Regarding the individual as a means to an end	The concept of self-ness Liberty and the individual
Anthropologic	Communication and culture	Communication and culture	Communication and culture Sociocultural consequences of behavior modification	Suppression of human identity
Legal	Legislation for consumer protection Law and natural resources	Normative regulation Applicable legal regimen	Criteria of professional responsibility: Ethical and legal	The right to privacy as a fundamental right of the individual Freedom of expression and the right to information
Sociologic	Relationship between production and consumption in contemporary society	Marketing research	Communications media and mass psychology	The individual and mass psychology

F. Central Theme: Labor and Society

Area	Problem nuclei			
	Society and bioethics	Institutions and bioethics	Professions and bioethics	Humanity and bioethics
Biologic-ecologic	The medicine of human activity Occupational diseases	Work-related accidents Unhealthful work	The physician as job selector Labor medicine Health examinations	
Psychologic	Work and society	Labor relations	Psychologic counseling Human relations Job selection Psychology and production incentives Experimentation in labor psychology	Labor relations and freedom Work: Self-realization or alienation
Philosophic	The problem of the individual and the problem of values The dignity of work as human fulfillment	The problem of standards The problem of liberty and responsibility	The problem of standards The problem of liberty and responsibility	Self-ness
Anthropologic	The anthropology of work: Problems regarding age and sex Work and free time		Work, identity, and professions	Work and identity
Legal	Human rights and the law The right to social security	The right to work and to social security Occupational accidents and diseases	Autonomy of the individual Rights to privacy Constitutional principles relating to work and social security	The right to work and professional associations
Sociologic	Labor relations in contemporary society	The sociology of organizations	The sociologist and manpower training	Social preparation of the individual

129

Bioethics: Implications for Medical Practice and Deontologic and Legal Standards in Brazil

Hélio Pereira Dias

Human existence, whether individual or collective, is fundamental to all the goods and interests protected by law. And since life, bodily integrity, honor, and liberty are the supreme values of human existence, their protection is a paramount duty of the State as it seeks to fulfill its role of preserving and perpetuating the species, maintaining ecological equilibrium, and promoting the peace essential to community survival.

Recent scientific discoveries and the extraordinary pace of scientific and technologic development have unquestionably increased man's power to control nature. But they have also increased the threat to life. Furthermore, the advances of science and technology have not generally been accompanied by comparable advances in morality and ethics—creating an imbalance that has tended to expose contradictions inherent in human nature.

In other words, major scientific discoveries, if well used, can greatly benefit humanity, but if misused they can also endanger or destroy it. Therefore, it is incumbent upon the moral conscience of the scientific community to know how to apply such discoveries properly. And it is incumbent upon those who establish the rules by which society lives, the technical and legal authorities, to establish rights and obligations that will lead to such proper applications being made.

Within this context, it seems clear that technical skills, which express the dialogue between the hands and the brain, must be subordinated to reason and knowledge, which regulate action so that human nature is not demeaned but is free to develop its full scope and potential. Here medical professionals pursuing their mission of preventing, treating, curing, and minimizing human suffering are at the center of attention. Their activity, involving as it does the supreme individual values of life and health (activity which because of its importance is subject to government supervision), creates very close links between medicine and the law.

At present, a wide range of medical actions posing possible risks to the rights of individuals, social welfare, and basic human conditions are attracting considerable public attention. Such actions cut across a wide range of fields—including genetics (e.g., genetic alteration of microorganisms, potential modification of human genes, release of genetically altered organisms into the environment); human reproduction (e.g., abortion, artificial insemination, birth control, sterilization); medical research (e.g., experiments involving human subjects); surgery (e.g., plastic surgery, transplant of organs and tissues, transplant of bodily parts, use of artificial organs); and termination of life (e.g., euthanasia)—as well as involving more general issues such as medical confidentiality, the deliberate withholding of medical assistance, and medical responsibility.

Much of the concern to date, and most of the studies being performed as a result, are directed at ensuring the observance of well-defined ethical standards derived from general principles that are compatible with humanity's best interests. Among other things, it seems clear that medical studies and research should be carried out using appropriate scientific and technical controls that simultaneously safeguard the interests of the researchers, their subjects, and society at large.

More broadly, free exercise of the medical profession involves actions that cannot pertain exclusively to the private sphere, given that from a legal standpoint health and life constitute undeniable and inalienable goods. Hence, it is imperative that medical activities be regulated and that standards enshrined in the so-called deontologic codes be improved. At present these standards appear increasingly unrealistic and subject to influence in many cases by marketing technologies that contribute to undesirable distortions of medical practice.

Morality, strictly speaking, is not the same as ethics. Morality involves acquired behavior or the manner in which behavior is learned by people in a social setting; while ethics, far from being a series of rules and instructions, is the theory or science dealing with moral behavior of people in society. Bioethics, then, is the application of this same theory to the practice of acts that affect human life—that may help to improve, preserve, or save it, or that can mutilate or destroy it.

In reality, the great prominence of medical ethics in recent years has not been due to any resurgence of moral, philosophic, or theologic principles; nor has it resulted from growing feelings of responsibility arising within a medical profession upset by the present health care situation. Rather, medical ethics has received greater attention because of mounting public concern about the behavior of health professionals, especially physicians. Indeed, it is often felt that codes of ethics are merely being used as a screen to conceal malpractice and medical errors; and some people have come to believe that these codes are nothing more than a device for maintaining physicians as a class immune from judgment by the community.

Every profession is anxious to appear efficient. In the health sector, professionals such as doctors once had to compete with healers, mothers, and others before they were able to establish their professional monopoly, exercise professional autonomy, and exclude interference from outside individuals and judgments. From this point of view, it is not so difficult to conclude that a physician should only be judged by other physicians, that any admission of medical error would amount to belittling the profession, and that medical errors are, above all, a product of the surrounding system.

As medicine and medical technology became increasingly specialized, however, physicians could no longer work alone. Instead, they began to work with and for the institutions that made their activities possible. And as medical care became increasingly expensive, the government and private companies came increasingly to bear the costs of treatment. Consequently, in large measure the physician came to trade his position as an autonomous professional for that of an agent of these institutions; and his work came to reflect distortions created by large corporations active in the sector.

Meanwhile, technologic advances in medicine, juxtaposed with our present disease-producing social crisis, have put the physician in a difficult position. On the one hand, many claims of technologic efficiency have the aim of promoting greater use of particular equipment, machines, and drugs to cure diseases. And on the other, there is a fundamental conflict—for it seems clear that no matter how sophisticated it becomes, medical assistance is not going to solve the basic social problems of the population.

The growing number of tests and other exploratory techniques now available, such as those used to assess people's genes in order to foretell future diseases in a person or that person's descendants, are currently causing concern. If it were possible to do something about such diseases or prevent them from harming the next generation, then these tests should be carried out. However, since some of these tests detect illnesses for which there is as yet no treatment, it is arguable whether the knowledge thus acquired is really useful or of anything but limited immediate value. Nevertheless, many scientists believe that an awareness of future health status (even if that status is bad) may help people to plan their lives better. In some cases, therefore, the benefits outweigh the costs, and the resulting good exceeds the risk. In addition, one must consider whether or not the person to be tested desires the test—because in some cases, such as when an individual is suspected of harboring the AIDS virus, the person may not wish to undergo the test.

Whatever the benefits, however, recent studies show that such tests are tending to become more common; and ongoing research on such problems as Alzheimer's disease, depression, manic disorders, schizophrenia, Huntington's disease (a rare and fatal brain disease), juvenile diabetes, and others is raising new and difficult questions in the fields of medicine and law, in matters of human intimacy and professional confidentiality, and in many detailed sorts of decision-making such as whether it is wise to tell somebody he is suffering from a serious disease, especially if it is incurable.

Deontology (from the Greek *deon*, duty), defined as study of the individual's moral obligations within the community, relates to moral action. Such action is understood to be action that is performed in the presence or with the participation of another person, that involves a choice of alternatives, and that depends upon the influence of feelings, the censorship of conscience, the means employed, the ends sought, and the formulation of judgments. In sum, such actions may be envisaged as depending upon a structure of interconnected motives, will, goals, and results.

In addition to being encompassed within this structure, moral action is also subject to ethical concerns of the individual himself (conscience), and also of class, community, nation, and history. As this suggests, morality in general, as well as morality relating to the health professions, is not the same at all times and places. That is, it changes as values change and as progress is achieved in integrating conscience and liberty into moral action.

Ethical Control: Discipline of the Health Professions

In Brazil, the Federal Medical Council and regional medical councils established by Decree Law No. 7.955 of 13 December 1945 are the bodies responsible for supervising medical ethics. They judge (and when necessary discipline) members of the medical profession, it being their duty to promote fully ethical conduct by the medical profession and to safeguard the prestige and good standing of the profession and its practitioners—in accordance with Law No. 3.268 of 30 September 1957 and the regulations authorized in Decree No. 44.045 of 19 July 1958. Other health-related professions are supervised in this manner by other federal and regional councils. Over the past three decades, three codes of medical ethics have been approved in Brazil. These are the Code of Medical Ethics approved on 11 January 1965, the Brazilian Code of Medical Deontology approved on 13 April 1984, and the current Code of Medical Ethics, approved on 26 January 1988. The latter, containing 145 articles, concerns itself with establishing fundamental principles regarding rights, responsibilities, prohibitions, and other matters affecting the medical profession— including relationships between the physician and the patient, the patient's family, and other physicians; professional confidentiality; remuneration; medical research; publicity; issuance of certificates and bulletins; and general standards. Again, other codes of ethics have been issued in recent decades for the other health-related professions—such as pharmacology, nursing, dentistry, etc.

Family Planning

In no circumstances whatever is it right for man to act contrary to the dictates of his conscience. It is quite possible that one may need to study a question further, or that one's conscience may be wrong, but it will never be right to act against one's conscience. Whatever one may do in an attempt to determine what the right action is, when the moment for that action comes there is always the matter of personal responsibility. Nobody, not even the Church, can exempt anybody from having to follow their conscience and accept responsibility.

Regarding human reproduction, the State cannot impose mandatory birth control. Without an inalienable right to marriage and procreation, human dignity cannot exist (*Populorum Progressio*, No. 37). However, public authorities, acting within the limits of their powers, can intervene by promoting relevant education and taking other appropriate measures, so long as they observe the requirements of the moral law and respect the liberty of spouses. The State should also see that those who need it receive appropriate information and education regarding the methods that Christian morality permits for purposes of responsible birth control. Poverty cannot be a reason for discrimination in this matter.

Because the concept of human dignity presupposes an inalienable right to procreation, parents have the right and the duty to decide how many children they will have—in other words, to exercise responsible parenthood and to use family planning. Indeed, responsible parenthood of this sort is necessary, not only for social welfare, but also for purposes of providing a balance between population growth and human and economic resources.

All too often, accelerating population growth complicates the problem of development; it is for this reason that studies and research in the area of human reproduction are urgently required.

However, population policy is only a part of general development policy, not an alternative to it. And final decisions involving practical action with regard to responsible parenthood depend on the individual conscience of each person; nobody should be forced or induced to act against his own wishes.

It should also be noted that family planning does not necessarily mean "limiting the number of children." A well-planned family may contain 10 or more children, provided that they live in hygienic and healthy conditions and have the necessary social and economic support to guarantee their education and livelihood.

It may be asserted that law, religion, sociology, and politics are all in agreement with the important concept of responsible parenthood. The Encyclical *Humanae Vitae*, broader and more enlightened than *Casti Conubii*, defends birth control as legitimate and in a number of places speaks of "responsible parenthood." Hence, disagreement among the various schools of thought is not about family planning itself, but rather about the methods used to provide reasonable spacing between pregnancies.

There is nothing illegal about family planning as such in any branch of Brazilian law. It is no crime to provide guidance to spouses regarding birth control practices, or for them to act on such guidance so long as the couple's liberty is respected. However, surgical sterilization, when not performed at medical direction, involves the destruction of the reproductive function, and therefore does grave bodily harm. There can be no justification for such action, even when it is based on the written consent of the wife or husband, since life and health are undeniable and inalienable goods.

The laws governing the organization of health systems in the states of Acre, Alagoas, Amazonas, Bahia, Ceará, Espírito Santo, Goiás, Pará, Paraíba, Piauí, Rio Grande do Norte, Rondônia, and Sergipe already contain the following stipulations:

☐ Measures to protect the health of mothers and children shall always have as their guiding principle the strengthening of the family, and any actions in this area must be grounded upon ethical and humanistic foundations.

☐ No steps shall be taken that may affect the offspring except on the basis of a medical recommendation to that effect designed to protect the mother's health and based on the freely expressed assent of the parties.

Article 226, Paragraph 7 of the 1988 Constitution of the Federal Republic of Brazil states the following: "Based on the principles of human dignity and responsible parenthood, family planning is the free decision of the couple, it being the State's function to provide educational and scientific resources to enable this right to be exercised, any form of coercion by public or private institutions being prohibited."

Abortion

According to the Brazilian Civil Code, the rights of the fetus are protected from the time of conception (Article 4). In addition, the Criminal Code (Articles 124 to 127) makes it a crime to cause an abortion, except in two situations described in Article 128, as follows: "Article 128— An abortion performed by a doctor shall not be punished when: (I) there is no other way of saving the mother's life; (II) the pregnancy results from rape and the abortion is preceded by the consent of the mother or, when she is incapable, her legal representative."

Hence, legal abortion performed by a doctor, known as "necessary abortion," is performed to save the life of the mother or to avoid the birth of an offspring resulting from rape. In this manner the Criminal Code recognizes two situations in which abortion is not a crime, one depending on a medical opinion and the other on emotional considerations. However, the wording of Article 128 is excessively simplistic and leaves scope for criminal abortion. Indeed, one can argue that the existing provisions should be amended to make it impossible for certain unscrupulous professionals to take advantage of them and practice illegal abortions on the grounds that heroic steps are being taken to save a life.

The draft Criminal Code (Special Section), published in October 1987 by the Ministry of Justice to encourage comment, provides for the possibility of so-called "eugenic abortion" when there are good grounds, certified by two doctors, for believing that the fetus shows signs of serious and irreversible physical or mental anomalies, provided that prior consent has been given by the pregnant woman or, when she is incapable, by her legal representative and, if she is married, by her spouse.

However, the legality of a necessary abortion does not depend on the consent of the pregnant woman or of third parties, since in the right circumstances it is fully protected by the law and by the precepts governing medical science. Nevertheless, current medical progress is steadily reducing the criteria justifying abortion as a means of preventing death of the mother.

Some people feel that the type of "necessary" abortion performed in connection with rape— also known as "sentimental" or "moral" abortion—can no longer be justified, because it gives the physician the right to take a life. And in such cases there are clearly no circumstances that could be deemed to make abortion a medical necessity. It is also said that it is extremely difficult to prove rape, and that for a doctor to terminate a pregnancy on these grounds is a simple way of obtaining an immediate abortion.

From the standpoint of the criminal law, there is no need for a conviction of rape to be obtained in order for the abortion to be permitted—it is enough for there to be convincing proof of the existence of a sexual offense. One reason is that charges are not brought in rape cases unless a complaint is filed, with two exceptions. That is, proceedings are brought via public action (Article 225 of the Criminal Code) if the victim or her parents cannot meet the costs of filing suit without using funds essential for their support, or if the crime involves abuse of a father's legal authority or abuse of a stepfather's, teacher's, or guardian's position. (In the former case, action by public authorities depends on representations made by the victim or her legal representative.)

Nelson Hungria, in his *Comments on the Criminal Code* (vol. 5, p. 313, 1958), says "If criminal proceedings are in progress against the accused rapist, it would be advisable for the judge and representative of the public prosecutor to be consulted, since their approval will not be refused if there is sufficient evidence for the preventive detention of the accused." And again: "In practice, to avoid abuses, the doctor should only act on the basis of conclusive evidence of the alleged rape, unless the offense is common knowledge or the rapist has already been convicted. In the meantime, if the doctor's knowledge of certain circumstances is such as to justify a reasonable belief regarding the possibility of rape, no blame will be attached to him should the allegations subsequently prove to be untrue. In such circumstances it is only the pregnant woman who will be criminally liable."

Regarding ethical codes, Article 54 of the Medical Ethics Code published in 1965 reads as follows: "The doctor must not perform an abortion except when there is no other way of saving the mother's life or when the pregnancy is the result of rape, and then always only after receiving the express consent of the mother or her legal representative. Par. (1): In either of these situations provided for in the law, the doctor may only act after conferring with at least two other colleagues. Par. (2): A record in triplicate shall be kept of this conference, one copy being sent to the Regional Medical Council and another to the clinical director of the establishment in which the operation is to be performed, with the third remaining in possession of the doctor who is performing the operation."

The Brazilian Code of Medical Deontology, approved by Resolution CFM No. 1.154/84 of 13 April 1984, merely prohibits doctors "from failing to comply with the specific legislation regarding cases of abortion" (Article 12) and from "performing, except in cases of urgency or emergency, any medical procedure without the prior consent of the patient or her legal guardian" (Article 24). The current Code of Medical Ethics, approved in 1988, omits any reference to abortion.

A number of increasingly insistent efforts have been made, using false arguments, to obtain support for an unacceptable legal protection of abortions, the most prominent claim being that clandestine abortions must be countered by legalizing or decriminalizing the practice. However, it can be argued to the contrary, on the basis of statistical evidence, that permissive laws do not eliminate clandestine operations, but instead produce a staggering increase in the ratio of abortions to live births.

Experiments and Medical Research

The Code of Medical Ethics currently in force in Brazil prohibits doctors from participating in any kind of experiment on human beings for military, political, racial, or eugenic purposes. It also bars experimental use of any treatment not yet approved for use in Brazil without proper authorization from the competent bodies and consent of the patient or person responsible. Such consent must be "informed" consent, in that the patient or person responsible must be duly informed of the relevant circumstances and possible consequences of the treatment before his or her consent is obtained.

The same code also prohibits any attempt by a physician to seek personal advantage or commercial gain from those financing medical research in which the doctor is participating. It requires that all medical research on human beings be approved and monitored by a committee that is not dependent upon or subordinate to the researcher in any way. It bars performing or participating in medical research that puts the patient at risk by suspending or stopping approved forms of treatment. And it prohibits any experiments involving new clinical or surgical treatments upon patients with incurable or terminal disease, unless there is reasonable hope of its being beneficial without imposing additional suffering.

More recently, in Resolution No. 1 of 13 June 1988, the National Health Council of the Ministry of Health issued regulations governing research in the health field. Specific matters covered include ethical aspects of research on human beings; utilization of new forms of treatment, diagnosis, therapy, and rehabilitation; use of under-age subjects, individuals not in a position to give informed consent, women of child-bearing age, and pregnant women; tests performed during pregnancy, childbirth, the puerperium, and lactation; research on individuals where something less than full and spontaneous consent may be assumed; research involving corpses, parts of the human body, organs, tissues, and organ and tissue by-products; pharmacologic research; research employing pathogenic microorganisms or biologic material that may contain them; research that entails the engineering and handling of recombinant nucleic acids; and research employing radioactive isotopes as well as devices and generators producing ionizing electromagnetic radiation. This National Health Council resolution deals with the activities of ethics and biological safety committees, as well as with research conducted by health institutions generally, and contains rules governing such work.

In this way, the resolution has filled a gap in Brazil by addressing the issue of medical research on human subjects. This issue has been arousing social controversy—because it may entail abuses, may represent a threat to man's physical integrity or health, and may involve illegal acts even after voluntary consent has been obtained. Failure to observe these regulations may constitute violations of an ethical-disciplinary or criminal nature (crime of direct or immediate danger, Article 132 of the Criminal Code), or of a health-related nature, contravening Law No. 6.437/77.

Euthanasia

The current debate over euthanasia is both necessary and inevitable. Even in Brazil, medicine has already reached that paradoxical point where it is possible to prolong life but not to bring an individual back from a vegetative state.

Euthanasia, a word whose meaning signifies "good death," "induced death," or, more simply, the "right to kill," finds no support in Brazilian law or in the postulates of medical ethics. In-

deed, euthanasia offends the national conscience, which cannot accept as lawful the right to die or the right to kill, since they contravene morality, customs, and public law.

On this point the current (1988) Code of Medical Ethics stipulates that a physician must use all the diagnostic and treatment resources at his disposal on behalf of the patient; it also prohibits him from employing, under any circumstances, means intended to shorten the patient's life, even at the request of the patient or whoever is legally responsible for him (Articles 57 and 66).

Furthermore, the Brazilian Penal Code punishes homicide, with which euthanasia can be equated because it involves the crime of "killing somebody." It is not suicide, although paradoxically it may have the characteristics of the crime referred to in Article 122 of the Penal Code, namely "assistance, inducement, or instigation to commit suicide." In addition, euthanasia is a civil offense because it causes harm to somebody (Civil Code, Articles 159 and 1.549).

In the light of all this, there is no possibility of legitimizing euthanasia or of giving a doctor or anyone else the right to perform it, even if he were invested with excellent motives—assuming that this were possible. Moreover, although attempts might be made to show that a doctor, in refraining from treating an incurable patient, was not committing euthanasia, the mere failure to provide treatment could lead to ethical and disciplinary action as well as civil and criminal penalties.

The purpose of the law is to promote the common good and ensure that each individual may fully enjoy his rights. These rights are supposed to include physical and moral safety, as well as effective protection against aggression and violence. Since life is our most prized possession, the law only performs its protective mission when it prescribes serious penalties for those depriving others of their lives. Consequently, the decriminalization of euthanasia, so as to permit advancing the deliberately "anticipated" death of a sick person on grounds of preventing suffering, even with the victim's consent (or that of immediate family members), offends greatly against both Christian morality and the law.

Transplants

Transplants of human body parts, organs, and tissues have raised a variety of technical, scientific, legal, moral, and theologic questions that must be dealt with by physicians, transplant donors, and transplant recipients. The subject is rife with all sorts of implications relating to life and death: the abnegation of the donor, the hopes of the recipient, the notion that part of a corpse may save a life, and so on. The most controversial issues relate to authorization for the transplant. Among other things, should the express authorization of a living donor be required or not?

In Brazil these issues are governed by Law No. 5.479 of 10 August 1968, which many people believe leaves much to be desired. The deficiencies cited relate mainly to the criteria used to determine death, the form in which donations are made available, authorization for transplants in cases of suicide and accidents, and the summary manner in which it deals with the range of operations involved. At present a number of bills are being discussed in the National Congress, but so far none has been approved.

In any event, it would seem that a sound code on transplants must establish five prerequisites—real necessity; professional confidentiality; exclusion of sensationalistic purpose; absolute confidence that the operation is not an experiment on human beings but only and indisputably a therapeutic action on behalf of the patient; and finally, reliable determination of the death of a potential donor, which is absolutely essential in such circumstances.

Medical Secrecy—Professional Confidentiality

Medical secrecy is strictly regulated by criminal law, the penal code, civil law, and medical deontology. However, there are permitted exceptions and a wide range of complications causing uncertainties that, in many cases, the law does not admit.

One reason for such complications is this: Clearly, maintaining confidentiality in the exercise of a profession is designed above all to protect and defend moral and material goods. Hence, the State should see to it that individuals find solutions while preserving this secrecy. In some cases, however, community interest needs to take precedence over individual interests, though it is not always easy to determine which those cases are.

According to the Criminal Code (Article 154), anyone who reveals facts of which he is aware as a result of his function, office, or profession without proper cause, and thereby actually or potentially harms another person, is liable to a prison term of three months to two years or a fine of 1,000 to 10,000 cruzados. On the other hand, a doctor who fails to inform the public authorities of a disease whose notification is compulsory is liable to a prison term of six months to two years or a fine of 500 to 3,000 cruzados (Article 269).

The criminal law also precludes "failure to communicate to the competent authorities . . . [a] public offense, of which he was aware in the exercise of medicine or another health-related profession, provided that the offense does not result from the act of representation and the communication does not expose the client to criminal proceedings. Penalty: fine of from 300 to 3,000 cruzados."

Meanwhile, the Civil Code (Article 144) states that "Nobody may be obliged to state facts regarding which, as a result of his status or profession, he should keep secret."

Chapter IX of the current Code of Medical Ethics approved in January 1988 and published in the Official Gazette on 26 January of that year prohibits the following physician actions:

☐ "Article 102—To reveal information he knows by virtue of exercising his profession—except for just cause, legal obligation, or express permission of the patient.
   Sole paragraph: This prohibition remains

in effect: (a) Even when the information is public knowledge or the patient has died. (b) When he gives evidence as a witness. In this situation, the doctor shall appear before the authorities and state why he cannot testify.

- ☐ "Article 103—To reveal professional secrets pertaining to a patient who is a minor, including to his/her parents or legal guardians, provided that the minor is capable of assessing the problem and arriving at a solution to it on his/her own, except when not revealing the information may harm the patient.
- ☐ "Article 104—To refer to identifiable clinical cases; to exhibit patients or their pictures in professional announcements or in the dissemination of medical matters on radio or television programs, in movies, or in articles, interviews, or reports in journals, magazines, or other publications.
- ☐ "Article 105—To reveal confidential information obtained during medical examinations of workers, even when requested to do so by managers of enterprises or institutions, unless keeping silent jeopardizes the health of the employees or the community.
- ☐ "Article 106—To provide insurance companies with any information regarding the circumstances of death of any patient except that contained in the death certificate itself, without the express authority of the legal representative or heir.
- ☐ "Article 107—To fail to instruct his assistants or ensure that they observe professional secrecy as stipulated by law.
- ☐ "Article 108—To facilitate the handling and inspection of dossiers, papers, and other notes of medical observations that are protected by professional secrecy by persons not similarly obligated.
- ☐ "Article 109—To fail to preserve medical secrecy in collecting fees by legal or other means."

In legal terms, if one is to determine that professional confidentiality has been violated, it is necessary to show that (a) a secret existed that was known to the violator by virtue of his function, office, or profession; (b) revelation of the secret could potentially harm someone; (c) there was no just cause for violating confidentiality; or (d) there was fraudulent intent.

From the standpoint of the criminal law, the willful factor in the crime occurs when the agent has a free and knowing desire to cause harm to another person (a directly criminal act) or when he risks causing harm even if not intending a harmful result (a potentially harmful act). In the latter case there is a basis not for legal punishment but for blame (for negligence, malpractice, or imprudence).

The notion that a just cause can be sufficient to overrule the commitment to confidentiality in keeping medical secrets depends, essentially, upon moral or social benefit that does or does not support such action, assuming considerable motivation capable of justifying the violation. In this context, a "secret" is understood to mean something known by one person or a limited number of people with an interest in keeping the knowledge hidden, because its revelation could cause harm. Similarly, "medical confidentiality" means the secrecy that the medical professional is obliged to maintain regarding certain facts he knows as a result of exercising his profession, with the aforementioned exceptions in special cases.

The principal reason for observing medical confidentiality is to gain the confidence of the patient, whose information is essential to ensure sound diagnosis and efficient treatment. And although justification on these grounds may seem less than absolute, there are those who maintain that a doctor's duty is absolute and leaves him no discretion.

Other more flexible positions derive from the modern notion that since life and health are goods protected by the State and medicine is rapidly becoming a true public service, the public interest should prevail over private interests. Therefore, in certain cases there is justification for breaking both traditional medical confidentiality and the portion of the Hippocratic Oath that says "What I may see or hear in the course of the treatment or even outside of the treatment in regard to the life of men, which on no account must be spread abroad, I will keep to myself."

To demonstrate changing attitudes toward stringent medical confidentiality it has become customary to cite current practices such as the televising of very complex operations or the publicizing of medical announcements through the mass media. Consideration must also be given to the fact that society has pertinent interests; what is at stake is the right of the community to mitigate the rigor of medical secrecy in its absolute form. Medical professionals have duties and obligations that are more important than their individual commitments, since their science and art are daily assuming an increasingly public character. To remain silent, for example, when an innocent person is condemned appears absurd, an unjust act of complicity.

Nonetheless, it should be noted that breaking the confidentiality that should govern the practice of medicine occurs only exceptionally, in very special situations, or when the law, recognizing a higher right to be protected, allows confidentiality to be broken.

Some authors like to enumerate situations in which laws made in the collective interest require that medical secrecy be broken, such as, for example: (a) in completing a declaration of birth or a death certificate; (b) to prevent a marriage, in the case of certain diseases that may endanger the health of one of the spouses or their offspring; (c) in declarations regarding communicable diseases; (d) when an illegal (criminal) act is involved; (e) in cases of child abuse, where injuries or diseases are involved that require care by the family and involve third parties; (f) in medico-legal examinations; (g) in dealing with criminal abortions; (h) in legal proceedings to collect medical fees; and (i) in providing information for hospital records.

Medical secrecy must be preserved principally to protect the interests of the patient, not just the reputation of medical science. On the other hand, it cannot be a crime to break medical confidentiality when there is a need to protect a more relevant contrary interest.

The legal basis for medical secrecy is the result not of a private interest contract but a public order stipulation. To remain silent against the interests of justice, for example, would be to give secrecy the character of complicity. As this shows, the idea that professional secrecy can never be broken cannot be reconciled with modern social realities or with public order—and so, in the face of pertinent social concerns, the precept becomes relative. Accordingly, modern legal thinking is not so strict as it used to be when such rigor is prejudicial to discovering the truth, or when it runs counter to what preserves the moral and social order and collective social welfare.

In practice, various situations arise that raise the issue of medical confidentiality. Along with the obligation to cure the sick, a physician is also obliged to protect other people against certain diseases. For example, a physician may learn that a patient with a contagious disease is reluctant to stop going to work—in which case he may be obliged to inform the competent authorities of the situation. Or, paradoxically, it may be necessary to break confidentiality to protect the patient's health or life. For example, a psychiatrist may determine that it is reasonably likely that a mental patient will try to kill himself. In such a case it is his duty to communicate this fact to the patient's family.

In general, however, the most complex questions tend to involve certain imperatives of law and justice. Within this area there are some cases in which the doctor must only respond to what he has been asked, and others that can only be resolved by the submission of his clinical report, which thereby releases him from any future responsibility.

Regarding epidemiologic surveillance, Article 10 of Law No. 6.259 (30 October 1975) provides that compulsory notification of diseases involves confidentiality binding upon the health authorities receiving the information. According to the sole paragraph of this Article, "Patients suffering from diseases whose notification is compulsory may only be identified, outside medical and health circles, in exceptional circumstances involving major risks to the community, at the discretion of the health authorities and with the prior knowledge of the patient or those responsible for him." Failure to observe this rule is a violation of the health regulations and makes the agent subject to the penalties provided for in Law No. 6.437 of 1977 as part of an administrative process providing ample safeguards to defend the identified patient. Here, then, is an instance in which the legislators decided to defend medical confidentiality while making its observance less than absolute in cases involving serious potential risks to the community.

In closing this overview of confidentiality issues, it seems appropriate to note the ethical questions raised by the spread of AIDS in Brazil. In particular, this has presented physicians with a conflict between protecting their patient's welfare by maintaining professional confidentiality and preventing the infection and death of other people by breaking it. This problem has led Brazil's Federal Medical Council to issue a recent statement asserting that "the desire of the patient who does not wish his condition to be revealed to family members must be respected. The ban on this secrecy being broken remains in effect after the patient's death, but special situations exist that can give rise to exceptions."

Bibliography

Alcântara, H. R. *Deontologia e Diceologia*. Editora LTR, São Paulo, Brazil, 1979.

Código Civil Brasileiro.

Conselho Federal de Medicina. *Código Brasileiro de Deontologia Médica, Brasil*. 1984.

Conselho Federal de Medicina. *Código de Etica Médica, Brasil*. 1965.

Conselho Federal de Medicina. *Código de Etica Médica, Brasil*. 1988.

Constituição da República Federativa do Brasil, 1988.

De França, G. V. *Direito Médico*. São Paulo, 1975.

Dias, H. P. *Direito de Saúde*. Brasília, 1982.

Encyclicals: *Populorum Progressio, Humanae Vitae, Casti Connubii*.

Hungria, N. *Comentários ao Código Penal, Brasil*. 1958.

Ministério da Justiça. Anteprojeto de Código Penal. Brasília, 1987.

Ministério da Justiça. *Código Penal Brasileiro (3rd ed.)*. 1986.

Ministério da Saúde. *AIDS recomendações técnicas e aspectos éticos*. Brasília, 1988.

Nobre Freitas. *O transplante de órgãos humanos á luz do direito*. Brasília, 1975.

World Health Organization. *Health Aspects of Human Rights, with Special Reference to Developments in Biology and Medicine*. Geneva, 1976.

World Health Organization. *Handbook of Resolutions and Decisions by the World Health Assembly and Executive Board (vol. 1, 1948–72)*. Geneva, 1973.

Current Bioethics Trends in Canada

Bernard M. Dickens

Training in Bioethics

Bioethics courses are now common in the philosophy programs of Canadian universities and are also found in related programs of religious studies. The Westminster Institute for Ethics and Human Values, associated with the University of Western Ontario, devoted its 1989 annual symposium to the subject of medical ethics education for the undergraduate medical student. This gathering found that bioethics training for students of medicine and related health professions was inadequate, although both undergraduate and graduate programs have been expanding.

Apart from the Westminster Institute, work in bioethics is conducted at a number of other centers. Modest bioethics training programs exist at the Universities of Calgary, Manitoba, and Montreal; and additional bioethics training is provided by the Joint Faculties Bioethics Project at the University of Alberta. Canada's oldest established bioethics center is the Center for Bioethics at the Clinical Research Institute of Montreal, while the most ambitious Canadian venture to date is found at McGill University, where the Center for Medicine, Ethics, and Law is promoting a number of imaginative research projects. Another bioethics teaching and research center began operating at the University of Toronto in the fall of 1989; following the experience of McGill, it is to provide bioethics teaching programs conducted at both undergraduate and graduate (including doctoral) levels and undertake research, particularly on macro-ethical issues.

In November 1988 the Canadian Bioethics Society was created by a merger of the Canadian Society for Medical Bioethics and the Canadian Society of Bioethics. The new society is expected to serve as a dynamic center promoting bioethics research as well as both academic and professional instruction in the subject.

It should also be mentioned that Canadian scholars and students of bioethics have long enjoyed access to programs in the United States and have collaborated with such distinguished organizations as the Hastings Center and the Kennedy Institute of Ethics at Georgetown University. However, special features of Canada's multicultural society and public health services are increasingly seen as raising distinctive issues that warrant the special attention of research, publication, and training programs.

Research Involving Human Subjects

In 1987 Canada's Medical Research Council (MRC) produced a new version of *Guidelines on Research Involving Human Subjects*, which superseded its 1978 version. The guidelines apply to all research that the MRC funds. Because such research goes beyond purely biological and biomedical projects, entering realms of other natural and social sciences, these guidelines take into account comparable guidelines issued by two other bodies, the Social Sciences and Humanities Research Council and the Natural Sciences and Engineering Research Council. (For instance, the latter council has interests in development and testing of prosthetic devices and implants.)

The MRC guidelines are initially applied to individual protocols by institutional (mainly university and hospital) research ethics boards. They are also applied in practice to innumerable projects that the MRC does not fund. This latter circumstance has raised the question of authoritative interpretation and application of the

141

guidelines, because the MRC is unable to express opinions on projects that it is not considering for funding.

To address the application of ethical principles to a full range of research involving human subjects, a new body has therefore been created. This body, the National Council on Bioethics in Human Research, was created as a semiautonomous agency in 1988 at MRC request, under the sponsorship of Canada's Royal College of Physicians and Surgeons. This council is charged with interpreting and promoting implementation of all relevant existing guidelines on the ethics of biomedical and health-related research involving human subjects, monitoring how institutions comply with such guidelines, and advising and consulting on ethics matters with bodies funding and undertaking human research. It will also foster educational programs among health and related professionals and the general public on ethical issues and concerns regarding human research. The Council held its first Workshop in April 1989, an event that brought together the heads of Canadian university committees overseeing application of the MRC guidelines and related ethical principles to research involving human subjects that takes place within their institutions and affiliated teaching hospitals.

Regulation of Reproduction

There have been relatively few developments in Canada regarding family planning, although some activities occurred in the fall of 1989 when the International Planned Parenthood Federation held its annual conference in Ottawa to celebrate the twentieth anniversary of the date when promotion of contraception in Canada became legal.

In 1986 the Supreme Court of Canada held that a purely contraceptive sterilization could not be authorized for a mentally handicapped adult on the basis of parental consent or judicial approval. At the same time, however, the court confirmed that the procedure is lawful when consented to by a mentally competent person. Spousal veto powers are also made unlawful in those provinces whose human rights laws prohibit discrimination on grounds of marital status, and may be more uniformly unlawful when they affect one's right to liberty and personal security, guaranteed by Section 7 of the Canadian Charter of Rights and Freedoms.

A number of hospitals had retained doubts about the legality of contraceptive sterilization, due to misinterpretation of the law. The 1986 decision removed these lingering doubts, and in early 1989 the Alberta Institute of Law Research and Reform issued a report (No. 52) entitled *Competence and Human Reproduction* that proposed means by which sterilizations might be undertaken on mentally handicapped adults.

Section 7 of the Charter of Rights and Freedoms also played an instrumental role in a January 1988 Supreme Court decision overturning a Criminal Code provision that had made abortion illegal. The court held the provision to be inoperative because it violated constitutional guarantees.

In effectively legalizing abortion in Canada, the Supreme Court observed that some sort of criminal limit on abortion might be constitutional, providing that it respected a woman's own priorities and aspirations and took effect at an appropriate stage of gestation, indicated as being at some time during the second trimester of pregnancy.

Abortion is legally regulated in Canada under provincial laws on the practice of medicine concerning such matters as unqualified and unethical practices. Abortion is otherwise regulated, as the Supreme Court observed, by personal morality. The Canadian Government took time in considering whether any new criminal abortion law should be proposed, and in the fall of 1989 it proposed new criminal law to prohibit abortion unless a doctor finds that a woman's physical, mental, or psychological health would be endangered by continuation of pregnancy. The proposal sets no gestational limits.

Before this, in February 1989, the Law Reform Commission produced for public discussion its Working Paper 58, entitled *Crimes Against the Foetus*. This was attacked by supporters of restrictions on abortion for proposing that abortion be quite liberally available up to the twenty-second week of gestation, and available thereafter if the fetus were held to be suffering from a malformation or disability of such severity that medical treatment could be legally withheld upon its birth. Supporters of allowing women to choose abortion attacked the report for proposing that abortion be available only to protect a woman's health, whether physical or psychological, and rendering a woman's reproductive choice subject to medical indications and authorization. In the new legislation proposed by the Government as a compromise among different preferences, few of the Law Reform Commission's recommendations were adopted.

In the outline of its program presented at the opening of the new parliamentary session in March 1989, the Government proposed establishing a Royal Commission on New Reproductive Technologies, which came into being in October 1989. The terms of reference of the commission have been widely drawn. The scope of the inquiry will cover infertility, artificial insemination, ovum and pre-embryo transfer, and *in vitro* fertilization, which is becoming increasingly available in Canada but is publicly funded only at a number of centers in Ontario. The inquiry will also cover surrogate motherhood, which is not necessarily dependent on medical technology. A growing phenomenon at some centers is interest in "full" surrogate motherhood, in which preembryos are created *in vitro* and implanted in a woman other than the ovum donor for surrender on birth to the source of the ovum and her sperm-supplying husband.

The commission was created in part at the urging of feminist activists who feel that the field of assisted reproduction warrants national attention and a nationwide approach. This view emerged partly in response to 1985 recommendations of the Ontario Law Reform Commission that appeared in its two-volume *Report on Human Artificial Reproduction and Related Matters*.

The most controversial recommendation in the report, proposed as an exercise in damage-control but sometimes misconstrued as advocating surrogate motherhood, supported a system of "surrogate adoption" dependent on judicial approval. The Canadian Fertility and Andrology Society and the Society of Obstetricians and Gynecologists of Canada are about to approve a code of ethics addressing artificial reproduction, but the proposed Royal Commission may cause other professional associations to halt or eschew independent initiatives in order to collaborate with the commission and respond to its final report and recommendations scheduled for the end of 1991.

The Science Council of Canada has work in hand on the medical, scientific, ethical, and legal issues raised by prognoses of genetic predispositions and is currently producing a report on this subject. The work involved is relatively comprehensive, and while its implications for human reproduction are potentially of considerable significance, human reproduction issues are only some of those to be addressed.

The issue of nontreatment of seriously handicapped newborns has aroused relatively little special concern in Canada, although ethicists and related professionals, including teachers, remain aware of the issues the topic raises and of regulatory responses in the United States, Europe, and elsewhere.

The Dying Process

In 1984 the Canadian Medical Association, the Canadian Nurses' Association, and the Canadian Hospital Association issued a *Joint Statement on Terminal Illness* intended to indicate the circumstances and conditions that made it ethical to write "do not resuscitate" orders. A protocol was thereby approved as a basic national guideline for those involved in care of the terminally ill. The joint statement was facilitated by the Law Reform Commission of Canada's 1983 report (No. 20) entitled *Euthanasia, Aiding Suicide, and Cessation of Treatment* and was reciprocally approved by implication in the commission's 1986 report (No. 28) entitled *Some Aspects of Medical Treatment and Criminal Law*.

The latter report went beyond patients in terminal conditions, however, and observed on page 12 that ". . . an individual may refuse treatment or have it stopped, even if doing so places his life in jeopardy. This is true, for example, of a Jehovah's Witness who refuses a blood transfusion or a patient suffering from a serious illness who desires to end treatment or to stop intravenous feeding. It is clearly important to ensure that the decision is that of a lucid person who is capable of making it. If this condition is met, the Commission considers that the decision should be carried out even though to an impartial observer it may not appear to be objectively valid." Consistent with the commission's thinking, in the spring of 1990 the Ontario Court of Appeal upheld an award of $20,000 in damages for battery to a Jehovah's Witness plaintiff who suffered blood loss in a serious traffic accident, even though the trial judge found that the blood transfusion she received while unconscious probably saved her life. (The defendant physician knew that the patient was carrying a signed Jehovah's Witness card refusing consent to blood transfusion.)

Associations of health professionals have been active in developing guidelines applicable to terminal care. In February 1987, for instance, the Canadian Medical Association issued a position statement on resuscitation of the terminally ill, and later in the year issued the report of its Committee on the Health Care of the Elderly. This latter report identified many strengths and weaknesses of the health care system in the geriatric field and recognized many critical areas, both medical and nonmedical, that affect the independence of elderly persons regarding terminal care decisions and other matters.

No Canadian jurisdiction has enacted legislation on natural death that legitimates "living wills"; but judicial decisions, including Supreme Court decisions, have given such statements considerable legal significance. Indeed, following the aforementioned Ontario Court of Appeal

decision on the claim of the Jehovah's Witness plaintiff, such refusals of treatment may now be said to have the force of common law. Several jurisdictions have enacted or amended laws on powers of attorney so as to permit such powers to apply when the principal who executed the power is no longer mentally competent. In these ways, advance medical care directives may be legally effective.

Death is increasingly defined in Canada to include whole brain death. This is legislated only in Manitoba, but following the Law Reform Commission of Canada's 1981 report (No. 15) entitled *Criteria for the Determination of Death* and its 1984 working paper (No. 33) entitled "Homicide," it is now widely accepted that death may be legally certified on the basis of this neurologic criterion.

Biotechnology

Since the Canadian Minister of State for Science and Technology issued the 1981 task force report entitled *Biotechnology: A Development Plan for Canada*, a number of agencies have published relevant papers. The most active agency has been the Science Council of Canada, which has produced papers including *Biotechnology in Canada: Promises and Concerns* (with the Institute for Research on Public Policy, 1981); *Biotechnology in the Pulp and Paper Industry* (1984); *Regulatory Policies of Biotechnology in Canada* (1984); and *Seeds of Renewal: Biotechnology and Canada's Resource Industries* (Report 38, 1985). Institutions in both the public and private sectors are responding to the industrial, commercial, agricultural, veterinary, medical, and other challenges and opportunities presented by biotechnology. Industrial and research activities tend to be based in the major population centers of Ontario and Quebec, but the potential for uniform regulation arises through federal law.

Accordingly, the Law Reform Commission of Canada has recently proposed commencing a study of regulatory law that would promote biotechnologic developments and also control applications of biotechnology where the public interest so requires. The project may stand by itself or be part of wider programs—such as one in administrative law that published the study paper *Pollution Control in Canada: The Regulatory Approach in the 1980s* in 1988, or the protection of life program that published the study paper *Pesticides in Canada: An Examination of Federal Law and Policy* in 1987.

Organ Transplants

Most provincial legislation in Canada relating to organ transplants is based on the Uniform Human Tissue Gift Act approved by the Uniform Law Conference of Canada in 1971. However, in 1987 the Uniform Law Conference of Canada, composed of those who chair the different provincial and territorial Law Reform Commissions, approved a new Uniform Human Tissue Act that was presented at the initiative of the Alberta Commissioners.

The new uniform draft act is currently under consideration for adoption in some Canadian jurisdictions. It retains the "opting in" basis of current legislation, except regarding the pituitary gland, which in some jurisdictions is subject to an "opting out" or "presumed consent" law. The uniform draft act generally reflects the conservative approach taken to amendment of prevailing legislation by the Alberta Commissioners, although it does include common law (legally unmarried) spouses among those able to consent to *post mortem* donations.

The Report of the Alberta Commissioners found no Canadian agreement on formalization of a national transplantation registry, although the Federal Government favored a national registry. The commissioners similarly considered that issues of donor and recipient selection should be addressed at the provincial rather than the federal level. Permission for commerce in transplantable human tissues was not proposed for consideration.

AIDS

The Canadian Federal Center for AIDS has proposed standards for anonymous unlinked seroprevalence studies. Such studies, currently being undertaken in Quebec, have been proposed in British Columbia and Ontario but are being obstructed there by laws that require, or are interpreted to require, that applicants for AIDS tests give their names, addresses, and perhaps health insurance plan numbers.

AIDS is a reportable disease in all Canadian jurisdictions, but it is unclear in some jurisdictions whether the AIDS-related complex (ARC) and HIV-positivity are reportable. Medical officers of health often seem reluctant to accommodate anonymous testing, although the climate of other informed opinion is turning strongly in favor of testing anonymity or strict confidentiality. At both federal and provincial levels, officers of governmental human rights protection agencies acknowledge that AIDS, ARC, and HIV-positivity are conditions of disability, and that to discriminate on the basis of them is unlawful. In January 1989 the Canadian Medical Association issued general guidelines on physicians' ethical responsibilities regarding management of HIV-positive patients and those at high risk of being positive, and also on the rights to compensation that arise in the case of occupational exposure to HIV. Recommendations for health professionals have also been issued by organizations such as the Canadian Dental Association and the Canadian Hospital Association.

Background and Current Status of Bioethics in Colombia

Fernando Sánchez-Torres

Bioethics first emerged as an intellectual discipline in the 1970s, so it is not yet even 20 years old. Rapid advances in medicine, boosted by the contributions of other biological sciences such as molecular engineering and biochemistry, have placed man toward the end of the twentieth century in a perplexing situation—and, Why not say so?—one of dangerous confusion. It was Van Rensselaer Potter of the United States, Professor of Oncology at the University of Wisconsin, who called attention to the need to anaylze these developments and measure their negative effects on individuals and society in his book, *Bioethics: Bridge to the Future* (1). This work gave currency to the term bioethics, which became a rapidly evolving discipline in some countries— although in others, such as Colombia, it has barely begun to be recognized.

The curiosity and daring of men of science who have plumbed the depths of biology, particularly in areas involving human reproduction, have created great expectations for their discoveries and the applications thereof. Now that science and technology have surpassed all estimates and predictions, it is impossible to imagine what the generations of the twenty-first century will know and see. But it is clearly worthwhile for the person who holds cherished spiritual values to be prepared for these new situations.

Within this context, it is the specific task of bioethics to examine the effects of the "authentic biological revolution"—as this collection of new developments has been called by the Span-

ish theologian Mariano Vidal (2)—in the light of moral principles and values.

Colombia is a country of about 28 million inhabitants with 21 medical schools, from which a little over 2,000 new professionals graduate each year. There are currently 23,000 doctors of medicine, a number that is not expected to exceed 45,000 by the end of the present century. Because of the way Colombia's health system is organized, however, 43% of the recently graduated physicians fail to find jobs; and, as may well be imagined, the competition is stiff in private practice. The need to survive under such conditions has made it tempting for physicians to go astray, forgetting the moral principles that underlie the ethical practice of medicine.

At the same time, Colombia is no stranger to advanced scientific and technological devices. Although it may not originate and produce them, it most definitely buys and uses them. New technology is the order of the day. It is not unusual to enlist computers, nuclear medicine, and sonar devices. Modern care facilities, both state and private, have sophisticated diagnostic and therapeutic equipment for performing various procedures—including computerized tomography, magnetic resonance imaging, and extracorporeal lithotripsy.

Organ Transplants

The practice of transplanting organs and other anatomic parts is growing steadily, as is the complexity of the procedures used. The city of

Medellín has become the hub of this activity. Both the San Vicente de Paúl University Hospital and the Santa María Clinic have the necessary technical equipment and human resources to perform various types of transplant surgery, and they lead the country in heart, liver, and kidney-pancreas transplants (3–5). Similar procedures are also performed in other cities, notably Bogotá and Cali. In Bogotá a homologous transplant of an adrenal medulla to the encephalon was carried out in 1987 as a treatment for Parkinson's disease (6). Currently, embryonic and fetal tissues are being used experimentally to treat this condition and also Alzheimer's disease.

This progressive surge in transplant activity created a need for the Government to take regulatory measures. In the *National Health Code* (*Código Sanitario Nacional*) designated Law 09 of 1979, "through which health measures are prescribed," Title IX deals with "the donation or transfer of organs, tissues, and organic fluids from cadavers or living persons for transplantation and other therapeutic users." Later, in 1986, the Ministry of Health issued Decree 2363, which supplemented this law. Among other things, this decree establishes a definition of "brain death." And most recently, in 1988, the National Congress passed Law 73, which refines some of the preceding provisions, especially those relating to organ donation, removal, and utilization.

Human Reproduction

It is especially in the area of human reproduction that research and technology have made far-reaching strides. Matters relating to abortion and contraception aside, the list includes development of sperm and ova banks, homologous and heterologous artificial insemination, *in vitro* fertilization and transfer of the embryo to the uterus, intrafallopian gamete transfer, examination of the amniotic fluid and biopsy of the chorionic villi for early detection of congenital alterations, *in utero* surgery, etc.

All of these new procedures are used in Colombia. Among other things, a "test tube baby" delivered in Bogotá in 1985 was the first such infant born in Latin America. From then up to March 1989 the Colombian Fertility and Sterility Center recorded 92 such births, 11 of which were produced from frozen embryos (7, 8).

Despite the medical, legal, social, and ethical implications of these new human reproductive procedures, however, the Government of Colombia has not yet issued any standards to regulate their practice. Therefore, in dealing with related ethical issues, Colombian physicians must rely on guidance issued by the World Medical Association, as set forth in Article 54 of Law 23 (1981), which is discussed below.

Terminal Patients

The establishment of intensive care units at university hospitals and private clinics in Colombia's major cities has unquestionably resulted in great benefits for the critically ill. At the same time, however, the tenet of some physicians, "while there's life there's hope," has also led to unjustified prolongation of suffering for those who can no longer be helped by medicine. Not infrequently, unconscious terminal patients, many of them brain dead, are subjected to heroic efforts and connected to machines to give them artificial life, creating false hopes for their families and unjustly burdening the budget available to cover the cost of the illness.

In response, at the initiative of individuals outside the medical profession in Colombia, movements have emerged to support the wishes of patients who want to be allowed to die in a dignified and peaceful manner. This is the origin of the Foundation for the Right to a Dignified Death, a nonprofit organization established in Bogotá in 1979 that has had a significant impact upon both the medical profession and society (9). It should be pointed out that in Colombia euthanasia, or mercy-killing, is considered a crime under the Criminal Code. It is currently being debated whether a physician who abstains from using extraordinary life-support measures, or even basic ones like provision of food and liquids, may be deemed to be practicing a passive form of euthanasia, which would be punishable under Colombian law.

Abortion

Abortion, without exception, is punishable by law. But virtually everyone, including the health authorities and police, know that the large cities harbor abortion clinics staffed by physicians and nurses, and no corrective action is taken. There thus appears to be a widespread conviction that abortion is a social necessity and that punitive measures alone will not solve the problem. Thus, a laissez-faire policy has been institutionalized.

AIDS

In Colombia, as in all countries, acquired immunodeficiency syndrome (AIDS) is a major concern of health authorities. As of April 1987 the Ministry of Health had registered 100 confirmed AIDS cases; by September of that year the number had reached 153; and by March 1989 the Ministry's Department of Epidemiology had recorded 350 cases. These figures could be low; for even though the reporting of AIDS is mandatory, its stigma may cause some cases to go unreported out of fear that the patient's identity will be discovered.

Government education and health agencies have undertaken broad information campaigns on AIDS prevention. As part of a program of community education, television broadcasts frequently include messages warning against sexual promiscuity and encouraging the use of condoms for couples in unstable unions. Also, Colombia's blood bank program exercises strict nationwide control over all blood and blood products to be used in transfusions by subjecting all donated blood to the ELISA test for antibodies to HIV.

The obvious ethical questions that AIDS poses for physicians and other health professionals have given rise to a number of conferences and forums within Colombia. Among other things, these have invariably concluded that from an ethical standpoint, patients cannot be abandoned or ostracized by those who are supposed to care for them solely out of fear of contracting the disease.

Bioethical Standards

Most Colombian physicians have taken an interest in the ethical questions raised by these and other contemporary situations. Forty years ago, when there were only six medical schools, the subject of ethics (deontology) was included in the curriculum but over time was gradually dropped. Similarly, in 1954 the Colombian Medical Federation approved a code of medical ethics that was soon forgotten.

More recently, following proliferation of the medical schools and development of new technology, the Medical Federation proposed a new code and urged the National Congress to give it legal status. After extensive discussion, the Legislature approved Law 23 of 1981, which "set forth standards in matters of medical ethics." Under this law, tribunals have been set up in the departmental capitals to deal with ethical and professional disciplinary matters arising as a consequence of medical practice.

Regarding education, Article 47 of this same law made the teaching of medical ethics in medical schools mandatory. And in 1987 the Colombian Association of Medical Schools established a program directed at teaching and explaining ethics to their students, and also at preparing instructors in this sensitive subject.

Other Matters

The period following promulgation of Law 23 saw emergence of considerable interest in both bioethics and medical ethics. At present it is common to find articles and commentaries on these subjects in medical and legal journals, as well as the daily press. In 1988 two books published on these subjects in Colombia received wide acclaim, these being *Etica médica* (*Medical Ethics*) by L. A. Vélez (*10*) and *Bioética: Principales problemas* (*Bioethics: Principal Problems*) by A. C. Varga (*11*). Before these volumes appeared, the only local source on the subject was G. Paz-Otero's *Deontología médica general* (*General Medical Deontology—12*).

In 1985, at the initiative of the present author, the Colombian Institute of Bioethical Studies was founded in Bogotá. This brought together distinguished professionals from various disciplines—including physicians, lawyers, priests, nurses, psychologists, and biologists. The Institute's main goals were to stimulate interest in bioethics, provide in-depth analysis of various problems posed by the "biological revolution," and disseminate the results of such analysis.

Since its founding, the Institute has only partially realized its aims. That is not surprising, since it is hard to maintain institutions on a strong and productive footing when they deal with matters that are not economically productive and lack official recognition and support. Nevertheless, the enthusiasm of the Institute's members bodes well for its survival and for a stable and productive future.

References

1. Potter, V. R. *Bioethics: Bridge to the Future.* Prentice-Hall, Englewood Cliffs, New Jersey, 1971.
2. Vidal, M. *Moral de la persona* (*vol. 2*). PS Editorial, Madrid, 1985, p. 176.
3. Villegas, A., et al. Experiencia con trasplante cardíaco en el Centro Cardiovascular Colombiano, Clínica Santa María. *Cirugía (Bogotá)* 1(3):117–124, 1986.
4. Restrepo, J., A. Velásquez, H. Aristizábel, et al. Experiencia con trasplante hepático en humanos. *Cirugía* 1(2):67–72, 1986.
5. Velásquez, A., H. Aristizábal, J. Restrepo, et al. Trasplante simultáneo de riñón y páncreas con pancreatico-duodenosistostomía. *Cirugía (Bogotá)* 3(3):144–148, 1988.
6. Bustamante, E., A. Matuk, E. Osorio, et al. Trasplante de médula suprarrenal al encéfalo para el tratamiento de la enfermedad de Parkinson. *Cirugía (Bogotá)* 2(3):127–129, 1987.
7. Lucena, E., J. Ruíz, J. Mendoza, et al. IVF and ET Program (abstract). In: *Proceedings of the Third World Congress on* in vitro *Fertilization and Embryo Transfer.* Helsinki, 14–17 May 1984, p. 73.
8. Lucena, E., R. Olivares, H. Obando, et al. Pregnancies following transfer of human frozen-thawed embryos in Colombia, South America. *Hum Reprod* 1(6):383–385, 1986.
9. Llano-Escobar, A. In Colombia, dealing with death and technology. *Hastings Center Report (suppl),* August 1988, p. 23.
10. Vélez, L. A., *Etica Médica.* Prensa Creativa, Medellín, Colombia, 1988.
11. Varga, A. C. *Bioética: Principales problemas.* Ediciones Paulinas, Bogotá, Colombia, 1988.
12. Paz-Otero, G. *Deontología médica general.* Editorial de la Universidad del Cauca, Popayán, Colombia, 1955.

Bioethics in Chile: Present and Future Status

Fernando Lolas

Although bioethics extends beyond the field of biomedical ethics, this brief account will be limited to the latter area, and more specifically to certain issues that are currently being examined.

As in other Latin American countries, the institutionalization and application of bioethical studies in Chile is still fragmentary. The inclusion of bioethics is uneven, both on the agendas of hospital ethic committees and in the curricula of university medical schools. And despite administrative instructions and requests by physicians, the discipline has not yet become well established.

The Chilean Health System

The Chilean medical profession enjoys a high degree of prestige, which Roa (1) attributes to its spirit of service and to a professional conscience in continuous evolution since establishment of the first medical school in 1833, a successor to the schools that first began providing similar instruction at the Royal University of San Felipe in 1756.

As of August 1988, Chile's National Medical Register listed 16,373 physicians—of whom 13,451 were residing in the country, 1,343 were abroad, 1,579 had died, and 68 had resigned (2).

At present, as a result of reforms made in 1979, the Chilean health system consists of essentially three components. One is the National Health Services System (Sistema Nacional de Servicios de Salud, SNSS), with 27 regional services, which provides free preventive care to the entire population and curative services to workers and indigents. Another is the National Health Fund (Fondo Nacional de Salud, FONASA), which administers the "free selection or preferred provider" system and reimburses expenditures by the SNSS. And the third consists of the Institutes of Health Security (Institutos de Salud Previsional, ISAPRES), which are enterprises that sell health insurance—with closed group, free election, and mixed plans—that were established in 1981. To these various services are added a private sector that varies in size depending on the geographic region of the country involved.

Changes the system has experienced in recent years, especially with regard to its financing, are pertinent to our discussion of ethics (3, 4).

Most public discussions of ethical issues in health have involved the Chilean Medical Association (Colegio Médico de Chile). This professional association, through its department of ethics, disseminates documents and standards, organizes sessions for reflection and analysis, awards annual prizes, oversees the actions of its members, and carries out research on conditions affecting the practice of medicine. Established in 1948 by Decree Law No. 9263, the society functioned as a public corporation until 1981. In that year Decree Law No. 3261 changed it to a professional association, and it was subjected to the new provisions of Decree Law No. 2757, which, among other things, provided for voluntary membership.

This measure, criticized by the association,

meant the loss of its professional-ethical control over all physicians, and also loss of its authority to set standards for fees and honoraria. The Chilean Medical Association has nevertheless maintained a certain moral position and has continued to carry out important activities in the field of ethics. To a certain extent it still regulates the relationships of physicians with other physicians, the public, and the State (2, 5–9).

Current Issues in Biomedical Ethics

The practice of medicine in Chile in recent years has been characterized by the following features pertinent to this discussion of ethics: the increasingly private and technical nature of health care on the one hand, and the increasingly proletarian nature of medical work on the other. These changes, evident in practically every developing country but very significant in Chile because of the situation prevailing since 1973, have shaped the medical community's principal ethical concerns.

This presentation will address two broad subjects: aspects of professional ethics (including interrelationships between physicians and their relations with the public and the State) and ethics of medical care (including the teaching and practice of biomedical ethics).

Aspects of Professional Ethics

Interrelationships between Physicians.

In recent years the ethical control of physicians by their peers has been an important issue. As already indicated, in 1981 Decree Law No. 3621 took jurisdiction over physicians away from the Medical Association and passed the power to settle disputes to the ordinary courts of justice. It thus removed the distinction between ethical misconduct and criminal misconduct.

Nevertheless, in its role as a professional association, the Medical Association retains the prerogative of investigating accusations made about its members, holding internal summary proceedings, and applying sanctions. The most important matters dealt with in recent times have included participation of physicians in torture, abuse of publicity, and establishment of parallel associations. Both the Medical Association Code of Ethics and other current regulations contain specific provisions concerning the relationships of physicians among themselves. Expulsion or temporary suspension from the association are provided for in the case of some violations; however, differences over the application of such provisions, regarding issues relating to freedom of association, have arisen between the Medical Association and the Supreme Court of Justice.

Although the institutional health structure has traditionally been "doctorcratic" in Chile, reserving managerial positions for professional physicians, the political and economic changes mentioned above have led to new problems. Participation of nonmedical economic entities (such as ISAPRES) in health activities has taken authority and autonomy away from the physicians' association and has resulted in censurable actions by some professionals. Likewise, the participation of physicians in government activities has led to disagreements on such matters as allocation of resources by the State and salary claims, and has prompted ethics-oriented legal proceedings, sometimes against high-ranking members of the profession.

The Medical Association Code of Ethics sets standards for those professionals who, as part of their functions, are involved in appointments or dismissals, and it prohibits them from replacing physicians who have been unjustly removed from their posts (Articles 38 and 39). In recent years there has been occasion to discuss and apply these principles.

The code also regulates remuneration or compensation for services rendered and expressly condemns charging commissions to fellow doctors (Article 41); in addition, it establishes the conditions under which professional advertising is permitted (Title VI). All of this needs to be understood within the context of an increasingly private and technical health system, one with growing participation by private profit-seeking nonmedical organizations in health activities.

An absence of legislation on medical specialties has led to creation of an Autonomous Commission on the Certification of Medical Specialties (*Comisión Autónoma de Certificación de Especialidades Médicas*—CONACEM), whose authority at this time is moral only. It should be noted that the preparation of specialists in Chile is supervised by the universities; however, there is active debate about the proper role and the obligations of the State in its interaction with the universities and with the Medical Association. From the standpoint of ethics in professional relations, treatment of this subject demands consideration of the association's actions in order to protect its hegemony over health care matters (*10, 11*).

In 1985, Article 25 of the Code of Ethics was supplemented by a set of standards regarding the medical care of prisoners and the participation of physicians in torture and interrogation. The Medical Association has investigated specific cases and has publicly denounced and censured some of its members. The degree to which ethics were violated in such cases has been hard to estimate (*12*).

Relations with the Public and the State.

Discussion of relationships between physicians, the State, and the public has tended to favor individualism in Chile and to hark back to the ideal "doctor-patient relationship." Ethical problems raised by medical secrets and confidentiality, *in vitro* fertilization, and cases of "difficult patients" (especially in psychiatry) are customarily dealt with from this standpoint.

At the same time, the heterogeneous nature of the current health system and the coexistence of various subsystems create discrepancies among a doctor's various functions that are not sufficiently explicit. For example, a physician might establish a "paternalistic" type of relationship with SNSS patients, a "contractual" type of relationship with private patients, and an "engi-neering" type of relationship as an adviser to an ISAPRES entity.

Title II of the Medical Association Code of Ethics, which deals with the physician's obligations toward his patients, reserves the "diagnosis, prognosis, and treatment of patients" exclusively to the physician and obligates the physician to treat any person who needs it. It stipulates that medical confidentiality (including confidentiality of the patient's name) is a natural right, requiring neither promise nor contract, and one which must be respected absolutely. Issues surrounding this matter of confidentiality exemplify recent ethical problems and show how ethical decisions need to be taken within a revised context of the doctor-patient relationship. Among other things, introduction of the State and profit-making business entities into the picture makes ethical review imperative. Along this line, the existence of automated data systems (including data banks controlled by nonmedical administrators), combined with the general public's increasing medical literacy and ability to interpret such data, means that the maintenance of medical confidentiality now depends on authorities outside the traditional doctor-patient dyad.

No less important has been the debate over the State's authority to procure confidential information relevant to criminal or terrorist acts. Although Article 19 of the Constitution of 1980 provides for respect and protection of private and public life, and Articles 246 and 247 of the Criminal Code recognize professional confidentiality, both the Code of Criminal Procedure and the Health Code regulate conditions under which these rights become relative. The issue arose recently because of conflicts—between a broadened national security doctrine (supported by the military government) and the traditional ways of interpreting medical confidentiality—in cases where the control of armed terrorism has been key. The various divergences existing between codes of ethics, the law, and political views are far from being worked out and will continue to be focal points of medical and public interest for years to come (*13–16*). In addition, new challenges are being posed by AIDS and other diseases now coming to the attention of Chilean physicians and health authorities (17–19).

Medical Care Ethics

Social "ethics," manifested through institutionalized practices considered legitimate and habitual components of the "medical rationale," does not necessarily coincide with legislated codes of ethics (20).

According to 1985 data, at that time the teaching of humanistic and psychosocial subjects accounted for no more than 6% of the total curriculum hours devoted to pursuit of a medical career (21). The nine medical schools existing in 1985 (the University of Chile had four independent schools that later merged into one) shared the same policy regarding length of instruction and teaching methods (22, 23).

Currently there is increasing interest in bioethics, and bioethics courses are being taught at the Catholic University of Chile and the University of Chile. The University of Chile's School of Medicine, the oldest in the country, established a course on medical ethics at the end of the 1960s (Armando Roa, University of Chile, personal communication, 1989). In 1988, as part of its centennial celebration, the Catholic University of Chile organized the nation's First Congress on Medical Ethics. These events, along with the ongoing work of the Medical Association, indicate that the subject of bioethics is gaining importance and will definitely be incorporated into undergraduate and graduate curricula (24). To date there has been no move to install a postgraduate program of medical studies devoted exclusively to bioethics.

Another development that points to the institutionalization of a bioethical rationale is the work of ethics committees. The Organic Regulations on Health Services promulgated by the Government in 1986, besides containing provisions on spiritual assistance for the sick (Title VI), established advisory committees under the director of each hospital whose members were appointed by the director. The replies to a questionnaire circulated on this subject indicated that most hospitals had no operating ethics committee, this function being assumed by the general technical committees, and that where such committees existed their functions and nature had not been well-defined (the replies either gave no information about their formation and operation or indicated that they tended to be confused with "cultural" committees). However, most of the medical schools and research institutes do have ethics advisory boards, which deal primarily with research involving human subjects. International legislation on this latter subject is widely disseminated.

Specific ethical issues relating to organ transplants (25), in vitro fertilization (26), AIDS (17–19), specific medical specialties (27–30), and conditions needed for the ethical practice of medicine have been dealt with repeatedly in meetings organized by the Medical Association or the universities (31). While the subject of bioengineering has generated great interest among both physicians and the public (32), to date its ethical implications have neither received comparable attention nor given rise to any specific legislation.

Future Outlook

Bioethics, which has displaced medical history as the basic medical discipline outside the natural sciences, is perceived in Chile as a necessary element in the teaching and practice of medicine. The most active participants in this field to date have been Chile's professional medical and university associations. Although this new discipline has not yet been fully institutionalized, the challenges posed by the political and institutional situation and changes expected soon in the medical system seem destined to promote its continued development. Within this context, it is possible that bioethics could prompt changes in the health care system and could contribute not only to a redefinition of medicine but also to less troubled and more effective relationships between medicine, law, and social practice (*33*).

Acknowledgments.

The author acknowledges with thanks the comments of Professors Armando Roa and Enrique Egaña of the University of Chile, as well as the materials and suggestions provided by Drs. María Luisa Cordero and Fernando Schürch of the Chilean Medical Association.

References

1. Roa, A. Grandes problemas éticos de la medicina contemporánea. *Rev Med Chile* 111(11):1183–1193, 1983.
2. Colegio Médico de Chile. Reglamentos vigentes. Santiago, 1988.
3. Castañeda, T. El sistema de salud chileno: Organización, funcionamiento y financiamiento. *Bol Of Sanit Panam* 103:544–570, 1987.
4. Viveros-Long, A. Changes in health financing: The Chilean experience. *Soc Sci Med* 22:379–385, 1986.
5. Colegio Médico de Chile. Normas y documentos de ética médica. Santiago, 1986.
6. Colegio Médico de Chile. *Primeras Jornadas de Etica Médica*. Santiago, 1984.
7. Colegio Médico de Chile. *Segundas Jornadas de Etica Médica*. Santiago, 1985.
8. Colegio Médico de Chile. *Terceras Jornadas de Etica Médica*. Santiago, 1986.
9. Colegio Médico de Chile. *Cuartas Jornadas de Etica Médica*. Santiago, 1987.
10. Chiorrini, J. Código de ética y moral profesional. *Vida Med* 34(1):20–21, 1983.
11. Academia Chilena de Medicina. Comentarios a la ley de creación de un sistema de prestación de salud (Ley No. 18.469, del 23 de noviembre, 1985). *Vida Med* 37(3):56, 1986.
12. Colegio Médico de Chile, Departamento de Etica, Consejo General. Participación de médicos en torturas. In: *Terceras Jornadas de Etica Médica*. Colegio Médico de Chile, Santiago, 1986, pp. 120–147.
13. Trejo, C. Secreto médico: Una perspectiva moral. *Vida Med* 40(1):34–35, 1988.
14. Pérez Olea, J. Sobre qué secreto, quienes lo controlan y cómo se resguarda. *Vida Med* 40(1):36–37, 1988.
15. Los médicos y el secreto profesional: Mesa redonda. *Vida Med* 41(1):14–16, 1989.
16. Kottow, M. La relación confidencial en medicina. *Vida Med* 40(6):342–343 and 374–375, 1988.
17. Seelmann, G. Proyección psicosocial del síndrome de inmunodeficiencia adquirida (SIDA). *Vida Med* 40(1):39–41, 1988.
18. Pavletich, A., and R. Sepúlveda. Aspectos éticos del SIDA. *Vida Med* 41(1):42–44, 1989.
19. Sepúlveda, C. SIDA: Un desafío científico y un problema de salud pública. *Vida Med* 41(1):30–33, 1989.
20. Rosselot, J. Dimensión social de la ética médica. In: *Terceras Jornadas de Etica Médica*. Colegio Médico de Chile, Santiago, 1986, pp. 53–76.
21. Goic, A., R. Florenzano, and A. Velasco. Análisis de la formación humanística y psicosocial en el pregrado de la carrera de medicina. *Rev Med Chile* 113:453–462, 1985.
22. Neghme, A. Visión panorámica de la educación médica en Chile: Problemas y perspectivas. Documento de trabajo No. 12/84. Corporación de Promoción Universitaria, Santiago, 1984.
23. Lavados, J. Síntesis final del seminario nacional "La enseñanza de la medicina en Chile." Documento de trabajo No. 11/84. Corporación de Promoción Universitaria, Santiago, 1984.
24. Egaña, E. Enseñanza de la ética en la formación del estudiante de medicina: Algunas connotaciones y proyecciones. In: *Terceras Jornadas de Etica Médica*. Colegio Médico de Chile, Santiago, 1986, pp. 27–42.
25. Roessler, E., and Y. Ellies. Etica y trasplantes renales. In: *Segundas Jornadas de Etica Médica*. Colegio Médico de Chile, Santiago, 1985, pp. 53–62.
26. Zegers, F. Fertilización *in vitro* y transferencia embrionaria. *Vida Med* 35(4):29–31, 1984.
27. Dörr, O. Fronteras éticas de la psiquiatría. *Vida Med* 40(3):158–165, 1988.
28. Castillo, P. Cirugía y ética. *Vida Med* 40(3):141–144, 1988.
29. Mezzano, D. Etica y transfusión. *Vida Med* 37(3):65–68, 1986.
30. Mardones, J. El problema ético en la prescripción de medicamentos. *Vida Med* 39(3):42–47, 1987.
31. Roa, A. La bioética ante la medicina del año 2000. In: A. Roa (ed.). *Hacia la medicina del año 2000*. Editorial Universitaria, Santiago, 1988, pp. 154–174.
32. Mönckeberg, F. (ed.). *La revolución de la bioingeniería*. Mediterráneo, Santiago, 1988.
33. Lolas, F. *Mehrdimensionale Medizin*. Zentrum für Medizinische Ethik, Bochum, 1988.

Dynamics of the Bioethics Dialogue in a Spain in Transition

Francesc Abel

If one analyzes the evolution of the bioethics dialogue from its beginnings—in other words, from the time when an interdisciplinary dialogue was instituted to seek a working methodology for resolving conflicts produced by the clash between biomedical advances and ethics—it is possible to see that in Spain the greater part of this evolution has occurred since 1975. It is also true that a lot of ground remains to be covered, especially if we take participation by our citizens in the public debate to be one of the cornerstones of the bioethics dialogue, something that seems both advisable and necessary before legislation is promulgated on bioethical issues with far-reaching social repercussions.

This chapter will begin by defining how it employs the term bioethics. Next, it will describe the characteristics of Spanish society during the transition from national Catholicism to a secular government in a relatively short period of time. It will then go on to broadly describe the most important bioethics centers in Spain today. And it will conclude with some of the author's personal views about the circumstances confronted by Spain's medical schools, physicians, and nurses and the roles these parties are playing in the bioethics debate.

Definition of Bioethics

In order to avoid other possible interpretations, it is advisable to begin by defining bioethics as that term is used here. Although bioethics can be defined as a discipline concerned with health ethics and health care, I prefer to regard it as the interdisciplinary study of problems created by biological and medical advances (at both the microsocial and macrosocial levels) and their repercussions on society and its value system, both today and in the future. This helps to clarify bioethics' dynamics while bringing into focus certain features that I feel to be essential: namely, the use of dialogue as a working methodology and the need for an interdisciplinary and interfaith approach.

As a prerequisite to participating effectively in such dialogue, one must receive training that fosters the ability to listen attentively, analytical rigor, and critical judgment. The difficulty that some persons perceive in accepting these elements while at the same time remaining faithful to their own principles and beliefs should not be an obstacle to dialogue. Indeed, for those coming to bioethics from a Christian perspective, it is inconceivable that one should fear either the truth or the unknown, or should fail to respect what is taught. This point deserves emphasis, because the individuals and centers pioneering the bioethics dialogue in Spain have been Catholic institutions working from a defined perspective, although not one that is monolithic. They have demonstrated a will to engage in dialogue with the health sciences and other ethical systems. Within these institutions today there is a clear perception of the need for dialogue and for a sharing of responsibilities in choosing the values that will help to guide the evolution of our society and all humanity.

Spanish Society in Transition

The following is a brief historical account that will help orient the reader unfamiliar with Spain's history since the 1930s. This account is limited to describing the Catholic Church's role in the transformation process (1). The period covered (1939 to the present) can be effectively divided into four shorter periods, those of 1939–1953, 1953–1965, 1965–1975, and 1975 onward.

1939–1953

At the end of the Spanish Civil War, the task of rechristianizing Spain was carried out with such fervor that for many, if you were not a good Catholic, then you were not a good Spaniard. The Church identified itself with the political regime. There was no lack of critical outcry, such as that by the exiled Cardinal Vidal i Barraquer, who warned Pope Pius XII not to let himself be dazzled by the external manifestations of official Catholicism.

Deep mistrust and fundamental problems that went unresolved delayed the signing of the Concordat between the Holy See and the Government of Spain until 1953. By virtue of the Concordat, the Government's religious nature was recognized, as was the fact that Spain's cultural institutions, from schools to universities, were Catholic. Paradoxically, the Concordat did not mark the beginning of a new phase of national Catholicism, but rather the Church's initial awakening to the legitimate aspirations of workers, intellectuals, and marginal groups, as well as to the idea of political liberties.

1953–1965

The intellectuals and the young clergy, receptive to the political currents in Europe and sensitive to social injustices, questioned the very foundations of the regime. The Spanish Civil War was reinterpreted, dispossessed of any messianic traits, and recharacterized as a fratricidal war. The crusading spirit began to be abandoned, and the young clergy confronted Franco's bishops who were more nostalgic for the past than they were able to take on the problems of social injustice.

The 1961 encyclical *Mater et Magistra* had a profound effect on the Spanish diocese, and there was gradual but unceasing evidence of a growing divergence between the diocese and the political regime. Agriculture, labor unrest, strikes, and the right of the Church to intervene in sociopolitical matters were the topics of numerous pastoral messages that infuriated a government unaccustomed to criticism.

1965–1975

During the years when political parties were prohibited, the Church, which had appropriate organizations, means, and opportunities, worked through select groups and followed the inspiration of its evangelical ideal to perform that function which, in other political situations, is performed by political parties and pressure groups: the promotion of human rights and liberties.

In 1966 the Spanish Episcopal Conference was established. Of the 77 bishops who made up this group, 83.1% had been named through prior presentation by the head of state, 10.1% predated Franco, and the rest had not passed through the formality of presentation because they were auxiliary bishops. Of the 77, 48 were over 60 years of age, 26 were between 45 and 60, and only three were under 45.

Around this time the Holy See encouraged resignation of older bishops, appointing young bishops and, above all, numerous auxiliary bishops in their stead. Because government approval was not necessary for the election of these latter bishops, the Holy See was able to choose them more freely, according to its own criteria. The spirit of Vatican Council II, especially the doctrinal decree *Lumen Gentium*, the pastoral letter *Gaudium et Spes*, and the decree on religious freedom *Dignitatis Humanae*, was received as a message of hope. As a result, by 1975 it could be said that the Spanish Church had an image that was new, bursting with life, and pluralistic.

1975 Onward

It was this Church which, after Franco's death in 1975, undertook the progressive reinstatement of its religious, nonpolitical role. On 27 November 1975, in a solemn liturgical act that accompanied the succession of Juan Carlos I to the throne of Spain, Cardinal Tarancón, the principal architect of the renovation of the Spanish Church, spoke the following words to the King: "The Church neither favors nor imposes a specific social model. The Christian faith is not a political ideology, nor can it be identified with any such ideology, given that no sociopolitical system can exhaust the riches of the gospel, nor is it part of the Church's mission to present specific government options. . . . The Church asks for no privileges. It asks for recognition of the freedom it proclaims for all; it asks for the right to preach the whole gospel, even when that preaching may be critical of the specific society in which it is spoken. . . . I ask, finally, Your Majesty, that we, as men of the Church, and you, as a man of government, may come together in a relationship of mutual respect for one another's autonomy and freedom, without this ever impeding mutual and fruitful collaboration from our respective fields" (2).

At that time Spain was prepared to learn the lesson of democracy. The basis for the dialogue had been established, but not all the tensions between the various plans for democracy that existed within the country had yet been resolved. It was possible to distinguish three pairs of democratic plans (3), which revolved around three distinct points of reference: (1) a purely political democratic plan (which did not seek to make any change in the socioeconomic and cultural model) and a comprehensive democratic plan; (2) a unitary democratic plan (which took little account of Spain's historically autonomous

units or "nations") and a profoundly decentralized plan (which acknowledged governmental unity but granted the various peoples a native social sovereignty which transcended the sovereignty of the State); and (3) a secular plan (which advocated the separation of Church and State, secularization of the values that guide public life, civil tolerance, and full respect for freedom of conscience) and a religious plan (defended by the supporters of ethical hegemony for Christian values in civil society and of the ecclesiastical presence maintained through social institutions of a religious nature).

The 1978 Constitution contained a formula for reconciling these various plans, as follows: There would be a social and democratic State of law, which would leave the door open for establishment of an advanced democratic society or a comprehensive democracy; the State would be autonomous, dovetailing the government's political unity with the right to self-government of nationalities and regions; and the State would be secular (but not laicist), granting religious freedom to individuals and communities.

Bioethics Issues and Regulations

This is the framework within which Spain's bioethics discussions must be viewed. It should also be noted that Spain's most important bioethics centers have appeared within private institutions, while the Government has moved more hastily to create legislation modeled upon European legislation or draft laws considered progressive, rather than legislation derived from a more profound ethic and consultation pertinent to diverse sociocultural groups. This is apparent from the procedures followed to develop legislation on bioethical problems.

The Spanish law of 1979 on organ removal and transplants (6-XI-1979) drew its inspiration from the Council of Europe's Resolution 29 on "Harmonization of Member State Legislation on Extractions, Injections, and Transplants of Substances of Human Origin" (11-V-1978). The legal standard, established by Royal Decree 426 of

22 February 1980, is consistent in structure and substance with the scientific uncertainties of brain death diagnosis and with fundamental ethical principles. However, this law's wording and development involve defects and complexities that although they seem destined to facilitate organ procurement have actually had the opposite effect.

In essence, rather than fostering free donation of organs, this decree sought to apply the principle (especially important when death was defined in terms of brain stem death) that any dead Spaniard was an organ donor if there was no evidence to the contrary (no known wish, explicitly stated by the subject while alive, not to give up his or her organs). As this provision was not well received, an attempt was made to correct it by imposing administrative restraints on organ donation, in such a way that physicians put themselves in a dangerous position if any removal took place without the prior completion of onerous formalities. All of these problems could have been foreseen and resolved, and the law could have more precisely addressed certain relevant scientific matters, if the Government had named an expert advisory committee and had weighed public opinion with respect to the draft law, after having provided adequate information to society.

An attempt was made to avoid these problems in developing legislation on assisted human reproduction (Law of 22 November 1988). On that occasion an expert committee was named, and its members engaged in a mannerly debate among themselves and with the Government. Unfortunately, however, the next step—public debate—was not taken, and the law was simply approved by a parliamentary majority.

I think it important to quote here one paragraph from the introduction of this law, where it outlines the elements needed to set the stage for discussions between those favoring different policies regarding techniques of assisted reproduction:

Gradual awareness is growing that these surprising discoveries are a most intimate invasion of the world of the origins and continuation of human life, and that human beings have been given the resources to manipulate and influence their own heredity, and to make changes in it. There does not seem to be any doubt that scientific and technological research should continue to expand and to move forward; nor should it be limited unless this is done according to well-founded and reasonable criteria which prevent this research from clashing with human rights and with the dignity of individuals and the societies in which they live, for these are inalienable rights. For this reason there must be an open, rigorous, and dispassionate collaboration between society and science, in such a way that, based on respect for the fundamental rights and freedoms of human beings, science may proceed unimpeded within the limits, according to the priorities, and at the pace which society indicates, while in both the sciences and society there must be continued awareness that, *strictly for the benefit of human beings it will not always be possible nor should it be attempted to do what it is within our power to do.*[1] These are matters of grave responsibility, which must not lapse or be left to the independent decisions of scientists, who in any case might refuse to decide them. In this order of things, the establishment of national multidisciplinary commissions—including broad social representation that encompasses the majority opinion of the population, together with experts in these techniques, and having the responsibility for follow-up and monitoring of assisted reproduction, as well as for providing information and advisory services on these techniques in collaboration with the corresponding public authorities—will facilitate definition of the limits of their application, as is occurring in other countries and as the Council of Europe recommended to its Member Governments in Recommendation 1046 of September 1986, thus helping in addition to supersede isolated national standards which, given the possibilities for further development of these techniques, will end by being ineffective or contradictory. From an ethical perspective, social pluralism and a divergence of opinion are frequently expressed with regard to the different uses that are made of assisted reproduction techniques. *The acceptance or rejection of these techniques must be debated based on what is considered accurate information, and must not reflect either the motivations of special interests or any ideologic, religious, or partisan pressures, being founded only upon an ethics of a civic or civil nature that is not immune to practical considerations and whose validity is rooted in an acceptance of reality in which the criteria for rationality and justification in terms of serving the general good have been* taken into account[1]—an ethics that reflects the feelings of the majority and the content of the Constitution, and which may be adopted without social tensions and be of use to legislators in taking positions or setting standards (4).

On 11 April 1985, between promulgation of the law on organ removal and transplants and the law on assisted human reproduction, the Constitutional Tribunal issued a judgment declaring constitutional the decriminalization of abortion in the following three hypothetical cases: grave danger to the life or health of the pregnant woman; pregnancy resulting from the crime of rape; and the probable existence of serious hereditary physical or mental defects in the fetus.

Before this judgment was issued, highly subjective information was disseminated through the mass media, and a heated debate began which was quite similar to that found in other countries where this topic had been debated. The Royal Decree on health centers for voluntary termination of pregnancy (21-XI-1986) liberalized the performance of abortion, doing away with controls and setting minimal conditions for the accreditation of centers for legal voluntary termination of pregnancy. A majority of the medical schools were opposed to this last measure, but their opinion was ignored by the parliamentary majority.

Other bioethics problems related to research with human subjects, hospital ethics committees, patients' rights, etc., are still depending on development of the General Health Law of 25 April 1986.

Bioethics Centers

Spain's bioethics centers should be viewed not so much as structures or institutions but as focal points for reflection and exploration. Various specialists from these centers are regularly asked to serve as *ad hoc* members on various government or ecclesiastic commissions that discuss biomedical projects and examine ethical questions.

The bioethics dialogue, as defined here, began in Spain in 1975, the year the Borja Institute on Bioethics was founded as an autonomous institute attached to the School of Theology of Barcelona. Nearly a decade later, in 1984, this institute became independent of the school and began operating as a private foundation recognized by the Autonomous Government of Catalonia.

From 1975 until 1985, bioethics leadership in Spain was exercised from this institute, which collaborated in establishment of the European Association of Centers on Medical Ethics and the International Study Group on Bioethics within the International Federation of Catholic Universities.

The so-called interdisciplinary dialogues organized by the institute have dealt with topics on the frontiers between the medical and biological sciences and ethics. The methodology used at these meetings has been as follows: Invitations are issued to a limited number of scientists, philosophers, and theologians, some 40 to 50 people in all. They share knowledge and weigh values from their distinct points of view. An attempt is made to clarify their differences, since it is felt that the interdisciplinary dialogue presupposes that the participants are competent within their own disciplines, and that their objective is less to convince than to suggest ways of focusing on issues.

Topics covered thus far in these dialogues have related principally to scientific and ethical aspects of the state of the human embryo, genetic engineering, the use of human embryos in research, natural law concepts, prenatal diagnosis, death with dignity, and euthanasia. Most of those involved have been interested largely in exploring more deeply, from a rational perspective, the arguments of Catholic morality presented by the Church in its doctrinal positions on biomedical advances.

The Pontifical University of Comillas, Madrid, has used a similar methodology to conduct bioethics dialogues at meetings on assisted fertil-

---

[1]The italics are the author's.

ization, AIDS, and euthanasia that it has organized since 1985. The university's bioethics department, directed by Javier Gafo, and the Department of the History of Medicine at the Complutense University, directed by Diego Gracia, are the most important university-based bioethics centers in Spain.

In recent years important teaching and research in bioethics has also been accomplished by the University of Salamanca and the Higher Institute of Philosophy (Friedrich Ebert Foundation) of Valladolid, the latter institution having organized the I National Congress on Bioethics in 1986.

Nevertheless, it would be inaccurate to give the impression that bioethics is centered only in certain universities. The professors of biology and ethics who have joined in the above-mentioned interdisciplinary dialogues serve as focal points for bioethics at their respective universities (Oviedo, Málaga, Córdoba, Granada, Bilbao, Lérida, etc.). Other institutes, such as the Institute of Ethical Sciences of Madrid, have also made excellent contributions to the current bioethics dialogue. At the same time, scientific and cultural foundations like the Valencia Foundation for Advanced Studies, have revealed the vitality and progress of bioethics through conventions and conferences.

Other important interdisciplinary dialogues have been organized by Professor Alberto Dou. In 1984 those participating in these dialogues established the José de Acosta Interdisciplinary Association, whose purpose is to "promote intellectual exchange between persons dedicated to the human sciences and those from the theological and philosophical disciplines, in order to promote a clarification of human problems and expressions of the message of Christianity which will encourage a dialogue between contemporary faith and culture on behalf of mankind in our time" (5).

Another bioethics focal point is the San Juan de Dios Maternal and Infant Hospital of Barcelona, where in 1974 the first hospital ethics committee, properly speaking, was established. This committee has served as its own model

through a process of reflecting upon and adapting to new demands that continue to arise as a consequence of biomedical progress and social pluralism in making ethical choices.

Finally, important meetings on bioethics and the law have been organized by the departments of criminal law of the Complutense University of Madrid and the University of Barcelona, in collaboration with professors from German universities; and important contributions in this same area have been made by the Vasco Criminology Institute of San Sebastián, as well as by the various university departments of civil and criminal law throughout Spain.

Unfortunately, our official medical organizations have hardly participated at all in the bioethics dialogue. Indeed, the medical profession has not yet perceived that, with rare exceptions, medical school training provides no special guidance for resolving the ethical problems that underlie medical decisions.

Benevolent paternalism, combined with occasional tyranny, has reigned for years over the physician-patient relationship in Spain. Physicians have been educated to believe that their duty is to "do good" for the patient, and that the patient's duty is to accept this. The ethic of the physician-patient relationship is thus converted into a characteristic "ethic of beneficence." The physician is a moral as well as a technical agent, while the sick person is a patient in need of both technical and ethical help. Being convinced of this, few physicians over the age of 50 have been willing to concede autonomy to their patients, while an ever more popular patient rights movement has been issuing magnificent declarations that, for lack of adequate official support by the pertinent administrative and legal bodies, remain mere good intentions.

The Health System and Medical Schools

Certain limitations and deficiencies within Spain's health sector pose serious obstacles for those seeking to evolve away from paternalism and toward recognition of patients as autonomous moral agents. Unless one recognizes these circumstances, it is hard to understand why the country's medical schools have played such a small role in the bioethics debate. Nonetheless, some attempt to increase that role was made in 1978 through revision and updating of deontologic codes, a process which was repeated in April 1990.

Almost the entire Spanish population is covered by the Social Security system, and thus is subject to that system's regimen—which does not allow patients to choose their physicians and is plagued by bureaucratic excess, patient backlogs at outpatient centers, and lack of time for developing the physician-patient relationship. Among other things, this has led to indirect pressure on the emergency care centers, where the patients are well cared for.

Within this context, it should be noted that the technical level and quality of care for inpatients at teaching hospitals are generally good and show a very high level of competence. Opportunities for specialization and use of highly sophisticated techniques by the most highly qualified professors attract both physicians and students. The result is a high concentration of physicians at a few hospitals located in major urban centers, combined with serious resource deficiencies and distribution problems in the rural areas. Not surprisingly, while inpatients tend to be highly satisfied with care received at the teaching hospitals and those administered by the Social Security system, they tend to be highly dissatisfied with care provided at the outpatient centers.

At the same time, physicians are generally dissatisfied. They feel that the Government places more responsibilities on their shoulders than they can handle. They are forced to listen to the patients' complaints, both founded and unfounded, about the limitations and deficiencies of the health care system. They have little time to care for patients at the outpatient facilities. And they feel discriminated against compared to other professionals in terms of salary.

Meanwhile, the Government seems unable to resolve the problem of growing health care costs, a problem sharpened by political and economic debate between political parties. What appears to be lacking is the courage, resolve, and political opportunity to embark on far-reaching reforms, the need for which is being articulated almost continuously.

The schools of medicine have experienced a weakening of their position with respect to government power. There are also signs of a split within them caused by lack of achievement and by the political interests of members of the profession. At the same time, an ongoing fight with the Government has developed—in an attempt to defend professional and economic interests and to reduce layoffs which have affected 20% of those in the profession.

The deontology committees at the medical schools perform a purely advisory function, and attempts to unite the professionals involved have been doomed to failure. On the one hand, there are certain reservations about "medical ethics" in view of the long tradition of trying to adapt them to Catholic morality—a morality associated with a social and political class inexorably tied to the Franco regime. At the same time, there tends to be more fear of legal problems than actual concern for professional ethics. Therefore, efforts by the medical schools' governing tribunals to contain abusive government interference in health matters have been checked by the interests of the same physicians at these institutions, who have demanded more legal protection and thus indirectly more legislation.

In contrast to the medical schools, the schools of nursing have organized and promoted debates on bioethics, and have shown positive interest in having nurses take part in discussions on bioethical topics. It is expected that nurses will have an important role to play on hospital ethics committees in the future—if, as anticipated, these committees are set up on an ongoing basis to protect the interests of patients and of the physicians themselves, who are increasingly threatened by lawsuits.

In this latter regard, the unhappy example of

the United States and its malpractice suits, with all of their conceptual, ethical, and legal ambiguities, hangs like a sword of Damocles over the increasingly beleaguered physician-patient relationship. The hope, therefore, is that these hospital ethics committees can ward off many of the potential distortions and abuses inherent in such lawsuits, while at the same time correcting the defects and abuses of medical paternalism.

References

1. Laboa, J. M. La Iglesia entre la democracia y el autoritarismo. In: *Al servicio de la Iglesia y del pueblo: Homenaje al Cardenal Tarancón en su 75 aniversario*. Narcea, Madrid, 1986, pp. 21–34.

2. Homily delivered at the Mass of the Holy Spirit held in the Parochial Church of San Jerónimo el Real on the morning of 27-XI-1975. *Ecclesia* 1768 (6 December):1556–1558, 1975.

3. Belda, R. Valoración ética del proceso democrático español. *Misión Abierta* 77:59–69, 1986, p. 63.

4. España, Jefatura del Estado. Ley 22-XI-1988, No. 35/1988: Reproducción Asistida Humana, Regula las técnicas. *Boletín Oficial del Estado* 24-XI-1988, No. 282, I.

5. Asociación Interdisciplinar José de Acosta. Article 2 of the Statutes of the Association. (Address: c/Alberto Aguilera 23, 28015 Madrid, Spain). 1984.

Current Trends in Biomedical Ethics in the United States

Daniel Callahan

Though there had been scattered interest earlier, the contemporary field of biomedical ethics in the United States really began to develop in the mid to late 1960s. During the 1960s a large number of advances occurred in basic research and clinical applications. That decade saw the advent of organ transplants, kidney dialysis, and prenatal diagnosis; widespread use of the respirator; the beginning of legal abortion; and development of some effective contraceptives. It also saw the establishment of two major health care programs that were partly or fully funded by the Federal Government: Medicare, providing health care for the elderly, and Medicaid, providing health care for the poor. The new technologic advances, it became clear, would generate difficult and historically unique moral problems. This circumstance, combined with the great explosion of activities and issues, stimulated birth of the field of contemporary biomedical ethics.

The first decade or so after those beginning years witnessed development of strong interest in the entire field. Courses began appearing in universities and medical schools; professional societies developed committees with special responsibility for ethical issues; medical journals began to carry articles on the topic regularly; and research on it also appeared in journals of philosophy, law, and social policy. In addition, a number of cases in biomedical ethics began to appear before the courts; various problems were also taken up by legislatures; and two important commissions were established by the U.S. Congress, one in 1974 and another in 1979.

The 1970s, in short, saw a great blossoming and unfolding of the interest that had been aroused for the first time in the 1960s. The net result was a decisive expansion and change in both the scope and nature of traditional medical ethics. At present, although the traditions of medical ethics certainly persist, they are now contained within the wider field of biomedical ethics—which is normally taken to include both traditional medical ethics and a wide range of ethical issues bearing on biological and social science research.

It could well take a page or more simply to list all the ethics topics that have come out of these developments in recent years. They include an array of matters dealing with the beginning of life (conception, abortion, prenatal diagnosis, genetic counseling and screening, fetal therapy, and so on) as well as a large number concerned with the end of life (care of the dying, termination of treatment, the distinction between ordinary and extraordinary care, the distinction between omission and commission in care of the dying, and so on). In between are topics dealing with all other stages of life—including organ transplants, artificial organs, research on human subjects, the AIDS crisis and the problems it raises for civil liberties and the public interest, issues of reproductive biology, surrogate motherhood, and so forth.

In sum, a simple list of all the topics dealt with in contemporary biomedical ethics would be long and rich. So it is perhaps not surprising that some years ago, when the Hastings Center took a comparative look at ethical problems in various fields and professions, it seemed as if there were more moral problems in medicine and biology than in all the other professional fields combined—including all of law, business, journalism, the armed forces, social work, public policy, and government.

When one tries to discern recent trends in the field of biomedical ethics in the United States, one is struck not only by how many of them have their historical roots back in the 1960s and 1970s, but also by how many have undergone significant transformation and development since that time. I would like in this presentation to talk about five major areas of great importance and comment on some recent trends within those areas.

Patient Rights and Autonomy

It was perhaps in this general area that the first and most significant developments took place in the late 1960s and 1970s. In 1967, for example, the Federal Government established the requirement for those receiving grant support that any research involving human subjects had to be screened by a special committee, not only to examine the potential hazards to patients, but also to make certain that informed consent had been given. That was the Federal Government's first important entry point into basic ethical questions relating to research.

Shortly thereafter, there emerged a great interest in the idea of "patient rights"—in the form of efforts to see that patients were accorded carefully prescribed rights and to ensure that those rights would place them in a position of parity vis-à-vis the rights of physicians. Various guidelines were developed along these lines, and a gradual agreement emerged to the effect that the relationship between doctor and patient should be that of moral equals, even though the doctor might possess considerably more technical knowledge.

In recent years, there have been few new theoretical or legal breakthroughs relating to this concept of patient rights and autonomy, but a lot of work has been done to establish the concept in the actual practice of medicine—a slow process. In general, repudiation of medical paternalism has given way to strong emphasis on patient autonomy.

At the same time, it is fair to say that some commentators believe the trend has gone much too far, not only reducing the legitimate authority of physicians but also failing to recognize the actual complexity and psychological circumstances of patient decision-making. Hence, while much of the 1970s and 1980s saw growth of patient autonomy, there has been a tendency recently to call into question some of the excesses in that direction.

Overall, at present it appears that the relationship between doctors and patients should be seen as one of equals, with each attempting to educate the other and each sensitive to the other's needs and rights. This implies a more balanced relationship than a heavy emphasis on patient autonomy might achieve.

The Sanctity Versus the Quality of Life

As a result of concern about termination of treatment, whether for elderly patients at one end of life or handicapped newborns at the other, there has been an ongoing debate about how we should understand the concepts "sanctity of life" and "quality of life." The former concept, with deep historic roots, is usually taken to mean that life should be preserved whenever possible—and that all doubt about appropriate treatment should be resolved in favor of life's preservation. The latter "quality of life" concept is of more recent vintage. While that phrase first emerged in the 1960s within the context of environmental issues, it soon migrated into the medical arena. There it has been used to help resolve the question of what is to be done when life might be preserved, but perhaps preserved at great psychological, moral, or spiritual cost to the patient. In that case, if the patient's "quality of life" is going to be low, is it always the obligation of physicians to preserve life?

Although questions relating to the sanctity of life have arisen particularly in regard to care of the dying, they have also come up in matters involving painful and difficult treatment, where a patient's life might be extended, say, by a cancer operation, but where his quality of life could be significantly compromised in the process.

It is sometimes thought that the sanctity of life concept requires that life be maintained under all circumstances, and it is sometimes also thought that the quality of life concept requires that the sanctity of life be always set aside in any conflict between the two principles. One problem is that neither concept has a very solid and fixed definition. This is particularly true of "quality of life," which because of its nontechnical nature and relatively recent vintage admits of great variation in meaning.

Increasingly, however, many are coming to believe it impossible to distinguish sharply between the two concepts. For instance, in considering the sanctity of life, one can reasonably ask what it means to be alive in some meaningful fashion, and one way to answer that question is to invoke the quality of life concept. Similarly, in probing the quality of life, one can reasonably ask why life itself matters, and one needs the sanctity of life concept to effectively answer that. In short, it may well be that the two concepts must work hand in hand, each modifying and complementing the other.

Obviously, recent years have seen a lot of concern expressed in the United States about potential abuse of the quality of life concept— especially when that concept might be used to end a life that in the judgment of others is not worth living. The specter of Naziism is commonly invoked, and there is great worry that the quality of life idea would come to totally dominate the sanctity of life concept. The recent effort to try to find a way for the two concepts to work together in a complementary way seems directed at countering that danger and making certain that neither is wholly able to dominate the other.

Interventions into Nature

Another subject of great importance, lacking an adequate title, might well be called "interventions into Nature." A longstanding theological and philosophical debate has revolved around the following question: How far, and in what ways, is it legitimate for human beings to intervene into Nature and manipulate Nature to their own ends?

Today the concern arises frequently in relation to genetic interventions into human beings' own nature, but it has been a question commonly posed throughout the entire history of medicine. One recalls that objections were raised to the use of ether and to many surgical procedures, and yet in time those interventions were accepted. By and large the inclination in the United States has been to allow such interventions unless one can decisively prove them likely to harm individuals or Nature.

Since that is rarely the case, the compromise solution has been to allow and facilitate such interventions, but to appoint supervisory or oversight bodies to make certain that appropriate guidelines are observed and that care is taken to do no damage. Overall, I believe, there was far more resistance to interventions into Nature in the 1970s than at the end of the 1980s. This may be largely because some of the potential harms invoked earlier (e.g., the dangers of recombinant DNA research) did not materialize. At present, while some groups regularly resist such interventions, there is little general resistance to them; and it seems that science can do almost anything it wants in our society so long as it complies with the extensive regulatory schemes set up to protect research subjects and the public.

Resource Allocation

During the 1960s and much of the 1970s, the topic of resource allocation was simply not important. By the end of the 1970s, however, medical care costs had mushroomed, and a major search was underway for ways to contain them. At the same time, it was increasingly being recognized that medical technology had the potential to produce an infinity of cures for an infinity of illnesses at an infinite price—but that in both theory and practice some limits would have to be set on health care resource allocation.

During much of the 1970s, considerable effort went into developing principles and procedures that would help achieve equity of access to care in the face of potential shortages. In general, those efforts were not very successful, largely because it was hard to get agreement on what would constitute just access to health care and what might comprise a minimally adequate level of care.

During the 1980s, as the cost pressures increased, the discussion shifted. Among other things, proposals were made to limit health care entitlements to the elderly on the basis of age, to force patients to spend more out of their own pockets, to set limits on various states' entitlement programs, and to limit the kind and extent of health care coverage provided by private enterprise.

At this point there is very little agreement on just how much should be spent for health care relative to other things, or on how best to limit costs. Although cost containment efforts have continued apace, the results have tended to be unimpressive. At present, it appears that there will be even more pressure to control costs in the future, together with a much more direct and open discussion of rationing. One state, Oregon, has in fact limited organ transplants significantly, and has established a state system of priorities to be used in providing health care. Other states seem likely to follow this lead.

Public Decision-making

One of the great changes that came out of the 1960s and 1970s was the far larger role assigned to the general public in making health care decisions and allocating health care resources. The earlier Hippocratic ethic really gave the patient no decision-making role at all, leaving everything to the physician. In contrast, today the U.S. public plays an increasingly active role in various ways—from individual patients taking part in decision-making about their own health care to legislators and administrators making broad decisions about health care policy and resource allocation.

The question remains, however, as to how much the medical profession should manage and regulate itself, and the extent to which it should be externally regulated by the Government. On the whole, physicians remain strongly opposed to government intervention, but that resistance seems considerably weaker now than it was 20 or 30 years ago. Among other things, many physicians now recognize that substantial public involvement can be expected so long as the public is paying a large share of health care costs.

One recent development of great importance in this area has been the emergence of hospital ethics committees. The purpose of these committees is to provide advice and counsel—not make decisions—about difficult moral problems that arise in the daily practice of medicine within the hospitals they serve. Some 60% or more of all American hospitals now have an ethics committee, the membership of which typically includes physicians, nurses, social workers, lawyers, and some outside lay people.

In general, these committees carefully scrutinize ethical issues, make themselves available as a resource, and render opinions on particularly difficult ethical subjects upon request. Beyond that, they help to organize educational programs and in some institutions help to write policy on relevant matters such as issuance of "do not resuscitate" orders.

What is striking about this overall trend is that the U.S. public now has a very significant and pervasive role in a great deal of health care delivery. This means that lay people are becoming increasingly familiar with the way medicine operates in this country, with its internal problems, and with difficulties inherent in the relations between doctors and patients, doctors and administrators, and hospitals and the broader political order. It is now generally accepted that the public will have a significant role in decision-making, and while physicians continue to mutter about the situation, they understand that it is probably a fact of life. An important question that has emerged of late, therefore, is how one can ensure that physicians maintain their own integrity and sense of responsibility while at the same time sharing considerable power and authority with nonmedical people.

These are five major areas of concern and some recent trends within them. There is one other trend that I would note, one that may be of great importance in the future. That is the increasing tendency to politicize health issues, a development that has drawn up strong factions against each other and has produced some very acrid and unpleasant public debate. While this has long been the case regarding abortion, it has recently become the case increasingly with regard to termination of treatment, some genetic issues, and allocation of health care resources.

With specific regard to biomedical ethics, in its early days this was a relatively small and quiet field. Most of the people involved worked closely with one another and most were on relatively friendly terms. As the field grew, however, the issues expanded beyond the sole domain of medical ethicists to include many religious and cultural interest groups and the general public. Hence, on occasion debates began to involve ordinary tactics of the political marketplace and some of the unpleasant rhetoric that goes with them. In general, one has seen much more of a tendency to choose up political sides, a greater polarization of the issues, and fewer efforts to develop compromise solutions. Nevertheless, despite the threat posed in this manner by political issues, the quest for consensus remains a central one for health care ethics in the United States.

Overview of Bioethics in Mexico

José Kuthy Porter and Gabriel de la Escosura

An ethical person is generally understood to be one who continually shapes his own behavior in terms of a reference group of positive human values, progressively defining himself in this manner to a point where he is seen as exemplifying those values and fostering them in others (1).

One of the most obvious reasons for the accelerated development of medical ethics today is that medicine's outstanding advances have given rise to ethical issues that are often hard to resolve; and the magnitude and complexity of these issues require contributions from disciplines other than medicine.

Among the advances involved, to name only a few of the most prominent, are techniques for successfully making organ transplants, implanting artificial organs, and artificially prolonging life, as well as genetic selection methods such as that afforded by the combination of amniocentesis and selective abortion. One should also mention the overuse of technological resources in studying patients, an occurrence that tends to mechanize medical care and entail the intervention of several professionals in caring for a single patient, all of which dilutes the personal nature of the physician-patient relationship.

In these and other ways, the complexities of modern medicine's instruments and scientific techniques can often turn against man, raising issues of an ethical nature that urgently need to be resolved. With this in mind, a group of physicians, humanists, sociologists, philosophers, and researchers has founded the Mexican Academy of Bioethics, "dedicated to promote the study, investigation, and reporting of medical and biological ethics" (2).

As set forth in the academy's bylaws, its members are physicians and health professionals with established reputations whose knowledge and experience can contribute to development of this field.

Of course, medical ethics goes beyond the dictates of precepts and the behavior of physicians toward ill patients in response to the relentless but sometimes dehumanizing advance of modern technology. For this reason, and in view of the unavoidable need for medical and biological research directed at improving techniques for preserving and restoring health, all workers in the health field should know the basic principles of medical ethics in order to maintain a moral outlook and slow the dehumanizing influence of science when it adopts attitudes and practices that cause physical or mental harm. Within this context, it seems clear that economic utilitarianism, a fundamental goal of medical practice, constitutes one of the greatest ethical threats to modern man.

Instruction

Although ethical principles have generally been observed in the practice of clinical medicine in Mexico, to date instruction in bioethics has been required by only a few of the country's medical schools; certain others offer it as an elective, while most do not offer it at all. It is therefore encouraging to note that an Institute for Humanism in Medicine was recently organized at the Medical School of Anáhuac University, in order to promote application of the principles of medical ethics in Mexico.

Like many other disciplines, bioethics can be a difficult and "heavy" subject if it is not related to real-life experiences in the world of medicine. Especially today, in our world of advanced technology, philosophical theory in isolation seems dull; but if it is tied to a course on the history of medicine or made a subject for discussion by the professors of all courses, it becomes more attractive because it can then be seen as a living discipline with practical applications.

In this regard, it is worth noting the following statement by the Director of the Medical School of the National Autonomous University of Mexico: "The teaching of ethics is related to respect for human dignity, and therefore should be imparted through the ethical example of each one of the professors; it sustains itself through the protection of human rights, which is why it should be expounded in a structured and absolutely independent manner with assurance by moral men that they will clarify the questions typical of youth; and it involves commitment, because failure to assume responsibility for attacking moral (and therefore ethical) problems, is to incur discredit . . ." (3).

Research on Human Subjects

Ethics has long been a fundamental part of the practice of medicine, especially with respect to the patient's welfare—a matter that should be the main object of the physician's actions. However, real interest in the ethical aspects of medical research on human subjects did not clearly emerge until just after World War II, with the 1947 Nuremberg trials of people accused of performing sadistic research on prisoners in concentration camps. When the accused were found guilty of behavior contrary to universally recognized human values, the foundations were laid for a new phase of medical ethics in which the fundamental principles were patient autonomy and respect for the dignity of man.

Another important step in this same field occurred in 1975, when the 29th World Medical Assembly approved an amended version of the 1964 Declaration of Helsinki, which reaffirmed existing codes of ethics and for the first time proposed creation of ethics committees at all hospitals where research on human subjects was conducted.

Mexico has encouraged development of many of the ethical rules relating to biomedical research that have been in force up to the present. In 1980 Mexico City was the site of the International Conference of the International Council of Medical Science Organizations. On that occasion Mexico's National Academy of Medicine concerned itself with developing and revising work performed with respect to "Proposed International Guidelines for Biomedical Research Involving Human Subjects" and offering solutions to problems raised in working sessions. The Academy also participated in a similar event organized one year later in Manila, the Philippines, which set the stage for drafting the final version of those standards.

Mexico's General Health Law states in Section 5 that "In the health institutions under the responsibility of the directors or respective representatives and pursuant to the applicable provisions, the following will be formed: a research committee, an ethics committee, and a biosafety committee" (4).

The regulations of the General Health Law pertaining to health research, which were published in 1987, precisely and broadly specify the ethical matters to be considered when conducting research on human subjects. Among other things, Articles 13 and 14 of Chapter 1 make the following points:

> In all research where human beings will be the subject of study, the criterion of respect for their dignity and protection of their rights and welfare should prevail.
> Research on human subjects should be conducted according to the following principles:
> 1. It will be in keeping with the scientific and ethical principles that justify it.
> 2. It will be based on prior experience with laboratory animals or on other scientific facts.
> 3. It will be conducted only when the knowledge sought cannot be obtained by other suitable means.
> 4. The likelihood of expected benefits should always outweigh the foreseeable risks.
> 5. Aside from exceptions stated in these regulations, informed consent obtained in writing from the subject of the study or his or her legal representative will be required.

6. It [the research] will be conducted by health professionals...with knowledge and experience in safeguarding the integrity of human beings, under the jurisdiction of a health care institution that is supervised by competent health authorities and possesses the human and material resources needed to ensure each research subject's welfare. And

7. It must have the authorization of the head of the health care institution and, when appropriate, the Ministry, in conformity with Articles 31, 62, 69, 71, 73 and 88 of these Regulations. (5)

The Ethics Committee of the General Hospital of Mexico has played an important role in establishing ethics committees in other hospitals throughout Mexico. It has also been involved, through the General Health Council (*Consejo de Salubridad General*), in translating into Spanish ethics handbooks for biomedical experiments—handbooks that are distributed in turn to other Spanish-speaking countries.

As a preliminary step in reviewing proposals for biomedical research on human subjects, it is important to note the desirability of considering the cost/benefit ratio, particularly in our area, in light of the present economic crisis. Therefore, it seems reasonable to propose that before any such research is conducted the following questions should be answered: How valid, from a scientific standpoint, is the research project, and what are its potential benefits? Is there justification for conducting the research at this time? Is the group on which the research will be conducted adequate and appropriate? What are the potential and identifiable risks involved? And, is the proposed research completely acceptable from the ethical point of view? (6)

Regulation of Reproduction

Mexico generally respects a couple's freedom to decide how many children they wish to have and promotes the idea of "responsible parenthood." At the same time, it fosters family planning methods with various measures, including mass social communication campaigns, even though not all these measures can agree with all the criteria applied by the array of diverse family and social groups constituting the Mexican population. The practice of abortion is illegal in Mexico.

Regarding genetic engineering, we believe it has a promising future. However, with regard to human reproduction it appears to have transcended the limits of what is normal in the field of gestation, and so the need for legislation on the subject is imperative. This is especially so regarding *in vitro* fertilization, intratubal transfer of gametes, and all methods related to interventions in human procreation. In this regard we support the moral criteria pertaining to the physician's intervention into human procreation that are contained in the work by Ratzinger and Bovone (7), which reads in part as follows:

The medical act should not be valued solely for its technical dimension, but also and above all for its purpose, which is the good of the people and their physical and psychological health. The moral criteria that regulate medical intervention in procreation derive from the dignity of the human person, from his or her sexuality, and from his or her origin.

Medicine that wishes to serve the integral well-being of the person should respect the specifically human values of sexuality. The physician is at the service of the person and human procreation; he does not have authority to instruct or decide upon them. The medical act is respectful of the dignity of persons when it is directed at helping the conjugal act, whether to facilitate its consummation, or to see that the normally performed act attain its end.

Regarding interventions on the human embryo, these shall be licit as long as they respect the life and integrity of the embryo, do not expose it to uncontrolled risks, and have as their goal its treatment or individual survival; in any case, however, the informed consent of the parents is required. Experimentation on embryos which is not directly therapeutic is unethical, because using an embryo or human fetus as an object of experimentation constitutes a crime against its dignity as a human being.

In vitro fertilization techniques make other forms of biological or genetic manipulation of human embryos possible, such as: plans and projects for fertilization between human and animal gametes, and gestation of human embryos in uteri unnatural to them. These procedures are contrary to the embryo's dignity as a human being and, at the same time, violate the right of a person to be conceived and born within and through a marriage. Also, attempts and plans for obtaining a human being without any connection to sexuality through "gamete fission," cloning, or parthenogenesis should be considered immoral because they are in conflict with the dignity of both human procreation and conjugal union.

Similarly, the freezing of embryos, although done to keep them alive, constitutes an offense to the respect due human beings, inasmuch as it exposes them to serious risk of death or of damage to their physical integrity, deprives them at least temporarily of shelter and maternal gestation, and places them in a situation in which they are susceptible to further injury and manipulation.

Some attempts to intervene in the area of influence of chromosomes and genes are not therapeutic, but seek to produce human beings selected in terms of sex and other preestablished qualities. Such manipulations are contrary to the personal dignity, integrity, and identity of the human being. They cannot in any way be justified by possible beneficial consequences for the future of humanity. Each person deserves respect in his own right; in this resides the dignity and right of the human being from the outset.

In conclusion, it is important to note that any intervention on the human body not only involves tissues, organs, and functions, but also, and at different levels, affects the person. Therefore, such intervention involves a moral significance and responsibility that is perhaps implied but nonetheless real. As Pope John Paul II reminded the World Medical Association:

> Each human person, in his unrepeatable singularity, is not made up just of the spirit, but also the body, and for that reason in the body and through the body one reaches the person himself in his concrete reality. Consequently, respecting the dignity of man implies safeguarding that identity of man, as the Vatican II Council affirmed. From this anthropologic vantage point one should find the fundamental criteria for deciding on procedures that are not strictly therapeutic, such as, for example, those that seek to improve the human biological condition. (7)

Death

The word death (*muerte*), from the Latin *mors* or *mortis*, means the cessation or end of life. From a biological standpoint it is the cessation of organ function in a living being, beyond a point where revival is possible. In law, natural death ends an individual's civil status in all personal legal relationships, both civil and penal, while all assets and obligations (including fines) are transferred to the decedent's heirs.

In forensic medicine, the clinical diagnosis of death is based upon cessation of respiration and circulation (functional death). For some time after death, certain other functions persist that can be easily demonstrated, such as electric excitability of the muscles, digestive functions, etc.; the point where such functions cease is termed "tissue death."

Technologic accomplishments and an extraordinary improvement in hospital care resulting mainly from new techniques for diagnosing and treating sudden illnesses that until recently led to death have given rise to situations that require a new approach to treating patients, the principal victims of such illnesses, as well as the patients' relatives who are the secondary victims.

In certain cases it is now possible to prolong a patient's vegetative life for many years—to a point where the extension of life is limited mainly by the economic means available. In such circumstances, the ideal thing would be for the patient himself to choose the time to die. This is a difficult concept to express juridically, however, especially since the patient's choice can have significant repercussions on third parties.

When a patient with a terminal condition is treated, those medically responsible face extremely difficult decisions. Use of artificial life-sustaining equipment and measures, such as respirators, hemodialyzers, etc., can create a serious problem, in that the patient may need them permanently. The decision to suspend use of such equipment under these circumstances is difficult for relatives, doctors, and the attending staff. At the same time, the treatments involved tend to be very expensive for the family, which is obliged to continue them not knowing how long they will be needed or how much it will be required to spend.

Therefore, the physician should be aware of what is involved in prolonging the life of a patient. If there is a reasonable probability that the patient will survive the disease, every effort is justified. But if the doctor knows that the patient will not survive, though sophisticated techniques and procedures might keep him "alive" indefinitely, he should assess what such prolongation of life means in terms of suffering for the patient and cost for the family. He should consider whether the large amounts of money and medical resources involved might better be used to treat several other patients with curable diseases—whose recovery would be emotionally and economically beneficial to their relatives and society.

At the same time, it must be accepted as an ethical principle that the physician has a medical duty to tell the patient and his relatives the truth regarding the patient's status, even when he has not been expressly asked. (8)

In general, the patient confronting certain death should be treated with a minimum of measures intended to prolong his "life" and a maximum of measures calculated to alleviate his suffering, even when this means high dosages of tranquilizers and analgesics. That is, we should treat the patient as we would like to be treated and not permit resuscitating maneuvers. We should also keep painful examinations to a minimum and not allow any laboratory studies for academic purposes or for confirmation of what is already a diagnostic certainty.

Organ Transplants

Mexico already has detailed laws that clearly determine what factors should regulate the use of tissues and organs for therapeutic purposes,

particularly for transplants. However, every day sees a greater demand for organs to transplant, and so there is a need for more volunteer donors and more careful registration.

The Ministry of Health and the Dr. Salvador Zubirán National Nutrition Institute have formally activated the National Transplant Registry, a facility created through joint agreement of the two institutions. This registry coordinates the distribution of organs and tissues throughout the country and maintains a register of the originating donors and patients awaiting organ transplants (9).

Regarding ethical issues relating to transplants, when the recipient and the donor are both humans, there is no doubt that the basic concept of transplanting organs is ethical. Indeed, the transplanting of animal organs to human recipients also appears ethical in concept, assuming that the procedure does not induce significant personality alterations in the receiver.

Allogeneic transplants between relatives involve a deep demonstration of the donor's love and generosity with respect to the recipient, motives that clearly indicate the deeply ethical nature of such transplants.

Allogeneic transplants between unrelated individuals, when the donor's sole motive is charity (as in the case of altruistic blood donations, for example) are richly deserving of social admiration and respect.

In addition, allogeneic transplants from a corpse to a living person, when the donor has just died and appropriate consent has been obtained, are obviously licit and ethical in concept. What is indispensable is an accurate determination that the donor is really dead before the transplant material is obtained; otherwise, the fundamental principle prohibiting homicide should prevail. (10)

Without trying to deepen the debate that has emerged regarding determination of the time of death, we would like to cite Kaufer (11), who states that "death should be considered the suppression of any manifestation of life by the organism as a whole, such that the time of death corresponds to the limit beyond which return and revival are not possible."

In accordance with this definition, once death of the cerebral cortex has been proven it is ethical to perform a transplant, so long as authorization has been obtained from the decedent's close relatives and anything that might be construed as "commerce" or "trafficking" in transplant material is avoided (12).

Especially in view of the fact that Mexico is a developing country, the matter of resource allocation for national transplant programs is important. This issue has a high ethical content because it concerns appropriate distribution of medical resources, particularly in the case of transplant procedures that are still in the experimental stage and that should remain exclusively within the domain of very specialized institutions. On the other hand, the virtues of more routine tissue and organ transplants—of corneas, bones, skin, bone marrow, kidneys, etc.— seem clear; the matter of limiting resources for such transplants has not yet come up for discussion in the developing countries; and we feel from an ethics standpoint that allocation of resources for these procedures is fully justified.

More generally, a presentation by Engelhardt to the Medical Society of Massachusetts (12) stressed that all expenditures made to achieve a life-saving therapy should be prudent—so that they can be justified in response to concern about whether the funds could have been spent better elsewhere. Specifically, Engelhardt asked whether use of such funds to improve prenatal care or reduce hypertension would have ensured greater survival or reduced morbidity in more people.

On the other hand, we believe that the judgment of different societies and social groups should be respected. For example, some societies may freely decide to assign relatively low priority to the transplant program so as to improve the quality of medical care for the poor. At the same time, certain societies with more abundant economic resources might decide to increase the funding and attention given the transplant program. We feel there is every reason to regard such choices freely made as valid.

AIDS

The acquired immunodeficiency syndrome (AIDS) was first identified in the United States in 1981. Since then the disease has been detected in most countries and all continents. In 1983 the first cases appeared in Mexico; since then the number of cases has grown rapidly, and at present it is estimated that this number is doubling every seven months (13).

It now appears that by 1991 there will be between 20,000 and 30,000 AIDS cases in Mexico. As in the United States, the disease in Mexico was initially limited to male homosexuals and bisexuals, but it soon began appearing in women, children, recipients of blood transfusions, and heterosexual males belonging to none of the known high-risk groups.

Extensive studies on AIDS have been performed in Mexico that deal with various clinical, bacteriologic, epidemiologic, economic, and health care aspects of the disease. However, there have been virtually no AIDS studies focusing on ethical questions—which is a principal reason why we recently conducted a survey of who was being informed of AIDS cases by the infectious disease specialists frequently encountering such cases. In a majority of cases the respondents indicated that only relatives interested in the health of the patients were informed, and that appropriate prophylactic measures were provided or practiced only in the case of HIV seropositivity being found in the closest family members.

In general, confidentiality is required. For clinical purposes, AIDS cases are reported to the National Information Center of the National AIDS Council (CONASIDA). This institution follows a procedure directed mainly at voluntary case identification. If the subject agrees, a card is filled out (the overwhelming majority of the subjects do not respond truthfully to the questions asked). Immediately thereafter a social worker reviews the data on the card and a psychologist briefly interviews the subject. Later a medical review is conducted and a blood sample is obtained from the subject. At all times the only means of identification used is a code on the card, which is filed at CONASIDA's information center. No attempt to identify the subject is made at any time, and maximum confidentiality is maintained.

When the subjects are seropositive, they are given their test results in private, along with recommendations and pertinent support.

CONASIDA has adapted an AIDS survey to Mexico that conforms to WHO recommendations and is based on experiences in other countries, primarily the United States (*14*). The results of this ongoing survey are computerized and analyzed by epidemiologists and infectious disease specialists. The medical records of AIDS cases are always registered with nothing more than a code, never with the names of the patients.

From the standpoint of medical ethics, it can be concluded that thus far no precise methodology has been applied with regard to AIDS patients. Therefore, work needs to be done in this area, proposals being needed for special treatment and other policies dealing not only with AIDS patients but also with related problems affecting their families and society at large.

References

1. Gaona Velasco, J. F. Etica y medicina. *Rev Fac Med* 29(3):123–124, 1986.

2. Bisteni, A. La bioética, realidad y necesidad. *Cardi* 5(7):161–162, 1987.

3. Cano Valle, F. Etica en la enseñanza de la medicina. *Rev Fac Med* 29(3):112–114, 1986.

4. Kuthy Porter, J. Etica en la investigación clínica: Simposium. *Gac Med Mex* 119(3):97–101, 1983.

5. México, Secretaría de Salud. Reglamento de la Ley General de Salud en Materia de Investigación para la Salud. Mexico City, 1987.

6. Kuthy Porter, J. Etica en la toma de decisiones en la investigación biomédica. Paper presented at the Reunión sobre Investigación en Medicina. Hospital General de México, Mexico City, 1988.

7. Ratzinger, J. Card., and A. Bovone. *Instrucción sobre el respeto de la vida humana naciente y la dignidad de la procreación: Respuesta a algunas cuestiones de la actualidad.* Congregación para la Doctrina de la Fe, Ed. Paulinas, Mexico City, 1987.

8. Sepúlveda, V. Derechos, deberes y decisiones en el ejercicio médico actual. *Gac Med Mex* 120(5):269–271, 1984.

9. México, Secretaría de Salud. Se fortalece la investigación y los aspectos jurídicos y éticos en el renglón del trasplante de órganos: Información general. *Bol Secret Salud*, October 1988.

10. García, I., and D. García. Aspectos morales y éticos del trasplante de órganos. In: E. Santiago Delpin and J. O. Ruiz Speare (eds.). *Trasplante de órganos.* Salvat, Mexico City, 1987, pp. 105–110.

11. Kaufer, C. El fenómeno de la muerte desde el punto de vista médico. In: E. Santiago Delpin and J. O. Ruiz Speare (eds.). *Trasplante de órganos.* Salvat, Mexico City, 1987.

12. Engelhardt, H. T. Allocating scarce medical resources and the availability of organ transplantation. *N Engl J Med* 311(2):66–71, 1984.

13. Cruz Ortiz, H., J. J. Jessurum, M. Romero, et al. Síndrome de inmunodeficiencia adquirida: Informe de las primeras veintinueve autopsias en la Unidad de Patología del Hospital General de México. *Rev Med Hosp Gen* 50(3):121–126, 1987.

14. Kensington, Maryland, Association of State and Territorial Health Officials' Foundation. Guide to public health practice: HTLV-III screening in the community. *MMWR* 31(31):501–513, 1982 and *MMWR* 34(31):477–478, 1985.

Bioethics in Peru

Roberto Llanos Zuloaga

Medicine is three-dimensional: It is a science, a profession, and a form of assistance. As such it has a decisive role to play in the technologic and axiologic changes in our culture. Bioethics is the rational response to the moral, political, and social problems posed by health care, with the sole purpose of producing benefits through biomedical interventions.

Biomedical technology has become extremely costly to apply, ambiguous in its authority, and uncertain in its efficacy, which is why it sparks great debates from an ethical point of view; its regulation is urgently required.

Peru is not excluded from those countries which are aware of this urgency. The three dimensions of medicine gave rise to bioethics or medical ethics, which viewed from another angle is the systematic study of human behavior in the field of the life sciences and health care, in the light of moral principles and values.

Education in Bioethics

Bioethics has existed as a discipline for 20 years, during which time it has gained ground, broadening its scope and increasing the depth of its theory and methodology. In the process, it has been taking on a distinctive identity, one that bears some resemblance to medical philosophy supplemented with elements of medical anthropology and medical epistemology, and has gained increasing recognition as a separate discipline.

The situation of bioethics in Peru, however, is somewhat different. Here it has not become so generally recognized or so widespread. There are still no signs on the horizon that the study of bioethics may give rise to an independent profession, and there is at present a conflict between two approaches to medical ethics—one of which places medical ethics under bioethics, while the other places it under professional ethics.

In the late 1960s, in Peru and the rest of the world, bioethics was taught in departments of philosophy and theology. Later there was a general tendency to incorporate it into the teaching of medicine. In Peru, however, it is still being taught in the same university departments as previously, and there are relatively few signs of major changes underway.

Ethics Committees

The Ethics Committee of the Peruvian Medical Association is in charge of reviewing all ethical problems that arise in the practice of medicine. There is also a National Commission of the Campaign against AIDS that concerns itself with regulations designed to prevent transmission of the AIDS disease agent and protect the quality of life of AIDS patients. In addition, it is expected that a committee on transplants will be formed to help regulate the operation of a recently passed law dealing with this subject. Moreover, virtually all major scientific bodies in Peru have bylaws providing for creation of ethics committees, though this does not necessarily mean bioethical principles are being applied.

Overall, Peru does seem to be reaching a stage where the discipline of bioethics is recognized to the extent that committees are being formed to put its theoretical principles into practice. It is to be hoped that this will serve to promote the quality of life of individuals, rather than mere indiscriminate "lifesaving," the former being appropriate for countries like Peru with growing populations and scarce resources.

Research on Human Subjects

Little research on human subjects is conducted in Peru, and the technology typically used in such research is not very advanced compared to that employed in highly developed countries. For example, it was only recently that Peru's first "test tube baby" was born, an event that precipitated considerable discussion about the ethical aspects of that medical practice.

When research on human subjects is conducted, the usual procedure of obtaining patient consent and publishing the aims of the experiment is not always followed. In this same vein, the author's experience suggests that Peru's requirements for pharmaceutical research on human subjects are less restrictive than those prevailing in European countries such as Germany.

Likewise, from a technical standpoint it is easier to get permission to sell a new medication in Peru than it is in Europe. On the other hand, research on new medications in Peru does not necessarily imply monetary compensation for the physician, a circumstance tending to diminish the reliability of the results obtained. For similar reasons, doubts have also been raised regarding quality control of medications being investigated in the country.

Like people everywhere, Peruvian patients tend to feel ambivalent when health professionals show a scientific interest in their diseases. They especially fear being research subjects when a multitude of analyses and technological interventions are performed. In this they are supported by the insurance companies, which are continually asking physicians not to order any more tests than absolutely necessary, even when the nature of the patient's disease stirs

scientific interest and requires further investigation.

Bioethics and Reproduction

There are several institutions in Peru concerned with human reproduction—among them the National Institute for Sexual Education (*Instituto Nacional para la Educación Sexual*—IMPARES) that seeks to foster responsible parenthood and encourages women to limit the size of their families. Their activities include periodic campaigns and publication of guides in Lima newspapers that help make women aware of their fertile days. Despite such work, the number of adolescents getting pregnant is very high (almost 15% in the capital), and many Peruvian women reach adulthood only after delivering two or three children and having perhaps one or two abortions.

A discussion is currently underway in the media regarding male vasectomies and their potential for regulating reproduction. This is a subject confronting numerous cultural prejudices—including the concept of *machismo*, which dictates that a male's image is better the more children he has. (Besides being popular among males, this attitude is shared by many Peruvian women.)

The birth control pill is quite expensive, and there are no plans for free distribution to women who request it. Very few institutions implant intrauterine devices at cost, meaning that in practice this method is available only to the middle and upper classes. The number of women receiving injections of slow-absorption contraceptives is very small. Condoms are sold almost exclusively in pharmacies; some, of uncertain quality, are distributed by roving street-vendors, as are herbs that "regulate" reproduction.

Abortion

Abortion is illegal in Peru except for medical reasons, in which case there must be two medical certificates (sometimes three) attesting to the need. There are no legislative bills pending on abortion, such as are pending in certain other countries, nor have the leading political parties chosen to deal with the issue in their health plans.

Despite this, illegal abortion is very common. So it is not surprising to find that certain herbs and medications are widely regarded as abortifacients, or that certain neonatal encephalopathies are suspected of being related to maternal attempts at abortion. Nor is it unusual to see newspaper stories reporting the deaths of young women as a result of abortion-related manipulations, or to find that women in critical condition from the same cause are frequently seen in the emergency rooms of large hospitals. The available evidence indicates that nearly all these abortions are performed without benefit of sterile procedure and pose grave dangers to the woman's life.

Other Gynecology Problems

In seeking to attain social and professional autonomy, it is not unusual for Peruvian women to find themselves working simultaneously as housewives, employees, supporters of dependent parents, and teaching assistants for their children. When they become ill or pregnant, they are obliged to establish priorities among their various duties in order to determine which must be set aside.

Even so, social attitudes toward gynecologic problems are such as to constitute a significant added burden. Practically any gynecologic problems that may arise are considered secondary and unrelated to the affected woman's work. The media do not commonly discuss the ethical aspects of gynecologic disorders. Medical procedures such as hysterectomy and tying the fallopian tubes produce heated family arguments and are regarded as socially unfashionable. Therefore, women who experience such procedures must keep quiet about them and must

generally overcome any psychological problems provoked or aggravated by these prevailing social attitudes on their own.

In Vitro Fertilization

This and comparable reproductive procedures are extremely expensive and out of reach of the general Peruvian population. Nevertheless, the recent delivery of Peru's first "test tube" baby spurred considerable debate in the media. Whatever the outcome of this debate, it has served to publicize various bioethical concepts related to human reproduction, as well as to improve public knowledge of reproductive anatomy and physiology. Thus, however indirectly, it may have helped to work against the many reproduction-related prejudices existing in our society.

Human Genetics

Genetic research is extremely costly and can only be conducted in Peru with the help of foreign institutions. For this reason, most genetic studies within the country have been of a theoretical nature. However, because of the frequency of Down's syndrome, a foundation will soon be created to encourage research in this field. Also, restricted application of prenatal genetic testing has begun, a development that could pose religious problems when detection of an abnormal fetus suggests the advisability of abortion.

AIDS

Ministry of Health regulations explicitly state that AIDS patients must be accepted by state hospitals. Nevertheless, Peru's special AIDS program has received unofficial reports that some hospitals or clinics are still turning away patients with this disease.

Termination of Life

In Peru, as elsewhere, there is currently debate about whether legislation permitting "compassionate murder" would create more problems than it would solve; whether "living wills," through which people can clearly express their desire to be allowed to die under certain conditions, should be accepted; and whether the shortage of medical resources and their high cost will push some people to choose to end their lives so as not to burden their families.

Resuscitation

The "living will," drafted like any other testament at a time when the testator is of sound mind, instructs the person's family and physician not to use extraordinary efforts to "resuscitate" him or her in the event of a terminal and irreversible disease. Besides debate over use of such documents, there is also discussion of whether the dying person's family should be able to have the physician turn off artificial life support apparatuses (resuscitators, artificial heart/lung machines, artificial kidneys, etc.). In considering this question, it is important to understand that "resuscitation" does not mean restoration of the brain to life, because although the patient's heart may stop beating briefly, his or her brain remains alive throughout the resuscitation process.

Interruption of Artificial Life Support

It is of course possible in some cases to maintain life processes artificially, even after the patient's conscious mind is dead. This has prompted discussion in Peru about whether or not the practice of applying machines, probes, cables, etc. to a human "vegetable" implies loss of respect for the human person. In this same vein, passive forms of euthanasia (such as suspended nutrient intake) have sparked debate in Peruvian medical circles. However, both the law and the Code of Ethics of the Peruvian Medical Association clearly forbid helping another person to commit suicide.

Organ Transplants

The new aforementioned law on transplants has raised questions about health professionals' role in defining death. Among other things, there is public concern that with death being defined in terms of brain function, physicians may be tempted to declare patients dead when they are not, in order to obtain the patients' organs for possible transplants.

Handicapped Children

Bioethical questions relating to handicapped children include, among other things, their acceptance by society, creation and availability of special schools, integration of the handicapped into regular schools, and creation of sheltered workshops. Of course, in nearly all cases society should not expect the affected children's diminished faculties to be recovered. It is rather a case of becoming accustomed to living with human beings not in full possession of their faculties. Experience has shown, however, that the proper setting and training can awaken rudimentary abilities in many handicapped children, enabling them to make good use of their potential.

Several years ago, Dr. Verna Alva stated that only 2% of the handicapped children in Peru received adequate health care. I personally believe that this figure remains essentially unchanged.

Several parents' associations and institutions have been making tireless efforts to help handicapped children deal with social prejudices. This is not easy in a country where many fear "catching" disabilities such as Down's syndrome, a fear reinforcing rejection of the handicapped.

Most private learning centers make it clear that they do not accept handicapped children, while the remainder use more subtle means to block admission. The situation is complicated by the fact that some schools administer an entrance examination to children applying for admission, and there are even "preparatory academies" for children applying to such schools. In addition, it is extremely difficult for pre-school-age handicapped children to be accepted among children without defects, and virtually impossible for handicapped adolescents to try to learn a trade together with other teenagers.

At present, the city of Lima with its seven million inhabitants has only one private learning center for adolescents with physical handicaps and normal intelligence, together with two or three sheltered workshops. Indeed, the whole country, with a population of roughly 20 million people, has only six or seven such centers.

Overall, Peru clearly needs many more schools for handicapped children. It also needs to train professionals in this field and to enforce labor protection laws for the handicapped.

ROUND TABLE

What Constitutes a Just Health Services System and How Should Scarce Resources Be Allocated?

Diego Gracia

Over the last century health has ceased to be a private matter concerning mainly individuals and has become a public problem, a political issue. The terms "health" and "politics," initially mutually exclusive, have become inextricably intertwined in the expression "health policy," until today it is hard to find any aspect of health completely detached from the immense bureaucratic apparatus of health policy.

Many consider the interference of politics in health excessive, while for others it is still insufficient; but both sides justify their points of view by appealing to the concept of distributive justice. Thus it is not surprising that one of the liveliest and most polemic chapters of bioethics today is that of justice in health.

When should a health service be considered just or unjust? What resources must be allocated to comply with the obligation of justice? How should one proceed when available resources are less than those theoretically needed? How can insufficient resources be justly distributed? These are some of the questions policy-makers, health promoters, and members of the general public ask repeatedly.

Perhaps any attempt to provide definitive answers will be pretentious; but this should not lead us to believe that such questions are useless or have no answers. Indeed, there are answers, but clearly not easy ones.

In my view, all answers acknowledging the issue's tremendous complexity must unfold on two distinct levels, which I shall call deontologic (i.e., addressing principles) and teleologic (i.e., addressing consequences). A coherent theory of justice is impossible if either of these is missing. Hence, what follows is divided into two sections, which correspond to the two parts of the title to this study: What constitutes a just health services system? and How should scarce resources be justly allocated? In the conclusion I will integrate the partial results of each section in an effort to suggest a comprehensive response to these questions.

The Deontologic Moment: What Constitutes a Just Health Services System?

The primary and basic meaning of "justice" is correction or adjustment of something in accordance with a model of what it should be. In this first sense, "just" means "adjusted," that which is adjusted to the model. Thus, we will say that an act is "just" when it is in accordance with the law, and that the law is "just" when it is an expression of moral principles. "Unjust," to the contrary, is that which is not adjusted to the general principle, norm, or criteria being applied.

That general principle of justice with which all other criteria and acts of man must be brought into line was defined by the Roman jurists as *suum cuique tribuere*, "to each his due." An act is just when each is given his due, and unjust otherwise. The problem lies in spelling out precisely what this means. Throughout Western cultures there have been no fewer than four different interpretations, which to some extent contradict one another; these have variously interpreted justice as "natural proportionality," "contractual freedom," "social equality," and "collective welfare." I will endeavor to characterize each of them as concisely as possible and to examine their impact upon the world of health.

Justice as Natural Proportionality

Historically, the theory of justice that has been the most widely applied is doubtless that which understands justice as "natural proportionality." Initiated by the Greek thinkers around the sixth century B.C., it went unrivaled until the seventeenth century.

According to this notion, justice is a natural property of things, whose name need only be known and respected. This is the meaning that the Greek philosophers attributed to the term *dikaiosyne*. As natural entities, things are just, and any type of maladjustment constitutes a denaturalization. Everything has its natural place, and it is just that it remain there. This applies not only to the cosmic order, but also to the political order. Plato's *Republic* tells us that in a "naturally ordered" society, which is thus "adjusted" or "just," there will be inferior men, artisans; there will also be guardians; and, finally, there will be rulers.[1]

In addition to this "general" justice, Greek philosophy distinguished other more concrete or partial meanings of the term. Aristotle differentiated at least two. They are called partial because they neither pertain to all of nature nor to the body politic as a whole, but are limited to relations among different members of society. One is "distributive justice," which governs relationships between the ruler and his subjects. The other, "commutative justice," regulates relationships between private persons. In the health world both are important, but especially the first (in the expression "justice in health," justice is always understood to mean "distributive justice").[2]

According to Aristotle, distributive justice regulates the distribution "of honors, or money, or anything else" among the members of society (1). If by our nature we were all identical, there is no doubt but that such distribution would not be considered just if it were unequal. But given the "natural" character of inequality and hierarchy in society, for the Greeks the distribution of honors, wealth, etc. cannot and should not be done on an "identical" basis, but rather "proportionate" to one's natural abilities.

Aristotle applies distributive justice to the distribution of "honors and wealth." The effect of this upon wealth is abundantly clear, but that of honors requires greater clarification. For all the philosophers of antiquity (understanding by this all those before the 17th century), the moral perfection achieved by each person in the community depended upon his place therein. The individual good of the sovereign was identified with the common good of all. The individual goods of the subjects, however, were not considered moral or good unless they were geared to achieving the common good of the sovereign. Hence the maximum individual good of the subject was obedience. This is the sense in which Aristotle understands the just or proportional distribution of "honors." The ruler is owed obedience and piety in the same manner as a father. This is the foundation of paternalism, a constant throughout the naturalist sociopolitical tradition.

The repercussions of these schemes upon medicine have been tremendous. The physician embodies the common good, while the patient seeks a particular good, health. But the patient cannot achieve this good other than through the general economy embodied in the physician.

---

[1]CF. *Rep.* v. 3, 21:415a–b.

[2]CF. *Et. Nic.* v. 4:1131b2b–1132a2.

Therefore, the only virtue that should be demanded of the patient is obedience. In the relationship between patient and physician, as in the relationship between parishioner and priest, or subject and sovereign, there is no place for commutative justice. The services of physicians, priests, and sovereigns are deemed so superior to those rendered by all other members of the community that it will never be possible to achieve equality in the exchange. Therefore, none of them is paid in accordance with the principle of commutative justice, but rather in "honor." The money they receive is an "honorarium."

The concept of justice as natural proportionality also has another health consequence of great importance. This derives from the fact that "proportionality" should be reflected in medical care, in accordance with an individual's social rank. This belief was already evident in Plato's *Republic*, which not in vain endeavored to describe the order of a "just" polis. There one can see how medical care should have a certain differential character, precisely by virtue of the principle of "distributive" justice. Slaves were attended by slave doctors; artisans had no access to lengthy or costly therapeutic procedures; and only the rich had complete access to the world of health.

All of this, written in the fourth century B.C., maintained its validity throughout the Middle Ages. Medieval society tried to follow platonic dictates insofar as possible, and medical care basically accommodated to these norms.

Thus was the theory of justice as adjustment to the proportional order of Nature, and thus it functioned in the field of medicine. Distributive justice led to the existence of three easily distinguishable levels of medical care throughout antiquity and the Middle Ages: that of the poorest strata of society (serfs, slaves, etc.); that of the free artisans; and that of the free citizens and the rich. Of the three groups' members, only those belonging to the latter fully benefited from the goods of the city, and only its members could have been and should have been just and virtuous. Perhaps that is why only they were beneficiaries of complete health care.

Justice as Contractual Freedom

In more recent times, political science has come to make basic alterations in the concept of justice, and also has come to insist increasingly on the importance of a social contract as the basis for all justice-related duties. In this way, justice was transformed from a mere "natural adjustment" into a strict "moral decision." The relationship of the subject and the sovereign was no longer based on "submission" but on free "decision." Man was seen as being above Nature, and as the sole and exclusive source of rights.

In his *Second Treatise of Government* (2), John Locke described what he regarded as basic rights of every man that derive from the mere fact of being a man. These are what are known as civil and political "human rights": the right to life, to health or bodily integrity, to liberty, and to property, together with the right to defend these rights when they are believed to be endangered.

In this view, these rights are the "individual good" and inalienable rights of every man. But in order for them to be converted into the "common good," a compact or contract known as the social contract must be entered into. Its purpose is to bring about "social justice," which is identified with the "common good," understood as "an established, accepted, known and firm law that serves by common consent as a norm of what is just and what is unjust" (3).

For Locke, social or legal justice has no aim other than that of protecting the rights that men have already had from the beginning, in such a way that they can never transgress those limits or oppose them. The social compact has the sole aim of protecting the natural rights (i.e., civil and political rights) of individuals. Political power, delegated as it is, has no realm other than that granted in the delegation—which, in turn, can have no object other than to protect natural rights and freedoms. All that transgresses these bounds is an unjustified and unjust abuse on the part of the State.

Obviously, this was a new concept of distributive justice, justice as contractual freedom. According to this theory, the distribution of honors and wealth is governed by several principles. One of them is the principle of acquisitive justice. According to this concept, work provides the primary title to property, since a worker puts something of his own into the object of his labor that is untransferable. Therefore, it is not Aristotelian proportionality that can tell us whether wealth has been distributed in a just fashion, but its manner of acquisition—and such acquisition will be just if it results from one's own work.

Together with this initial principle goes another, that of the just transfer of property—whether by gift, purchase, or inheritance. (Regarding the latter, according to this principle children have a just right to inherit the property justly acquired by their parents.)

The result for Locke is a minimalist notion of the State. Specifically, the State's only legitimate purpose is to facilitate people's exercise of their natural rights to life, health, liberty, and property. When the State does not do so, or does so poorly, i.e., when the laws do not respect the natural limits, or the State steps beyond its bounds and dictates laws that go beyond the powers granted to it in the social contract, such laws are unjust.

In sum, according to liberal thought, justice is understood to consist of "contractual freedom," as embodied in a contract that assures and protects individual freedom. This contrasts sharply with the old idea of natural adjustment.

This approach to the problem of distributive justice had a great impact upon all liberal thought, perhaps most notably that of the classical economists—including Adam Smith, David Ricardo, and Robert Malthus. Although liberal economics was gradually replaced by so-called social market economics as time passed, since 1970 the old liberalism has been regaining relevance, not only in economics (through Hayek, Friedman, and others), but also in ethics. Thus, philosopher Robert Nozick vigorously defends distributive justice as contractual freedom in his book *Anarchy, State, and Utopia* that was published in 1974 (4).

All this has been and continues to be of enormous importance to the world of medicine. According to liberal philosophy, the health market should be governed, like all others, by the laws of free trade, without the intervention of third parties. This has been the guiding concept of so-called "liberal" medicine, which insists that the physician-patient relationship must accommodate itself to free-market principles, and therefore should not be mediated by the State. In this light, any state intervention is considered artificial and harmful.

Throughout the nineteenth century, one can see how medical deontology in every country condemned the physician to become a wage-worker; and even today, when health insurance pays for almost all health care in many countries, there are still countries such as France where the patient continues to pay the physician directly, rather than having such compensation handled by Social Security or the State (5).

Within this model of liberal medical practice as it existed in nineteenth century Europe, one can distinguish three types of medical care. The first was for the well-to-do, who had sufficient resources to pay physicians' and surgeons' fees. The second was for a much larger middle-class group that used private insurance to cover the special expenses of surgery and hospital stays. And the third was for the poor, who had no chance of gaining access to the liberal health care system on their own, and who were provided for by so-called "benevolent" institutions. The moral obligation of benevolence, however, was not based on the moral principle of justice, but upon the concept of charity. Hence it was much more lax. Indeed, this "benevolence" generally involved poor and miserly financing that produced conditions that were miserable or clearly bordered upon misery. The literary works of the era are rife with testimony starkly depicting the impoverished character of all such benevolent health institutions (6).

In recent years, the liberal theory of justice has found new health applications. Confronting possible excesses by a "benevolent" State, the new liberals have returned to the thesis that health is an individual right that should be protected by the State, but only "negatively," not in a positive fashion. The State has the obligation in justice to hinder anyone attacking another's bodily integrity, but not to provide health care for all citizens. This is the difference between the negative right to health and the positive right to health care.

Within this context, compulsory health insurance cannot be demanded according to the principle of distributive justice, once distributive justice has been defined in the sense of Locke and Nozick. Thus H. Tristram Engelhardt concludes that "a fundamental human right to health care, even to a decent minimum of health care, does not exist."[3] The reason, says Engelhardt, is that the right to health care exists only where it has been discovered or legislated as such.

In current discussions of health justice, the liberal point of view has found major proponents, though important nuances of difference exist among them. For example, Daniel Beauchamp considers that the clear negative right to health may compel the State to provide certain health services—because physical integrity is threatened not only by a physical attacker but also by harmful factors of a collective and social nature, which are in some way controlled by the State. Since these disease-related factors are caused by society, the State has the obligation to attend to them through a wide-ranging health care program.[4]

A third approach to the matter of distributive justice from the standpoint of liberal theory has been proposed by Baruch Brody. This au-thor begins by accepting Locke's criterion of work as the basis of appropriation; but he understands it as a principle of "acquisition," not of "property." Such a change must be introduced, Brody argues, because the value of a good (farmland, for example) is determined not only by the work done on it but also by the value of its natural resources.

Work, therefore, confers ownership of the value added, but not of the natural resources, which belong to all. In all probability, he continues, it is not possible to distribute these resources among everyone; and so those who exploit them should compensate all others for the benefit they receive for using something that is not theirs.

Accordingly, the social contract must always stipulate the following: that the natural resources in the land belong to those who possess them; but such persons, to compensate, owe a rent to all others that is proportional to the resources used. This rent may be charged in the form of taxes and used to finance a social security fund distributed equally among all. This would constitute redistributive justice. Health care should be considered part of this redistributive justice, but not as a separate and autonomous right, there being no specific right to health care, but only a generic right to the redistribution of certain wealth (7).

Justice as Social Equality

The third of the great theories of justice, which regards justice as social equality, involves numerous variants, some more "utopian," others more "scientific." Of them all, Marxism stands out because of its importance. For Marx and Engels the only advantage of the liberal State is that it does away with the despotic and absolutist State. All else—the attempt to convert the State into a permanent institution based on the theory of civil and political rights—is meaningless.

It is absurd to hypostatize rights as liberal thought does, because neither those rights nor

[3]H. T. Engelhardt, Jr., *The Foundations of Bioethics*, Oxford University Press, New York, 1986. Cf. also H. T. Engelhardt, Health Care Allocations: Responses to the Unjust, the Unfortunate, and the Undesirable, in Earl E. Shelp (ed.), *Justice and Health Care*, Reidel, Dordrecht, 1981, pp. 121–137.

[4]Cf. D. Beauchamp, Alcoholism as blaming the alcoholic, *International Journal of Addiction* 11:41–52, 1976; Public health and social justice, *Inquiry* 13:3–14, 1976. For a critique of this position, cf. T. L. Beauchamp and R. R. Faden, The right to health and the right to health care, *Journal of Medicine and Philosophy* 4:125–126, 1979.

the State based upon them go to the core of human existence. Rather, they are mere superstructure built on an infrastructure defined by the material conditions of life—in particular private property's control over the means of production. For Marx the modern constitutional State, based upon respect for civil and political rights, perpetuates inequality and injustice, because it perpetuates private property's control over the means of production.

This, in turn, makes possible a new definition of distributive justice. Those things that should be distributed equitably are not the means of production but the means of consumption. The problem is defining what is meant by "equitably." Marx solved this problem by adopting an idea of Louis Blanc, which is: "From each according to his ability, to each according to his needs."[5] If we return from here to the classic definition of justice offered by Justinian, "*Justitia est constans et perpetua voluntas just suum cuigue tribuens*" ("justice is the perpetual and constant will to give to each his due"), we see that the change lies in the way in which one defines what is "his due." For liberal thought it is "that which pertains to oneself," while for Marx it is "what one needs." Distributive justice is not adequate if it does not give to each "according to his needs." Only in this way can justice coincide with equality.

With communist justice thus defined, let us now see how it has been applied to health. For that purpose health has been defined as an "ability" and illness as a "need." This interesting pair of definitions makes health a production good and illness a consumption good. Since the State should give to each according to his needs, it has an obligation to provide free and comprehensive health care for all its citizens. This was done in Russia immediately after the 1917 Revolution, drawing on the medical insurance system

(known as the *zemtsvo*) that had existed in Czarist Russia since 1867. In the process, the Soviet State strengthened the *zemtsvo*'s coverage and effectiveness, turning it into a fundamental part of the new socialist order. This Soviet public insurance system has been the model for all those that have been established since in its sphere of political influence.

Justice as Collective Welfare

The socialist thinking that has exercised the greatest influence in Western countries has not been orthodox Marxism but what is called "democratic socialism." As its name indicates, it has advocated a mixed system combining elements of liberal democracy and the social State; and it has given rise to the so-called "social rights State," in particular the "welfare" State.

Using this approach, justice is not defined as mere contractual freedom, but neither is it defined as social equality. Instead, it is understood to mean "collective welfare." The quantitative novelty of the new system is found in the concept of welfare.

During the last century we have been witnessing the birth of a welfare economy, a welfare State, and also, naturally, a welfare ideology. This ideology has its own concept of justice. And since that concept of justice may be the one that is most widespread in the Western countries today, it is worth taking the time to review briefly its origins and nature.

Initially, the principal aim of democratic socialism was to correct the liberal theory by introducing a principle of redistributive equality. Therefore, it did not seek to annul the liberal theory's list of human rights, but rather to round it out with others—namely, economic, social, and cultural rights. The former rights of the liberal theory were called "negative" human rights, since they preceded formation of the State and could be demanded before the existence of any positive law. The latter were considered "positive" human rights, because they could be implemented only by the State, and therefore had no value other than that confer-

[5]K. Marx, Kritik der Gothaer Programms, in *Marx-Engels Werke (vol. 19)*, Dietz, Berlin, 1976, p. 21; cf. R. C. Tucker, Marx and Distributive Justice, in *The Marxian Revolutionary Idea*, W. W. Norton, New York, 1970, p. 48, and G. G. Brenkert, *Marx's Ethics of Freedom*, Routledge and Kegan Paul, London, 1983, p. 246.

red on them by positive law—hence the need to demand them in the political, social, and labor struggle.

In essence, this is what leftist trade unions did in Europe in the second half of the nineteenth century. Democratic socialism arose confronting democratic liberalism. While the latter promoted the *minimal State*, the former tried by all means to establish a *maximal State*, i.e., a State that would promote and protect not only the negative rights but also the positive ones, establish a fair workday, prohibit exploitation of women and children, demand a minimum wage, and protect the unemployed, the sick, the retired, widows, and others from misfortune. Thus arose consciousness of everyone's right to education, adequate housing, well-paid work, unemployment compensation, a pension, and health care.

The importance of this movement for health is clear. While liberalism discovered the *right to health*, socialism cast light on a new right, the *right to health care*. The first is a negative right preceding the social contract, and the State can do nothing but protect it; the second is a positive right that the State must actively guarantee. The first is a specification of the principle of *freedom*, while the second is deduced from the principle of *equality*.

Nevertheless, it should be noted that equality, for socialism, is the condition that makes possible all authentic freedom. Thus it turns out that both rights are derived, albeit by different routes, from freedom. Here one must distinguish between two types of freedom, "freedom from" and "freedom to." However much one may be "free from" external coercion, one cannot live in society under adequate conditions if one does not have "freedom to" work, have a family, raise children, etc., such freedoms being granted by economic, social, and cultural rights. For this reason, socialism began to consider the "freedoms from" as purely formal human rights vis-à-vis the "freedoms to," which were seen as "real" rights.

In the realm of health, this attitude has led people to conceive of health care as something

that can justly be demanded. This in turn has prompted a radical change in the way governments deal with health problems; for in this light health can no longer be considered merely a private matter; rather, it becomes a matter of public concern and hence a political issue. This marks the beginning of "health policy" as a chapter in social and welfare policy. The social justice State, which in the Western countries has become identified with the welfare State (or benevolent State), must have as one of its top priorities protection of the right to health care. Otherwise, the development of the entire Western system of compulsory health insurance would be incomprehensible.

Because the pressure for the aforementioned economic, social, and cultural rights was brought to bear by the labor movement, at first these rights were only applied to workers. (This is why the first compulsory health insurance systems covered only workers.)

Bismarck, Germany's Iron Chancellor, was a pioneer in this area. In the early 1880s he established an extensive social security system to help protect workers against the consequences of accidents, illness, and old age. The medical insurance component of this system, known as the "fund for the ill" (*"Krankenkassen"*), was the first compulsory health insurance and a key foundation-stone of the modern welfare State.

This example was followed shortly thereafter by Great Britain, which approved a Pensioners' Law in 1908 and a National Insurance Law in 1911 that gave rise to a system similar to that of the *Krankenkassen* in the area of health. In 1915 Sweden followed suit with a law on pensions and retirees, which helped create a society that Marquis Childs later dubbed "the Sweden of the just average."

But the definitive take-off of social security and health insurance systems came about as a result of the 1929–1931 economic crisis. As a more or less late response to this crisis, almost all the European states imitated the German health insurance model and instituted health protection for the working class.

The United States entered into a similar process from 1932 to 1943, but concrete gains were very limited—resulting in what Hirschfield has called "the lost reform" (8). In 1946 a general employment law was passed that recognized the Government's responsibility to maintain "maximum employment, productive capacity, and purchasing power." Later, in 1953, the Department of Health, Education, and Welfare (HEW) was established, and this was later used by President Lyndon B. Johnson for his "war on poverty." The medical programs known as Medicare (compulsory health insurance for the elderly) and Medicaid (payment of health care expenses for those considered by local authorities to be needy) were established under the auspices of HEW.[6]

In England, events took a different course. In 1942 the British economist William Beveridge prepared a report for the British Government entitled *Social Insurance and Allied Services*, in which he proposed establishment of a National Health Service that would provide for all citizens' health needs. In 1945 and 1946 the Labor Government issued very advanced social legislation that did not accept the private elements in Beveridge's plan, but that was otherwise based largely upon the Beveridge report. This legislation included the National Health Service Act, which went into effect in 1948. Thus appeared the first National Health Service in the Western world that was obligated to provide coverage for the entire population under all circumstances.

Ever since then, the Western countries' national health systems have had to choose among the three existing types—the liberal, or U.S. system; the socialized, or British system; and the German, or intermediate system—or else they

have had to come up with a more or less original mix of the three. In any event, protection of health as a social right became general as health came to be considered a basic aspect of any social welfare policy; and so the "benevolent" or "welfare" State had to include health care among its priorities.

Beginning in the 1970s, coinciding with the new economic recession, the need for all these welfare policies came to be questioned. Was health care, as had been claimed for decades, a demandable right by virtue of the principle of justice? The polemic was unleashed in the United States, which had never accepted the need for the so-called National Health Systems. In 1971 John Rawls' well-known work, *A Theory of Justice*, appeared. This defined justice not as natural proportionality or contractual freedom or social equality but as "fairness."

By fairness Rawls meant something equally distant from Aristotle, Locke, and Marx, and very close to some of the fundamental ideas of Kantian ethics. In Rawls' view, the naturally moral human being may construct a "well-ordered" society with the following two characteristics: (1) It will be effectively regulated by a public concept of justice; i.e., it will be a society in which all accept, and know that all others also accept, the same principles of right and justice. And (2) the members of a well-ordered society will be free and equal moral persons, and will see themselves and others as such in their political and social relations. Therefore, on the basis of the moral person, one can think of a well-ordered society governed by the principles of freedom and equality.

Rawls' thesis is that a society can only be considered just when it complies with the following principle: "All social values—freedom and opportunity, income and wealth, as well as the social bases and respect for oneself—must be distributed equitably, unless unequal distribution of some or all of these values is to the advantage of all, especially the neediest" (9). Within this context, Rawls' primary social goods are civil and political rights as well as economic, social, and cultural rights.

---

[6]Cf. R. H. Elling (ed.), *National Health Care: Issues and Problems in Socialized Medicine*, Aldine-Atherton, Chicago and New York, 1971; T. R. Marmor, *The Politics of Medicare*, Aldine, New York, 1973; R. Stevens and R. Stevens, *Welfare Medicine in America: A Case Study of Medicaid*, Free Press, New York, 1974; J. M. Feder, *Medicare: The Politics of Federal Hospital Insurance*, Lexington Books, Lexington, 1977; P. Starr, *The Social Transformation of American Medicine*, The Brookings Institution, Washington, D.C., 1982; S. I. David, *With Dignity: The Search for Medicare and Medicaid*, Greenwood Press, Westport, 1985.

In effect, his theory of justice is an intelligent reformulation of social democratic thought. His is thus an intermediate theory between pure "liberalism" and pure "egalitarianism" that understands justice as "fairness."

This theory has been extremely successful. Indeed, no other theoretical study on justice has had such a great impact in this century. Among other things, Rawls' work has had major repercussions for medicine. Whether they accept or criticize Rawls' work, all major studies related to justice in health in the past 15 years have taken his work as a point of departure.

One of the authors who has attempted to apply Rawls' theory of justice to health has been Norman Daniels. In his opinion the right to health care is a primary good subsidiary to the principle of equal opportunity proposed by Rawls. Only in that way, Daniels believes, can an adequate theory on the "right" to health care be constructed whose only possible correct meaning is that of the "justice" of medical care, or "just" medical care.

But, Daniels continues, this demands a precise definition of the "needs" for medical care. Daniels attempts to answer this question using as criteria the "typical functioning of the species." This makes it possible to define conditions that require care, in accordance with the principle of distributive justice to all, as those involving "deviations from the natural functional organization of a member of the species" (10), but not those involving other deviations. For instance, appendicitis should be covered under this approach but not an aquiline nose that could be altered by plastic surgery.

Considering health to be a primary social good that should be added to Rawls' original list has enabled another bioethician, Ronald M. Green, to make some important contributions to justice in health, especially in relation to our duty to safeguard the quality of life of future generations.[7] This latter subject, which received scant attention until recently, is growing progressively more serious—to a point where in the next few years it may become the key topic of discussions on bioethical justice.

Theories other than Daniels' and Green's that should be cited include that of Charles Fried, according to which it is not possible to justify health care as a right derived from the principle of distributive justice, but only as a duty derived from the principle of benevolence. Fried believes that this duty to be benevolent generates a right to assistance that is naturally related to all others, and therefore creates a secondary right of distributive justice. This confers on the State the right and obligation to come to the aid of those most in need of health care until a decent minimum of care is provided.[8]

Other specific models could be added. But it may be more important to reflect on certain common characteristics. One, perhaps the most significant, is the authors' persistent appeal to the bases of Kantian ethics. The entire Rawlsian tradition is based on ethical Kantianism, which is not difficult to justify, as all of the authors cited do, on the grounds that every society is obligated to comply with certain "moral minima."

These moral minima, which Adorno called *"minima moralia"* (11), relate to the concept of justice, i.e., to what the State owes its citizens by virtue of the principle of distributive justice. Some, like Rawls, place these "minima" on the list of "primary social goods"; others, like Amartya Sen, place them elsewhere (12). But all agree on two fundamental points: (1) These moral minima are demandable by virtue of the princi-

[7]Cf. R. M. Green, Health Care and Justice in Contract Theory Perspective, in R. M. Veatch and R. Branson (eds.), *Ethics and Health Policy*, Ballinger, Cambridge, 1976, pp.

111–126; R. M. Green, Justice and the Claims of Future Generations, in E. E. Shelp (ed.), *Justice and Health Care*, Reidel, Dordrecht, 1981, p. 196; Intergenerational distributive justice and environmental responsibility, *Bioscience* 27:260–265, 1977; *Population Growth and Justice*, Scholars Press, Missoula, Montana, 1975.

[8]Cf. C. Fried, Rights and health care: Beyond equity and efficiency, *N Eng J Med* 293:241–245, 1975; C. Fried, Equity and rights in medical care, *Hastings Center Report* 6:29–34, 1976; and Es posible la libertad? In S. M. McMurrin (ed.), *Libertad, igualdad y derecho: Las conferencias Tanner sobre filosofía moral*, Ariel, Barcelona, 1988, pp. 91–132.

ple of justice; and (2) such minima totally or partially cover the area of health care.

The Teleologic Moment: Allocating Scarce Resources

As previously noted, however, justice in health has another equally important dimension. That is because the term "justice" is ambiguous; it has two sides. One looks to principles, the other to consequences. For the first instance, we say something is not just when it violates a deontologic principle, such as that of truthfulness. But in the second we use the term in clearly teleologic contexts; for example, we say that something which fails to attain the maximum benefit at the minimum cost appears to be unjust. If the director of a hospital has a certain sum of money, he must consider how he can spend it so as to produce the maximum health benefit for the community being served. Only then should he feel he has acted justly. Hence, justice involves not only respecting moral principles but also maximizing good consequences.

This second, consequence-oriented aspect of the ethics of justice is extremely important. It also tends to be easier to apply than the principle-oriented aspect, since the issue of consequences is readily quantifiable using mathematical procedures such as those used, for example, by economists. Indeed, this aspect of the ethical doctrine has been developed primarily by economists—including Adam Smith, David Ricardo, and John Stuart Mill.

In this regard, economic rationality is essential to ethical rationality. Among other things, the idea of justice is not completely removed from the economic criterion of "maximum utility" or the so-called "Pareto optimality." Unfortunately, situations to which such criteria can be applied are not very common. Moreover, as originally formulated, the Pareto optimality had only "retrospective" value, being useful only in judging situations already past. It was K. J. Arrow who provided a "prospective" version,

which Allan Gibbard has applied to the problems of justice in health.[9]

Another approach was taken by two British-based economists, John Hicks and Nicholas Kaldor, who developed a broader criterion than Pareto's. This made it possible to accept an act as efficient or efficacious not only if it *was* good for someone, but also if it *could* improve everyone's situation, although in fact it might not. Today this idea of Kaldor and Hicks survives in the form of cost-benefit and cost-effectiveness analyses.[10] In addition, other indices have been derived from these, the best known of which is probably "quality-adjusted life years" (QALY) (13).

The importance of these methods was not recognized until recently. In the 1970s, just as a serious worldwide recession was beginning, economists began to speak of the health cost "explosion." Until then health expenditures had been rising, but at a pace resembling that of economic growth in the developed countries; so the rise was considered normal. Only when the economic recession began and the gross national product stagnated or declined did it become clear that containing health expenditures was very difficult, if not impossible.

This was the moment economists had been awaiting—to chide physicians and policy-makers for irrational health resource management. Until then, the deontologic moment had been thought sufficient for establishing health policy, but at this point the consequences of such an approach became apparent. A radical change in

---

[9]Cf. the excellent work of A. Gibbard, The Prospective Pareto Principle and Equity of Access to Health Care, in President's Commission for the Study of Ethical Problems in Medicine and Biomedical and Behavioral Research, *Securing Access to Health Care: The Ethical Implications of Differences in the Availability of Health Services* (vol. 2), U.S. Government Printing Office, Washington, D.C., 1983, pp. 138–140 and 153–178.

[10]The bibliography on these indices is vast. Cf. P.S. Wenz, CBA, Utilitarianism, and Reliance upon Intuitions, in G. J. Agich and C. E. Begley (eds.), *The Price of Health*, Reidel, Dordrecht, 1986, pp. 71-89; and R. Audi, Cost-Benefit Analysis, Monetary Value, and Medical Decision, in G. J. Agich and C. E. Begley (eds.), *op. cit.*, pp. 113–131.

policy was needed, according to the economists, one that gave priority to the teleologic moment. Health expenditures, like all others, should be made in accordance with the laws of economic reality. All else was pure squandering, which could lead only to disaster.

This disaster began to be perceived as uncomfortably imminent in the 1970s. In 1978 economist J. M. Simon used data published by the MacKinsey Institute to calculate that health expenditures by the rich countries had increased by 1 supplementary percentage point of the gross national product of each country from 1950 to 1960; by 1.5 supplementary points from 1960 to 1970; and by 2 supplementary points from 1970 to 1980. These figures clearly illustrate the rapid growth of health expenditures as a share of domestic product.

However surprising it may seem, this rate of growth is actually no surprise at all, since in our century we have changed from treating health care like a production good to treating it as a consumption good. In 1857 German statistician Ernst Engel formulated three laws on the evolution of consumption, which are as follows: First, food spending as a share of the family budget decreases as income increases. Thus, food expenses in France accounted for 64.2% of the family budget in 1950, 27.9% in 1970, and 25.9% in 1976. Second, the percentage of the budget spent on buying goods such as clothes and furniture, and on paying rent, tends to remain constant. These expenditures evolve in proportion to income. Thus, they accounted for 27.1% of the family budget in the France of 1950, as compared to 29.4% in 1960 and 31% in 1970 and 1975. And third, the share of the budget spent on services, cultural goods, and leisure (hygiene and health, culture, education, vacations, transportation, communication and telecommunications, insurance, etc.) tends to increase as income increases. In France these expenditures accounted for 26.7% of the total budget in 1950, 34.5% in 1960, 41.1% in 1970, and 43.2% in 1975 (14).

The fact that health is a consumption item

obeying Engel's third law explains why there are no theoretical obstacles to health expenditures increasing more quickly than a country's total wealth. (In the United States, per capita health expenditures have tripled since 1950.)

Nevertheless, the figures prompt certain questions. Can other social and public services be allowed to go underfunded in order to attend to health demands? Is every health expenditure ethically justified and demandable in justice? Must the right to health and the right to health care be covered in all of their unending dimensions, or are there some limits to demand, beyond which nothing can be demanded in justice? If so, what are those limits?

These questions, which have become urgent since the 1973 economic crisis, have led to a massive influx of economists and their teleologic criteria into the health field. This would seem all the more necessary because technologic advances of the preceding decade had shot costs upwards, partly because such advances permitted people who in any other epoch would have died without recourse to be kept alive for long periods.

The young Karen Ann Quinlan lived in a permanent vegetative state for over 10 years. Was there an obligation by virtue of the principle of justice to provide her all sorts of medical care? The question has considerable social import, for hers is but one example of a practice that has become commonplace for medicine— the practice of acting in an anti-Darwinian direction.

If Nature, according to Darwin, selects the most apt and condemns to death the weak and unadapted, medicine does exactly the opposite. This constantly increases the number of chronically ill with no hope of recovery (disabled children, the retarded, the incapacitated elderly, etc.) and contributes very substantially to the "cost explosion." So the question comes around again: Is there an obligation grounded in justice to attend to all these patients with all the resources involved in their care? Up to what point should they be treated? When does the obligation cease to be perfect (or one of justice) and become imperfect (or one of charity)?

For economists and health managers this series of questions has a relatively clear answer. The cost explosion can only be halted by "cost containment," and this must be done in accordance with the criteria of economic rationality. Thus, distributive justice must be governed by the cost-benefit ratio, so that there is never any obligation to do something "irrational" in justice (understanding rationality to mean economic rationality). In other words, that which is just is identified with some approximation of the economically optimal.

This has several implications. First, however "limited" health resources (they will always be limited whenever health consumption is unlimited), it is not just to divert funding from other budget areas to health if the cost-benefit ratio is better in fields other than health. Thus, for example, education or housing policy may have a higher cost-benefit ratio, in which case what is just is to invest in those areas.

Second, within the health realm the limited resources should be earmarked for activities that yield a relatively great health benefit at a relatively low cost. For example, if one must choose between a vaccination campaign and heart transplants, in most cases the cost-benefit ratio will accord greater priority to the vaccination program, even though this may lead to damage and even death for some people.

Third, certain health benefits and services cannot be demanded in justice, given their low cost-benefit ratios. This was the case until a short time ago with respect to heart, lung, and liver transplants; at present it appears to be the case regarding brain-dead patients, permanent vegetative states, etc.

These examples help to show why economic rationality is important in health care and how it provides a new and essential perspective on the issue of justice in health. Today we know that one cannot construct a coherent theory of justice with deontologic principles alone. The teleologic complement, which weighs and assesses consequences, is also needed.

All this makes it easy to see why bioethical studies of what is now known as "cost containment" and "distribution of scarce resources" are important. Such studies include the interesting work that Haavi Morreim has been carrying out on the problem of justice in U.S. health,[11] and also the impressive group of works by various authors partaking in the lively current debate over the limits of the younger generations' duty of justice vis-à-vis the elderly.[12]

But this does not resolve all the problems. It is still unclear whether economic rationality must be reconciled with the rationality of the principles of justice, or whether it should supplant the rationality of justice, leaving utility as the sole criterion. When the latter happens, when utility becomes the only criterion capable of defining an action as just or unjust, then we have another theory of justice, the utilitarian theory so common in our culture since the times of Jeremy Bentham.

In his *Fragments on Government*, Bentham established that the objective of any ruler can be none other than to bring about the greatest happiness of his subjects; and to do so he has no recourse other than to be guided by the principle that "the greatest happiness of the greatest number is the measurement of what is just and

[11]Cf. E. H. Morreim, Cost containment: Issues of moral conflict and justice for physicians, *Theoretical Medicine* 6(3):257, 1985; E. H. Morreim, Stratified scarcity and unfair liability, *Case Western Reserve Law Review* 36(4):1033–1057, 1986; E. H. Morreim, Cost containment and the standard of medical care, *California Law Review* 75(5):1719–1763, 1987; E. H. Morreim, Clinicians or committees: Who should cut costs? *Hastings Center Report* 17(2):45, 1987; E. H. Morreim, Cost constraints as a malpractice defense, *Hastings Center Report* 18(1):5–10, 1988; E. H. Morreim, Cost containment: Challenging fidelity and justice, *Hastings Center Report* 18(6):20–25, 1988.

[12]Today the bibliography on this topic is quite extensive. Cf., among others, the following: L. Olson et al., *The Elderly and the Future Economy*, D. C. Heath, Lexington, 1981; A. Pifer and L. Bronte, *Our Aging Society*, Norton, New York, 1986; D. Callahan, *Setting Limits: Medical Goals in an Aging Society*, Simon and Schuster, New York, 1987; N. Daniels, *Am I My Parents' Keeper? An Essay on Justice Between the Young and the Old*, Oxford University Press, New York, 1988; N. Daniels (ed.), Justice between generations and health care for the elderly, *The Journal of Medicine and Philosophy* 13(1):5–116, 1988.

what is unjust" (*15*). There can be no other criterion of distributive justice. As a promoter of the *res publica*, the politician must seek to achieve the greatest benefit at minimal cost, so as to maximize utility. This is very important today in medicine, since health has become a public matter, a political issue.

But is it not unjust to govern health policy solely and exclusively by criteria of economic utility? And conversely, is it not equally unjust to "reject" the utilitarian and consequence-oriented dimension of health as rendering health policy "absolute"? More specifically, is justice in health *solely* consequence-oriented, or is it *also* consequence-oriented? This is the last point we will address.

Conclusion: The Two Moments of Justice in Health

This brief review of the contemporary debate on justice in health illustrates just how complex the matter is. One reason for that complexity is that workable theories in this field, to explain events, must perforce articulate the two moments cited, the deontologic or principle-oriented moment and the teleologic or consequence-oriented moment.

In the Western world, there seems to have been a certain convergence of the various deontologic theories contesting the explanation of distributive justice—such that the theory which understands justice to be synonymous with collective welfare is clearly the most generally accepted. The fact that almost all human rights declarations and the constitutions of many Western countries place the slate of economic, social, and cultural rights alongside civil and political rights suggests that the deontologic theory of justice cannot be understood today as "natural proportionality," or as "contractual freedom," or (at least in most of our countries) as "social equality," but rather as "collective welfare."

Agreement is even clearer regarding the teleologic moment. Health promoters and policy-makers have an obligation to maximize the "public utility" of available resources, for which purpose they must act in accordance with economic principles and criteria. And although economics is neither alien to nor separable from deontologic principles, it has developed a wide range of techniques and procedures of a strictly teleologic nature, which are the ones that may prove most useful to those in government in their endeavors. Hence, to deny the consequence-oriented moment of justice in health would be as dangerous as rendering that moment absolute.

Once the duality of moments is accepted, the mode of their articulation must be established. How do they relate to one another? In some cases they "complement" one another, and then there is no doubt that one's moral duty is to respect all the principles involved and optimize all the consequences. Unfortunately, however, such cases do not abound and may well be exceptions. Indeed, what is most common in ethics is not complementarity but conflict, conflict between principles and consequences as well as between different principles.

How should such situations be resolved? Ideally, the two categories should be reduced to a single one, since properly speaking there are no conflicts between principles and consequences, but only between principles. That is because we use the consequences as criteria for ranking the principles.

Generalizing this procedure, one arrives at conclusions very similar to those proposed half a century ago by David Ross. According to these, deontologic principles (e.g., those involving each and every human right—civil and political, economic, social, and cultural) may be considered "*prima facie* duties." When these primary duties do not enter into conflict among themselves, then they are morally binding, and therefore also constitute "actual duties." But when two or more are incompatible in a concrete situation, such that respecting one necessarily harms another, then they must be ranked.

This can be done in several ways. In some cases one can establish the order among them using solely deontologic criteria; thus, civil rights are generally accorded a higher rank than social rights. But these cases are the least of it. In general, to establish a proper hierarchy one must bear in mind the so-called teleologic principles relating to the consequences of the various possible acts. This ranking of deontologic principles partly in accordance with the second moment of the theory of justice makes it possible to resolve conflicts among principles and convert the "*prima facie* duties" into "actual duties."

Any of the methods just presented for solving conflicts among the different constitutive elements would appear theoretically correct. However, this does not mean the selected method would be adhered to in real, everyday practice. Indeed, it is likely that the greatest problem of justice in health facing our countries today is that of the failure of actual practice to conform to the theoretical principles set forth above. Health policies are usually devised with almost exclusively utilitarian criteria in mind, paying little heed—less than should be paid—to the principles of equity. To put it more graphically, it could be said that economics and politics have done away with ethics. In this sense I believe that what the Hastings Center said in a study about the ethics of cost-benefit analysis (CBA) holds across the board: "The traditional approach of CBA excludes formal considerations of the distributive effect, of the equity and justice variety. Although economists disagree on how to resolve this problem, it is likely that considerations of equity will continue to be underestimated in practice" (*16*).

This is the concluding point of our analysis: that in the obligatory dialectic between principles and consequences, the latter receive little attention in theory, and the former continue to be underestimated in practice. In other words, in issues related to distributive justice in health, ethics appears to have ignored economics and politics, which in turn have decided to ignore ethics, if not supplant it; and this appears to constitute a serious form of injustice.

References

1. Aristotle, *Et. Nic.*, V. 2: 1130b31s.
2. Locke, J. *The Second Treatise of Government.* 1690. Bobbs-Merrill, 1952.
3. Locke, J. *Dos ensayos sobre el gobierno civil.* Aguilar, Madrid, 1969, pp. 94 and 103.
4. Nozick, R. *Anarchy, State, and Utopia.* Basic Books, New York, 1974, p. 149.
5. Hartzfeld, H. *La crisis de la medicina liberal.* Ariel, Barcelona, 1965.
6. Laín Entralgo, P. *La relación médico-enfermo: Historia y teoría.* Revista de Occidente, Madrid, 1964, pp. 198–314.
7. Brody, B. Health Care for the Haves and Have-nots: Toward a Just Basis of Distribution. In: Earl E. Shelp (ed.). *Justice and Health Care.* Reidel, Dordrecht, 1981, pp. 151–159.
8. Hirschfield, D. *The Lost Reform.* Harvard University Press, Cambridge, 1970.
9. Rawls, J. *A Theory of Justice.*
10. Daniels, N. *Just Health Care.* Cambridge University Press, Cambridge, 1985, p. 28.
11. Adorno, T. W. *Minima moralia: Reflexiones sobre la vida dañada.* Taurus, Madrid, 1987.
12. Sen, A. Igualdad de qué? In: S. M. McMurrin (ed.). *Libertad, igualdad y derecho: Las conferencias Tanner sobre filosofía moral.* Ariel, Barcelona, 1988, pp. 134–156, esp. pp. 152–154.
13. La medición del nivel de salud. *Jano* (712):511–576, 1986.
14. Gracia, D. Medicina social. In: *Avances del Saber.* Labor, Barcelona, 1984, p. 200.
15. Bentham, J. *Fragments on Government.*
16. The Hastings Center. Appendix D: Values, Ethics, and CBA in Health Care. In: Office of Technology Assessment. *The Implications of Cost-Effectiveness Analysis of Medical Technology.* U.S. Government Printing Office, Washington, D.C., 1980, p. 175.

Justice Issues in Health Care Delivery

James F. Drane

When one speaks of freedom, or truth, or love, people have a common-sense understanding of what the terms mean. The same is not true of justice. Even in Aristotle's time the term justice communicated more ambiguity than clarity. One reason is that justice sometimes refers to the whole of one's moral life (the just man), while at others it is taken more narrowly as referring to what is lawful. In the context of health care, justice has still another meaning, this being what philosophers call "distributive justice," fair distribution of scarce goods throughout a community.

For all its pretense of clarifying complexities, philosophy has not yet succeeded in clearing up the muddles surrounding the term justice and its different meanings. Despite this, the topic of justice in health care has been at the center of medical ethics concerns for many years. For medical ethicists, the decade of the eighties was dominated by debates over allocation of scarce resources and distributive justice, and this is not expected to change in the 1990s. Indeed, if the next decade in medical ethics is thought of in musical terms, we can foresee that the justice debate will be the unifying theme, with differing theories of justice creating a point-counterpoint refrain that will be repeated no matter what issues are considered.

Health Care Delivery becomes a Problem

Every country has justice problems in the sense of difficulties achieving just distribution of scarce health care. The United States spends US$600 billion a year on health care, and even those of us who cannot comprehend such figures know that is a lot of money. The health insurance costs of an individual American can easily reach US$400 a month, while the annual cost of private health insurance coverage for a family may exceed US$12,000.

As this suggests, even rich nations find health care costs spiralling out of control and are compelled to wrestle with justice questions as competing claims exceed available resources. Technology, third party payers, physicians' specialization, patient expectations, the number and type of hospitals, and the structure of financing systems all push health care costs higher and force hard thinking about what justice requires in the distribution of health care services. And what is true of wealthy nations regarding the affordability of health care costs is even more true of struggling and developing ones.

As pressure mounts on health care delivery systems, demands for restructuring and reform grow louder. Indirectly, these demands are also calls for hard thinking about philosophic, political, economic, and ethical issues. One can go along with a properly functioning health system without critical reflection on its underlying principles; but when signs of collapse appear or restructuring is called for, hard thinking cannot be avoided.

A principal reason is that rebuilding or even reforming a threatened medical care delivery system has to take into consideration different claims about justice. When people responsible for health care institutions address the need for change, they have to consider competing health care models, and behind every model are theories about what makes health care delivery right or just or good. Hence, reflection about health care structure and resource allocation always involves questions about justice.

Such reflection is sometimes ideologic, in the sense of being driven by a set of fixed beliefs accompanied by strong emotions. Associated with ideologic solutions are familiar rhetorical phrases: "Doctors have a right to freedom of choice." "Patients have a right to health care." "Free enterprise and competition will solve medicine's problems." "In every advanced nation today the State provides health care for all." Most people who hold opinions about health care are not philosophers, but behind many strongly endorsed solutions lie philosophic theories. Hence, intelligent reflection or debate about health care is advanced by an understanding of background philosophic theories and the ethical terms associated with them.

The Role of Justice Theories

Because contemporary cultures are pluralistic, no one set of values is accepted by all members, and no one theory of justice dominates. Consequently, different theoretical foundations support different models of health care organization. When health care policy-makers alter delivery systems, they often seize on some aspect of one or another justice theory in order to justify

their decisions. This doesn't mean that philosophic theories of justice dictate how a particular culture will structure the concrete dimensions of its health care system; nevertheless, such theories do influence the organization of health care.

Socialist theory combined with concrete pressure from workers unhappy with a traditional health care system led to major structural changes during the nineteenth century in Germany and later in the Soviet Union. Pragmatic political considerations did as much as theory to restructure health systems toward what today we call socialized medicine, but theory played a part. Moreover, it still plays a part, even in the less theory-driven capitalist countries, most of which have come to adopt a modified version of the socialist model. As community after community, and nation after nation, faces continuing problems with health care, different political groups call for different types of restructuring and support their calls for change with arguments derived from theories of justice.

The reason such theoretical arguments are important is that human beings require justification for what they do. Theories of justice do not generate full-blown health care delivery systems, but they do provide all-important justifications for them, while supporting or condemning particular pragmatic solutions. Indeed, it may be that theories play their most powerful social role in criticizing and condemning that which is unjustifiable and unfair. It is within this context that theories of justice, political pressure groups, think-tanks with private agendas, and hard-nosed empirical studies on the consequences of different options all play a role in the challenging search for a workable health care delivery system that is also just.

Types of Justice Theories

Different theories of justice tend to agree about abstract classic formulae such as "*cuique suum*" ("give to everyone his due" or "treat like cases alike"). But such agreement produces no agreed-upon particular answers to questions about what really is due, or in what particular respect cases or people are equal. Competing theories of justice therefore attempt to specify what is everyone's due, what is basic equality, in order to be more specific and fill in the empty classic formulae with content. In this way material and concrete principles flesh out the formal and abstract ones.

These former material principles of justice either specify what is due everyone (in terms of benefits like health and burdens like taxes) or else specify how people are equal and how they should be treated equally. In other words, these principles establish the basic standards for distribution of burdens and benefits.

Of course, not all these material theories of justice agree with one another. At one end of the spectrum are principles like "to each according to individual need," and at the other are ones like "to each according to fair acquisition in a free market economy." And between the two extremes are theories that contain mixed elements. No one theory of justice convinces everyone, and yet elements of different theories enjoy very broad public support.

Libertarian Theories

Justice according to Libertarian theories is not an independent moral principle with separate content. There are separate moral principles like truth, fidelity, beneficence, etc., with their own meanings, but justice is reducible to the principle of autonomy or freedom. If the exercise of freedom (primarily economic) is protected and guaranteed, then according to these theories justice is done.

As this suggests, Libertarians question the very existence of a distributive justice that would presume to take any goods away from anyone who earned them fair and square: "The term distributive justice is not a neutral one. Hearing the term 'distribution,' most people presume that some thing or mechanism uses some principle or criteria to give out a supply of things. Into this process of distributing shares, some error may have crept. So it is an open question, at least, whether *redistribution* should take place; whether we should do again what has already been done once" (1).

Libertarian theories are often mixed with theories of merit or theories based on a person's contribution to society. They assume that hard work and ability ought to be rewarded, and that a person's freedom to decide how to spend these rewards ought to be protected. The exercise of a free market is assumed to do the distributive task and take care of distributive justice. Though free market distribution is deemed to create inequalities regarding access to health care, Libertarians do not consider these unjust and do not believe they should be remedied by tax plans or any other type of redistribution.

This reduction of justice to personal freedom involves an important assumption about individual responsibility for ill health. Libertarians frequently use examples provided by smokers, gluttons, and sky-divers to make their point. State involvement in health education is more acceptable to them than State-supported health care. They tend to emphasize the efficiency created by application of free-market principles to health care delivery. And they naturally prefer private health insurance systems in which each person purchases the amount of health care he or she wishes, or can afford.

Libertarianism is applied to health care in a systematic way by H. Tristram Engelhardt, Jr. (2). Following Nozick, Engelhardt believes that justice is done when people are not coerced, not even by a government collecting taxes to carry out projects endorsed by the majority.

Engelhardt distinguishes between illness and disease caused by another person, which he calls "unfair," and the same conditions not so caused, which he calls "unfortunate." Within this context, *retributive* justice, which requires government intervention and even forced retribution in case of injury, is consistent with Libertarian principles. Another supporter of Libertarianism, Charles Freed, does not object to some government involvement in health care delivery so long as the patient is the one who makes the choice (3). In addition, even within the Libertarian framework some government involvement in health care is needed to address public threats like AIDS, TB, malaria, sexually transmitted diseases, etc.; and neither Engelhardt nor any other Libertarian objects to economically advantaged people acting charitably toward the poor.

Engelhardt summarizes his support of a Libertarian view of justice as follows:

A market [Libertarian] approach maximizes free choice in the sense of minimizing interventions in the free associations of individuals and in the disposition of private property. In not intervening, it allows individuals to choose as they wish and as they are able what they hold to be best for their health care. It makes no pretense at cost containment. Health care will cost as much and will receive as much commitment of resources as individuals choose. The percentage of the gross national product devoted to health care will rise to a level determined by the free choices of health care providers and consumers. If some element of health care becomes too expensive or not worth as much as a competing possible expenditure, individuals will engage in cost containment through not purchasing such health care, and its price will tend to fall. Finally, there will be no attempt to achieve equality, though there will be considerable room for sympathy and for the loving care of those in need. A free market economy, through maximizing the freedom of those willing and able to participate, may create more resources than any other system and thus in the long run best advantage those most harmed through the natural lottery. By creating a larger middle class, the market may tend to create greater equality at a higher standard of living and of health care than would alternative systems. Further, charity can at least blunt severe losses at the natural and social lotteries.[1]

Engelhardt's endorsement of a Libertarian view of justice is far from being flat-footed. His or anyone's application of Libertarian philosophic assumptions to the issues of health care delivery depend upon factual circumstances, especially the extent to which the free market is

now or will remain the best provider of a high standard of living and of health care. Even Engelhardt recognizes the advantage of a mixed or two-tiered system that provides at least some health care for all while allowing affluent people to purchase additional health care if they desire:

My analyses of the principles of autonomy and beneficence and of entitlements to property support a two-tiered system of health care. Not all property is privately owned. Nations and other social organizations may invest their common resources in insuring their members against losses in the natural and social lotteries. On the other hand, . . . not all property is communal. There are private entitlements, which individuals may freely exchange for the services of others. The existence of a two-tiered system (whether officially or unofficially) in nearly all nations and societies reflects the existence of both communal and private entitlements, of social choice and individual aspiration. A two-tiered system with inequality in health care distribution would appear to be both morally and factually inevitable.

The serious task will be to decide how to create a decent minimum as a floor of support for all members of a society, while allowing money and free choice to fashion a special tier of services for the advantaged members of society. The problem will be to define what will be meant by a "decent minimum" or "minimum adequate amount" of health care . . . .[2]

Having said this, Engelhardt returns to the centrality of autonomy and free choice, as he insists that different communities and nations will generate different views of that minimum which can be provided by public support. Some will not be able to provide any health care out of the public treasury. In more affluent societies like the United Kingdom, a decent minimum will not include dialysis for patients over 55 years of age (which is provided in the United States). Heart transplants are not included in the U.S. minimum.

Particular systems of health care exclude others. Particular systems of health care are particular in choosing certain goals but not others, in ranking some goals higher and others lower. That patients in one system will receive care that they

---

[1]H. T. Engelhardt, Jr. (2), p. 357.

[2]H. T. Engelhardt, Jr. (2), pp. 361–362.

would not in another, that patients who would be saved in one system die for lack of care in another, is not necessarily a testimony to moral malfeasance. It may as well be the result of the different choices and visions of different free men and women. As we have seen, there are limits to our capacity as humans to discover correctly what we ought to do together. We humans must instead settle for deciding fairly what we will do together, when we cannot together discover what we ought to do. Even gods and goddesses must choose to create one world rather than another. So, too, must we.[3]

Equalitarian Theories

If justice for Libertarian theorists is essentially the protection of autonomy, for the Equalitarians it is essentially equality. Justice is done when resources are allocated to those in greatest need, so that disparities are overcome and as much equality as possible is achieved. If Libertarian theories are grounded in modern or postmodern secular visions of life, Equalitarians tend to share a more religious vision—one in which people are called upon to do more than recognize the lottery-like dimensions of a life that distributes benefits and burdens unequally. The religious task, and the task of justice, is to work to overcome natural and social inequalities through rational altruistic policies.

Libertarians and Equalitarians agree that health care costs, like defense expenditures, can absorb the resources of any nation. (People never seem to have enough health or enough defense.) The ethics of health care allocation address the problem of deciding who has an ethical claim on scarce resources. Every community and nation is forced to contain health care costs, so the ethical question is how the cost containment should occur.

Equalitarian theorists insist that scarce resources be used where there is the greatest need, rather than where free market forces determine. Bioethicists who espouse this view include Robert Veatch (4), James Childress (5), Jean Outka

(6), Paul Ramsey (7), and many others. Moreover, many of the structural health care changes proposed in the U.S. during the 1960s and 1970s relied heavily upon equalitarian arguments coming from politicians and political economists; and the concept of equal access to health care based on need still enjoys broad support worldwide.

Critics talk about the ambiguity of "need." Even if those citizens in greatest need could be identified, channeling care to the most needy could quickly exhaust any budget.

Veatch responds by setting out a view of what constitutes a moral community that differs radically from Engelhardt's. For Veatch, every person's welfare must count equally if a group is to qualify as a moral community. Inequality is not accepted as an "act of God." Morality is seen in terms of meeting needs and achieving impartiality. Social decision-making, both in health care and in other areas of social life, must take equal account of all persons; and only by so doing does a community move beyond egoism into a moral perspective.

"The Equalitarian understanding of the principle of justice is one that sees justice as requiring (subject to certain important qualifications) equality of net welfare for individuals" (3).

What Veatch means by equality is neither equal ability nor equal merit of individual claims. His understanding of justice as equality is that people have a claim that the total net quality of their lives be equal as far as possible with the net quality or welfare of others. Consequently, when benefits are distributed, those least well off will be the ones most favorably impacted if the benefits are distributed justly. Just distribution should have the goal of equalizing welfare as its primary objective. Gross inequalities are fundamentally wrong, and their remediation should be the aim of any just social policy. Thus, equalitarian justice requires that social practices and policies strive for an equality of net welfare.

Within this framework, simple equal distribution of health care would be foolish. If the goal of justice is to produce a chance for equal net

---

[3]H. T. Engelhardt, Jr. (2), pp. 368–369.

welfare, distributing care to those in need is critical. Therefore, Veatch does not favor giving the same amount of care to all but rather providing health care in proportion to need, focusing especially upon the most needy.

But Veatch, like other theorists, also faces up to the hard facts of economics, bureaucracies, and conceptual ambiguities. In so doing, he sums up how his Equalitarian theory of justice finally influences what is actually done by health care planners and how his theory differs pragmatically from Libertarian theories:

> With a fixed budget, reasonable people will come together to decide what health care services can be covered under it. The task will not be as great as it seems. The vast majority of services will easily be sorted into or out of the health care system. Only a small percentage at the margin will be the cause of any real debate. The choice will at times be arbitrary, but the standard applied will at least be clear. People should have services necessary to give them a chance to be as close as possible to being as healthy as other people. Those choices will be made while striving to emulate the position of original contractors taking the moral point of view. The decision-making panels will not differ in task greatly from the decision-makers who currently sort health care services into and out of insurance coverage lists. However, panels will be committed to a principle of justice and will take the moral point of view, whereas the self-interested insurers try to maximize profits or efficiency or a bargaining position against weak, unorganized consumers.[4]

Equalitarian-Libertarian Theories

John Rawls, in his influential work *A Theory of Justice* (8), asserts that society is a grouping of people dedicated to advancing the good of all. Rawls maintains that the basic "goods" involved are liberty and equality; and he arrives at the basic values of both by lowering a veil of ignorance that functions as an epistemologic device.

Specifically, Rawls asks what rational people would choose if, behind "a veil of ignorance," they were asked to decide on principles for a just

society. No one knows what his or her station or particular lot would be, and on this basis decisions about the just structure of society can be made. In other words, Rawls believes that a just society would be one ruled by the principles that rational people devise in a state of rational blindness or veiled ignorance.

Using this approach, Rawls finds that the first emerging principle is that of liberty. A just society, Rawls insists with the Libertarians, is one of maximum liberty. Liberty is basic for a just society because it provides the basis for individual or personal self-esteem. No rational person, according to Rawls, would sacrifice basic liberty, even for material possessions. Hence, "each person is to have an equal right to the most extensive total system of basic liberty compatible with a similar system of liberty for all."

But rationality behind the veil of ignorance also reveals another basic principle of a just society. Natural and social lotteries generate inequalities; and rational people ignoring their place in society would want to minimize these inequalities. Therefore, a just society would be one that minimizes the accidents of history and biology by espousing the ideal of equality.

This Rawlsian principle of equality or fair distribution, as asserted by unencumbered reason, means that justice (working through just social institutions) should improve the lot of the least advantaged as much as possible. In order to overcome the inequalities of life's lotteries, the equality principle requires compensation for people who suffer handicaps. It also redresses naturally unequal distributions of benefits by making inequalities acceptable only if they benefit the least advantaged. The just society, then, would be one ruled by the dual principles of liberty and equality—such that justice translates into freedom and fairness.

Many different thinkers refer to some aspect of Rawls' theory for support and justification. Veatch, for one, uses a Rawlsian framework—both a contract theory of justice and a variation on the veil of ignorance device (which Veatch calls the moral point of view). He refers to

---

[4]R. M. Veatch (4), p. 265.

Rawls' theory as a "maximum" position and takes a more radical equalitarian stance to distinguish his own viewpoint. That is, Rawls' just society tolerates inequalities so long as they provide relatively greater benefits to those with less. Veatch wants just policies to focus on achieving equality in a more direct and straightforward way.

Applied to health care, Rawls' equality principle requires that health delivery systems grant the least well off access to a certain level of medical care and services, so as to maximize their benefits. In this manner, this principle provides a standard against which particular health care systems can be tested. The thrust of Rawls' theory is that a just society (or institution or health care system) is one that ensures maximum liberty and works against inequalities.

Although Rawls does not himself apply his theory to health care delivery issues, other philosophers do. Among the most prominent is Norman Daniels (9), who argues that health care should be provided so that more persons would be free to take advantage of society's opportunities. Daniels insists that there should be no obstacles—either financial, racial, geographic, or sexual—to initial access when health needs are present; for he argues that without minimal health care for all, the idea of equal opportunity simply will not work.

Daniels also moves from this philosophic argument to more concrete policy issues, recommending planning strategies that will make his justice standard politically feasible. He insists that a rough measure of equal opportunity—enough to revise and carry out one's life plan—be present at each stage in life, even for the elderly. This of course requires financial planning, because the elderly will consume proportionally larger amounts of health care resources. Daniels therefore makes tax recommendations aimed at providing such benefits without creating conflicts with younger generations (10). The underlying theoretical foundation for these restructuring plans is the Rawlsian theory of justice.

Utilitarian Theories

All the above-mentioned theories could be described as deontologic. Justice in every instance is identified with a principle that establishes what is right or just independent of consequences. But not all theories of justice are based on principle. Specifically, the fathers of Utilitarianism, Jeremy Bentham (11) and John Stuart Mill (12), attempted to move away from an ethics driven by principle; they set out to reform legal and social institutions on the basis of objective calculations about social benefits.

In general, Utilitarians believe that right or just actions are not those that conform to principles but those that produce desirable results or minimize undesirable ones. Regarding health, individual responsibility to do good and avoid evil, social responsibility in the sense of duty to create a decent society, and the economic resources available all have to be balanced in order to fashion a system of health care that is just according to Utilitarian theory.

According to this approach, justice obliges people to prevent evils such as diseases and poor health as much as possible. But health care justice provides no independent ethical standard. Indeed, the term "utility" at the heart of Utilitarianism may be defined as meaning the greatest good for the greatest number; and within this context, Utilitarians see justice as merely another term for talking about this objective. When it comes to making health care policy or reforming a health care system, rather than striving to make the system promote an independent standard of justice such as equality or freedom, Utilitarians look for trade-offs, compromises, partial allocations that maximize benefits and minimize costs while striking a balance among competing groups. It should be noted, however, that these benefits and costs are measured for the greatest number and not for any special population (like the most needy).

Nonphilosophers who work with health care issues (politicians, economists, social policy planners, government health care administrators, etc.) most often assume an underlying Utilitarianism. They work to design or reform the system so that many different interests are balanced, positive outcomes for most people are achieved, and burdens are spread evenly throughout society. Those innocent of philosophy may even identify the Utilitarian approach with common sense, missing the underlying assumptions and problems of their perspective.

The principal problem is that achieving the greatest benefits for the greatest number is not as simple as it looks. In particular, there is the problem of how to quantify benefits and burdens in order to make just choices. Things like pain, death, and disability are hard to quantify; and comparing benefits and burdens means comparing much that is subjective rather than objective.

Objective cost estimates can be attempted, however approximate they inevitably turn out to be. But if Equalitarians can rightly be faulted for not giving enough attention to economic costs, the Utilitarians can certainly be faulted for overestimating the objectivity of their cost analyses. Indeed, cost balancing often loses contact with individuals who are helped or harmed. Policies that produce the greatest net benefit for most people may involve terrible costs for small groups who are unattended. It is precisely these least advantaged that the Equalitarians and Rawlsians insist on helping.

Utilitarians side with Equalitarians about the moral superiority of altruism over Libertarian egoism, but differ with them about how to make concrete health care allocations.

In general, Libertarians seem more sensitive than Utilitarians about redressing harms or injuries. That is, Libertarians require government action to redress injuries caused by others, whereas Utilitarians might excuse such injury if it were accompanied by great social benefit.

The highest compliment theorists of other persuasions pay to Utilitarian theories of justice is the use they inevitably make of Utilitarian strategies for cost-assessment of alternatives. John Rawls himself uses such strategies (13).

Tom L. Beauchamp (14), a widely published

bioethicist, applies a Utilitarian perspective to the issue of justice in health care allocation. In so doing, he denies making any practical application of deontologic theories of justice: "Policies governing practical matters of great complexity cannot be directly and consistently derived from highly abstract principles. Such derivations cannot be achieved in law, and even less can they be achieved in philosophy. There is no single, consistent set of material principles of distributive justice that reliably applies when concrete issues of justice arise" (15).

Beauchamp's starting point is in the midst of financial exigencies and political pressures. These can be measured and balanced, and only by doing so can one move toward a just health care policy. For Beauchamp, cost-benefit analysis rather than moral principle is the method of choice for arriving at justice (16).

There is no positive right to health care for Beauchamp, and yet he does recognize some sort of social obligation to provide health care goods and services. How much service and care depends not upon the obligations created by principles, but rather upon careful measuring and balancing of costs and benefits. Within this context, Utilitarian theory might support a decent minimum of health care for all or might not, depending on the fiscal circumstances and political pressures involved.

If deontologists fault Utilitarians for the ambiguities associated with weighing hard-to-quantify human benefits and burdens, Utilitarians and Beauchamp fault deontologists for the ambiguities associated with defining just what they mean by "need," a "decent minimum," and "socially caused" disease. If people want to talk about rights to health care services, Beauchamp insists that the focus be placed on limitation of such rights and specification of the health care services that can be afforded. For him the "major issues about rights to health and to health care turn on the justifiability of social expenditures rather than on some notion of natural, inalienable, or pre-existing rights."[6]

---

[6]T. L. Beauchamp and R. R. Faden (15), p. 130.

Socialistic Rights Theory

A radical Marxian critique of all the preceding theories, especially Libertarian theory, might go something like this: Talk about justice and health care by philosophers in capitalistic systems is purely formalized discourse—the reflection of an underlying economic structure that is itself unjust. All the above theories are nothing more than justifications of the injustices present in the underlying capitalistic infrastructure.

For Marxists, the so-called universal rights to civil liberty, life, happiness, property, etc. are negative, guaranteeing only that people will be left alone to pursue their own individual objectives. But to be truly free and fully human, citizens need positive rights, including those proclaimed by the Marxist Manifesto in 1948: rights to work, housing, education, and health care.

This approach equates formal justice with giving everyone his due, and Marxist theory insists that meeting basic human needs is everyone's due. Hence, in Marxist theory basic needs create the foundations of basic rights, including the right to health care. Marx did not like referring to "rights," because he felt this reflected the way capitalist ideologies view citizens. But according to Marxist theory every citizen should be guaranteed health care "according to his needs," and the whole society should bear the cost. Thus, in effect, there is a positive right to health care.

Anyone who thinks theories of justice and philosophies of life really don't count for much needs to consider the influence of Marxist theory on health care organization around the world. Immediately after the Russian Revolution of 1917, Marxists took advantage of a socialized medical system that had been developed by the Czars to meet the needs of liberated serfs, one that had been in place in Russia since 1867. That is, the Marxist Government expanded this health care system to provide coverage first for all workers and then for all citizens. Article 20 of the U.S.S.R.'s 1936 constitution granted every citizen social security including health care and guaranteed that free medical care would be provided through a large network of hospitals. The Soviet system became a model for other countries, both within the Soviet sphere of influence and beyond.

In 1917 Mexico made industries responsible for the health needs of their workers and committed the Government to a social security system which included health care. In 1919 Germany established a similar sort of government-run health system. And in subsequent years other countries took action along similar lines.

In 1948 the American Declaration of the Rights and Duties of Man was signed at Bogotá, Colombia. This hemispheric declaration included health care among the basic human rights. Later that same year Article 25 of the United Nations Declaration of Human Rights spoke of health and health care as basic human rights. These declarations of the right to health care neither established a socialized system of free care nor specified how governments would respond to proclamation of this right. But the idea of health care as a right—one usually claimed against the government, at least as a last recourse—has had an enormous influence on health care throughout the world.

To the eighteenth-century negative rights have been added nineteenth-century positive rights, including the right to some form of health care. Even in capitalistic countries with liberal political systems, talk about a right to health in the sense of not being impeded in the pursuit of health or not being deprived of health by injury, has given way to talk of a positive right to some form of health care. In 1981 the President's Commission for the Study of Ethical Problems in Medicine and Biomedical and Behavioral Research reflected this trend in the U.S. It did not go so far as to declare a right to health care, but it did speak of a social obligation to provide a decent minimum for all. Society, in the sense of the collective American community, has an obligation according to this prestigious and influential commission to ensure equitable access to adequate health care for all. It endorsed a two-tiered system in which those who are poor and old will be provided for by the Government and those who can purchase more health care via insurance are free to do so.

Political groups, however, and particular philosophers do speak of health care in terms of a positive right (17). A positive right attains legal status when, for example, a Medicare or Medicaid law grants a health care entitlement or when the constitution of a nation extends its social security act to cover the health care needs of every citizen. In the U.S. there is no constitutional right to health care, but there are limited medical care rights (i.e., for veterans, the elderly, and the poor). The argument among philosophers is whether or not a moral right exists, and whether justice requires health care coverage. Allen Buchanan, a philosopher from the University of Arizona, argues for a right to an adequate (not maximal) level of health care with the tools of linguistic analysis without making any reference to the historic grounds for such a right (18).

Philosophers, legislators, and health policy experts in the U.S. continue to argue for some type of national insurance which would relieve the scandal of so many citizens not having access to health care services. They call attention to the fact that in the U.S. an institutional commitment to equality exists in education and in the legal system. Law and education are one-tiered, government-supported, and accessible to all. But when it comes to health, the rhetoric of free enterprise and the illusion that it will somehow provide the best health care for all continues to influence health policy. Philosophers making arguments for a right to health care play a role, but ultimately rights language and appeals to justice are translated into strongly Utilitarian categories.

Conclusion

If theories of justice do not generate just health care systems but do influence their adjustment and reform, then it makes sense to take such theories seriously. Theories of justice have in the past had enormous influence on the way

health care is delivered, and they continue to play an important role today. The literature of medical ethics during the 1980s was dominated by justice issues, and the same will most likely be true during the present decade. Health care systems are under enormous pressure, both in capitalistic and socialistic countries. The AIDS epidemic threatens to overwhelm even the best organized systems in the most advanced nations. Pressures are felt everywhere to expand or improve or reform existing health care systems; and theories of justice inevitably become part of the reflective process and accompanying debate.

Most people agree that no one theory is adequate to the complexity of a just health care delivery system. So a climate of compromise and respect for different perspectives has to be created. And no matter what the system, scarcities have to be confronted. Each system has its own way of handling these, and each has its special drawbacks. Nationalized or socialized systems put a cap on how much of the available resources will be spent on health care. Then the salaries of health care professionals are capped. Costs are controlled further by deciding what not to treat. Finally, available care is rationed, usually by permitting lines to develop (making people wait saves money).

Not all socialist systems are the same. Some have more to spend than others. But government-imposed restrictions are difficult to take when people die who could live. Thus, as time goes on, socialist systems create greater and greater numbers of critics. Usually they start out with high marks and great popularity, but both decline as the years go by and the deficiencies mount.

Capitalist systems are more consumer-driven, but increasingly employers have to pay the bills. Pure capitalistic care, in the sense that each individual buys what care he or she wants or can afford, seems impossible, and inevitably the government becomes a provider, at least for the poor and elderly. Even so, situations develop that most citizens consider blatant and morally unpalatable injustices.

The cost of caring for so many uninsured cannot long be absorbed by hospitals. In many

U.S. cities the public hospitals are near collapse under the weight of the poor and people whose only access to health care is through the emergency room. In places like New York or Washington, D.C., even people with insurance sometimes cannot gain needed access because the available beds are filled. Moral community cannot endure with a health system in which life and death depends upon wealth, and only the very wealthy can be adequately treated.

Different types of economic systems thus create different types of health care delivery problems but force people into the same reflections upon what is right or just. In this way, health care delivery problems make reflection on theories of justice inevitable.

If cooperation can take place across ideological lines in matters of politics, economics, and defense, then it is not too much to hope that health care planners (even those endorsing different theories of justice) can find common ground and cooperate to make the health care that all people value so highly a reality. Or more modestly, perhaps at least theorists and planners can cooperate to keep innocent people from dying when resources are available to save them, if only these resources were part of a more just system of distribution.

References

1. Nozick, R. *Anarchy, State, and Utopia.* Basic Books, New York, 1974, pp. 149–150.

2. Engelhardt, H. T., Jr. *Foundations of Bioethics.* Oxford University Press, New York, 1986.

3. Freed, C. *Right and Wrong.* Harvard University Press, Cambridge, 1978, pp. 120–122.

4. Veatch, R. M. *A Theory of Medical Ethics.* Basic Books, New York, 1981, p. 265.

5. Childress, J. F. Who shall live when not all can live? *Soundings* 53:339–354, 1970.

6. Outka, J. Social justice and equal access to health care. *Journal of Religious Ethics* 2:11–32, 1974.

7. Ramsey, P. *The Patient as Person.* Yale University Press, New Haven, 1970.

8. Rawls, J. *A Theory of Justice.* Harvard University Press, Cambridge, 1971.

9. Daniels, N. Health care needs and distributive justice. *Philosophy and Public Affairs.* Spring, 1981.

10. Daniels, N. *Am I My Parents' Keeper.* Oxford University Press, Oxford, 1988.

11. Bentham, J. *An Introduction to the Principles of Morals and Legislation.* Hafner, New York, 1948.

12. Mill, J. S. *Utilitarianism.* Bobbs-Merrill, New York, 1957.

13. Rawls, J. Two Concepts of Rules. In: M. Bales (ed.). *Contemporary Utilitarianism.* Anchor Books, Garden City, 1968.

14. Beauchamp, T. L., and J. F. Childress. *Principles of Medical Ethics.* Oxford University Press, New York, 1979.

15. Beauchamp, T. L., and R. R. Faden. The right to health and the right to health care. *Journal of Medicine and Philosophy* 4(2):127, 1979.

16. Beauchamp, T. L. Morality and Social Control of Biomedical Technology. In: H. T. Engelhardt, Jr., and S. F. Spicker (eds.). *The Moral Uses of New Knowledge in the Biomedical Services.* Reidel, Boston, 1980.

17. Brock, D. Justice, health care, and the elderly. *Philosophy and Public Affairs,* Summer 1989.

18. Buchanan, A. E. The right to a decent minimum of health care. *Philosophy and Public Affairs* 13(1), Winter 1984.

Bioethics: A New Health Philosophy

José Alberto Mainetti

I should like to offer a few comments and join author Gracia in briefly discussing the question of "What constitutes a just health services system and how should scarce resources be allocated?"

A Health Dilemma

Health, understood as "absence of illness" achieved through an approach to medicine that appears to harmonize the scientific, artistic, and spiritual, has ceased to be a private matter. Today health is a public matter whose object is "welfare," and whose approach is one based on a kind of medical care that produces conflict between industry, trade, and politics.

Health advances aimed at improving the quality of life may have become the most significant advances in the recent history of mankind. However, the price of success has been high and has produced a variety of problems. Possible benefits have come to conflict with the ethical and economic limits of the system, which is undergoing a crisis of values related to well-being and financial resources.

All this has made medicine the new Pandora's box of industrial society. Medicine has many fine attributes, but at the same time is the source of many evils. It nurtures the sort of hope that mankind used to place in ambrosia—the "bread of health and immortality" capable of being transformed into the bread of disease and madness. In both life and mythology such transformations are disconcertingly commonplace—as illustrated by the fate of Asclepios, who was punished for engaging in anti-Darwinian behavior, because his revival of the dead was depopulating Hades.

Within this context, the metaphorical Pandora's box of the modern health system is commonly found in the intensive care unit, where the desire of men to fight death ends up as denial of the right to die, reduced quality of life, and increased health expense. In this manner the technologic requirements of modern medicine produce questionable benefits and sometimes lead to tragic situations causing people to redefine medical objectives. The discipline known as bioethics attempts to organize these objectives by appealing to the moral principles of autonomy, welfare, and justice.

Health and Justice

The economic recession of the seventies resulted in a greater awareness of the price of health care, and an explosion of health costs without results terminated belief in the equation "health care equals health." Since then, in a situation where health has been treated as a consumer good in an increasingly ailing and aging society, and where technology, malpractice, and social security abuse have made the expansion of medical services expensive, there has been a general increase in health service use and health expenditures accompanied by a dearth of available resources that have to be carefully allocated. The matter of paying for health is now at the center of health policy, and is, in turn, a very significant aspect of politics generally in the aftermath of the crisis of the "welfare" State.

The result has been to make the theory and

practice of justice encompass health concepts and health care. The problem of distributive justice, the main element of health policy in bioethics, involves both ethics and economics. It is a question of principles and results, a deontologic and utilitarian matter with general and specific levels in terms of resource application. The three main doctrines of social justice (based on equality, liberalism, and redistribution) are founded on alternative systems of access to health care (socialized, free, and mixed).

In addition to these theories, however, justice must be applied. Justice, understood to be the most appropriate means of allocating scarce resources, provides the basis for proportional analysis of costs and benefits. Such analysis, based on laws of economic rationality and principles of profit and utility, seeks to derive the maximum benefit from possible actions. In short, the question of justice as it applies to health is curiously reminiscent of the first physiologic concept of health—Alcmene's concept of isonomy or equilibrium and equal rights, which is also related with the order of the cosmos seen as justice in Anaximander, that outstanding political and legal model of the natural philosophy of the Ionians.

Economic Ethics

The nature of health as a social good makes health care a cornerstone of justice in terms of "moral minimums"—a cornerstone in the sense of health policy that reconciles financial rationalization with ethical rationality and deontology or equity criteria with the "right" to medical care. In short, health is justice that should be administered, and for that reason ethics should not ignore economics and vice versa. To paraphrase Kant, ethics without economics is useless, economics without ethics is blind.

If available resources are to be rationally used, a cost-benefit analysis of just health care must be undertaken. Relative to other goods, and within the health context, this should articulate the applicable criteria of descriptive or quantifiable economics (as opposed to esoteric and prescriptive economics) and relate them to the moral principles of liberty and equality.

"Minima moralia, ethical economics or moral economics" is a topic that might be proposed for an imperative dialogue between economics and medical ethics within the framework of health policy. Questions of justice, efficiency, and equity with regard to health care should no longer be of interest only to health care officials who work at the social level of large-scale allotment of resources. These questions should also interest physicians in charge of small-scale allotment of resources, since the socioeconomic reality of health cost has an important bearing on clinical decision-making. The challenge to the Hippocratic ethos, expressed as serving the interest or welfare of the sick person, presents physicians with the need to control care costs without infringing upon their obligations to their patients. Perhaps the most dramatic question involved in this new "Doctor's Dilemma" is that of how to earmark scarce resources for medical treatments such as hemodialysis and organ transplants: "Who should live when all cannot live?"

Pro Domo Sua

Justice is at the heart of the new health philosophy proposed by bioethics. Indeed, bioethics itself is a product of the postindustrial welfare society and that expansion of "third generation human rights" (toward peace, development, the environment, and respect for humanity's common heritage) which marks the transition from a state of law to a state of justice. The question no longer involves just "negative" individual rights to health or even the broader general right to health care, but also the obligations of a just and responsible "macrobioethics" confronted with life-threatening situations (e.g., population growth, genetic issues, ecological catastrophe, nuclear strategy) and the need to preserve the rights of future generations. This transgenerational perspective reveals the worth of the biological and bioethical revolution, as well as of health promotion, education, and environmental, antinuclear, biogenetic, epidemiologic (AIDS!), and preventive medicine.

The Constitution of the World Health Organization states: "The health of all peoples is fundamental to the attainment of peace and security and is dependent upon the fullest cooperation of individuals and States." This broadened policy view of medicine and ethics has intensified since the meeting at Alma-Ata and other international forums where developing countries appealed for greater access to health care. In brief, it appears that if health is understood holistically as welfare and medical care is regarded as the appropriate technical vehicle for achieving welfare, then it seems reasonable to ask in the name of international justice whether the richest nations of the world do not have a moral obligation to offer other nations more health resources than those they are currently providing.

It is also fitting to examine the heart of Latin America's bioethics vision using the example provided by Argentina. After the United States and Canada, Argentina is the country of the Region that spends the most on health (8% of the gross domestic product). Most Argentines could not accurately describe their lives in economic terms as "first-class," but many might say that Argentina's health care and attention to the dying are indeed "first-class," if one applies the paradoxical guideline of "rescue" medicine as opposed to the community health or preventive care model. Unfortunately, this latter assertion would not be true, because the quality and cost of medical care pose major problems within the context of present national disorder. We must therefore ask why inefficiency and inequity exist in the area of health services. It is within this context that bioethical rationality could come to provide the intellectual and moral stimulus needed to effectively transform the system into one where the theory and practice of the new health philosophy of bioethics will no longer be a marginal consideration.

APPENDICES

International Codes of Ethics

The Hippocratic Oath

I swear by Apollo Physician and Aesculapius and Hygeia and Panacea and all the gods and goddesses, making them my witnesses, that I will fulfill according to my ability and judgment this oath and this covenant:

To hold him who has taught me this art as equal to my parents and to live my life in partnership with him, and if he is in need of money to give him a share of mine, and to regard his offspring as equal to my brothers in male lineage and to teach them this art—if they desire to learn it—without fee and covenant; to give a share of precepts and oral instruction and all the other learning to my sons and to the sons of him who has instructed me and to pupils who have signed the covenant and have taken an oath according to the medical law, but to no one else.

I will apply dietetic measures for the benefit of the sick according to my ability and judgment; I will keep them from harm and injustice.

I will neither give a deadly drug to anybody if asked for it, nor will I make a suggestion to this efect. Similarly, I will not give to a woman an abortive remedy. In purity and holiness I will guard my life and my art.

I will not use the knife, not even on sufferers from stone, but will withdraw in favor of such men as are engaged in this work.

Whatever houses I may visit, I will come for the benefit of the sick, remaining free of all intentional injustice, of all mischief and in particular of sexual relations with both female and male persons, be they free or slaves.

What I may see or hear in the course of the treatment or even outside of the treatment in regard to the life of men, which on no account must be spread abroad, I will keep to myself, holding such things shameful to be spoken about.

If I fulfill this oath and do not violate it, may it be granted to me to enjoy life and art, being honored with fame among all men for all time to come; if I transgress it and swear falsely, may the opposite to all this be my lot.

(Reprinted from Ludwig Edelstein, ''The Hippocratic Oath: Text, Translation, and Interpretation,'' Bulletin of the History of Medicine, *Suppl. 1, p. 3, by permission of Johns Hopkins University Press.)*

Declaration of Geneva (Oath of Professional Fidelity)

Adopted by the Second General Assembly of the World Medical Association (Geneva, September 1948) and amended by the 22nd World Medical Assembly (Sydney, August 1968) and the 35th World Medical Assembly (Venice, October 1983)

At the time of being admitted as a member of the medical profession:

I solemnly pledge myself to consecrate my life to the service of humanity;

I will give to my teachers the respect and gratitude which is their due;

I will practice my profession with conscience and dignity;

The health of my patient will be my first consideration;

I will respect the secrets which are confided in me, even after the patient has died;

I will maintain by all the means in my power, the honor and the noble traditions of the medical profession;

My *colleagues* will be my brothers;

I *will not permit* considerations of religion, nationality, race, party politics, or social standing to intervene between my duty and my patient;

I *will maintain* the utmost respect for human life from its beginning even under threat, and I will not use my medical knowledge contrary to the laws of humanity;

I *make these promises* solemnly, freely, and upon my honor.

(Reprinted by permission.)

International Code of Medical Ethics

Adopted by the Third General Assembly of the World Medical Association (London, October 1949) and amended by the 22nd World Medical Assembly (Sydney, August 1968) and the 35th World Medical Assembly (Venice, October 1983)

Duties of Physicians in General

A *physician shall* always maintain the highest standards of professional conduct.

A *physician shall not* permit motives of profit to influence the free and independent exercise of professional judgment on behalf of patients.

A *physician shall*, in all types of medical practice, be dedicated to providing competent medical service in full technical and moral independence, with compassion and respect for human dignity.

A *physician shall* deal honestly with patients and colleagues, and strive to expose those physicians deficient in character or competence, or who engage in fraud or deception.

The following practices are deemed to be unethical conduct:

a) Self-advertising by physicians, unless permitted by the laws of the country and the code of ethics of the national medical association.

b) Paying or receiving any fee or any other consideration solely to procure the referral of a patient or for prescribing or referring a patient to any source.

A *physician shall* respect the rights of patients, of colleagues, and of other health professionals, and shall safeguard patient confidences.

A *physician shall* act only in the patient's interest when providing medical care which might have the effect of weakening the physical and mental condition of the patient.

A *physician shall* use great caution in divulging discoveries or new techniques or treatment through nonprofessional channels.

A *physician shall* certify only that which he has personally verified.

Duties of Physicians to the Sick

A *physician shall* always bear in mind the obligation of preserving human life.

A *physician shall* owe his patients complete loyalty and all the resources of his science. Whenever an examination or treatment is beyond the physician's capacity, he should summon another physician who has the necessary ability.

A *physician shall* preserve absolute confidentiality on all he knows about his patient, even after the patient has died.

A *physician shall* give emergency care as a humanitarian duty unless he is assured that others are willing and able to give such care.

Duties of Physicians to Each Other

A *physician shall* behave towards his colleagues as he would have them behave towards him.

A *physician shall not* entice patients from his colleagues.

A *physician shall* observe the principles of the "Declaration of Geneva" approved by the World Medical Association.

(Reprinted by permission.)

Code for Nurses: Ethical Concepts Applied to Nursing

Adopted by the International Council of Nurses in May 1973

The fundamental responsibility of the nurse is fourfold: to promote health, to prevent illness, to restore health, and to alleviate suffering.

The need for nursing is universal. Inherent in nursing is respect for life, dignity, and the rights of man. It is unrestricted by considerations of nationality, race, creed, color, age, sex, politics, or social status.

Nurses render health services to the individual, the family, and the community and coordinate their services with those of related groups.

Nurses and People

The nurse's primary responsibility is to those people who require nursing care.

The nurse, in providing care, promotes an environment in which the values, customs, and spiritual beliefs of the individual are respected.

The nurse holds in confidence personal information and uses judgment in sharing this information.

Nurses and Practice

The nurse carries personal responsibility for nursing practice and for maintaining competence by continual learning.

The nurse maintains the highest standards of nursing care possible within the reality of a specific situation.

The nurse uses judgment in relation to individual competence when accepting and delegating responsibilities.

The nurse when acting in a professional capacity should at all times maintain standards of personal conduct which reflect credit upon the profession.

Nurses and Society

The nurse shares with other citizens the responsibility for initiating and supporting actions to meet the health and social needs of the public.

Nurses and Coworkers

The nurse sustains a cooperative relationship with coworkers in nursing and other fields.

The nurse takes appropriate action to safeguard the individual when his care is endangered by a coworker or any other person.

Nurses and the Profession

The nurse plays the major role in determining and implementing desirable standards of nursing practice and nursing education.

The nurse is active in developing a core of professional knowledge.

The nurse, acting through the professional organization, participates in establishing and maintaining equitable social and economic working conditions in nursing.

(Reprinted by permission.)

Principles of Medical Ethics Relevant to the Protection of Prisoners against Torture

Developed by the Council for International Organizations of Medical Sciences and adopted by the United Nations General Assembly

Principle 1.

Health personnel, particularly physicians, charged with the medical care of prisoners and detainees have a duty to provide them with protection of their physical and mental health and treatment of disease of the same quality and standard as is afforded to those who are not imprisoned or detained.

Principle 2.

It is a gross contravention of medical ethics, as well as an offense under applicable international instruments, for health personnel, particularly physicians, to engage, actively or passively, in acts which constitute participation in, complicity in, incitement to, or attempts to commit torture or other cruel, inhuman, or degrading treatment or punishment.[1]

Principle 3.

It is a contravention of medical ethics for health personnel, particularly physicians, to be involved in any professional relationship with prisoners or detainees the purpose of which is not solely to evaluate, protect, or improve their physical and mental health.

Principle 4.

It is a contravention of medical ethics for health personnel, particularly physicians:

a) To apply their knowledge and skills in order to assist in the interrogation of prisoners and detainees in a manner that may adversely affect the physical or mental health or condition of such prisoners or detainees and which is not in accordance with the relevant international instruments;[2]

b) To certify, or to participate in the certification of, the fitness of prisoners or detainees for any form of treatment or punishment that may adversely affect their physical or mental health and which is not in accordance with the relevant international instruments, or to participate in any way in the infliction of any such treatment or punishment which is not in accordance with the relevant international instruments.

Principle 5.

It is a contravention of medical ethics for health personnel, particularly physicians, to participate in any procedure for restraining a prisoner or detainee, unless such a procedure is determined in accordance with purely medical criteria as being necessary for the protecion of the physical or mental health or the safety of the prisoner or detainee himself, of his fellow prisoners or detainees, or of his guardians, and presents no hazard to his physical or mental health.

Principle 6.

There may be no derogation from the foregoing principles on any ground whatsoever, including public emergency.

(Official text from resolution A/RES/37/194, adopted by the General Assembly of the United Nations, 9 March 1983.)

---

[1] See the Declaration on the Protection of All Persons from Being Subjected to Torture and Other Cruel, Inhuman, or Degrading Treatment or Punishment (UN General Assembly resolution 3452 (XXX), annex), article 1 of which states:
   "1. For the purpose of this Declaration, torture means any act by which severe pain or suffering, whether physical or mental, is intentionally inflicted by or at the instigation of a public official on a person for such purposes as obtaining from him or a third person information or confession, punishing him for an act he has committed or is suspected of having committed or intimidating him or other persons. It does not include pain or suffering arising only from, inherent in, or incidental to, lawful sanctions to the extent consistent with the Standard Minimum Rules for the Treatment of Prisoners.
   2. Torture constitutes an aggravated and deliberate form of cruel, inhuman or degrading treatment or punishment."
Article 7 of the Declaration states:
   "Each State shall ensure that all acts of torture as defined in article 1 are offenses under its criminal law. The same shall apply in regard to acts which constitute participation in, complicity in, incitement to, or an attempt to commit torture."

[2] Particularly, the Universal Declaration of Human Rights (UN General Assembly resolution 217 A (III), the International Covenants on Human Rights (UN General Assembly resolution 2200 A (XXI), annex), the Declaration on the Protection of All Persons from Being Subjected to Torture and Other Cruel, Inhuman, or Degrading Treatment or Punishment (General Assembly resolution 3452 (XXX), annex), and the Standard Minimum Rules for the Treatment of Prisoners (*First United Nations Congress on the Prevention of Crime and the Treatment of Offenders: Report by the Secretariat* (United Nations publication, Sales No. 1956.IV.4), annex I.A).

International Research Codes of Ethics

The Nuremberg Code

International Tribunal of Nuremberg, 1947

Permitted Medical Experiments.

The great weight of the evidence before us is to the effect that certain types of medical experiments on human beings, when kept within reasonably well-defined bounds, conform to the ethics of the medical profession generally. The protagonists of the practice of human experimentation justify their views on the basis that such experiments yield results for the good of society that are unprocurable by other methods or means of study. All agree, however, that certain basic principles must be observed in order to satisfy moral, ethical, and legal concepts:

1. The voluntary consent of the human subject is absolutely essential. This means that the person involved should have legal capacity to give consent; should be so situated as to be able to exercise free power of choice, without the intervention of any element of force, fraud, deceit, duress, overreaching, or other ulterior form of constraint or coercion; and should have sufficient knowledge and comprehension of the elements of the subject matter involved as to enable him to make an understanding and enlightened decision. This latter element requires that before the acceptance of an affirmative decision by the experimental subject there should be made known to him the nature, duration, and purpose of the experiment; the method and means by which it is to be conducted; all inconveniences and hazards reasonably to be expected; and the effects upon his health or person which may possibly come from his participation in the experiment.

The duty and responsibility for ascertaining the quality of the consent rests upon each individual who initiates, directs, or engages in the experiment. It is a personal duty and responsibility which may not be delegated to another with impunity.

2. The experiment should be such as to yield fruitful results for the good of society, unprocurable by other methods or means of study, and not random and unnecessary in nature.

3. The experiment should be so designed and based on the results of animal experimentation and a knowledge of the natural history of the disease or other problem under study that the anticipated results will justify the performance of the experiment.

4. The experiment should be so conducted as to avoid all unnecessary physical and mental suffering and injury.

5. No experiment should be conducted where there is an a priori reason to believe that death or disabling injury will occur; except, perhaps, in those experiments where the experimental physicians also serve as subjects.

6. The degree of risk to be taken should never exceed that determined by the humanitarian importance of the problem to be solved by the experiment.

7. Proper preparations should be made and adequate facilities provided to protect the experimental subject against even remote possibilities of injury, disability, or death.

8. The experiment should be conducted only by scientifically qualified persons. The highest

degree of skill and care should be required through all stages of the experiment of those who conduct or engage in the experiment.

9. During the course of the experiment the human subject should be at liberty to bring the experiment to an end if he has reached the physical or mental state where continuation of the experiment seems to him to be impossible.

10. During the course of the experiment the scientist in charge must be prepared to terminate the experiment at any stage, if he has probable cause to believe, in the exercise of the good faith, superior skill, and careful judgment required of him, that a continuation of the experiment is likely to result in injury, disability, or death to the experimental subject.

(Reprinted from Trials of War Criminals before the Nuremberg Military Tribunals under Control Council Law No. 10, *vol. 2 (U.S. Government Printing Office, Washington, D.C., 1949), pp. 181–182.)*

Declaration of Helsinki Recommendations Guiding Physicians in Biomedical Research Involving Human Subjects

Adopted by the 18th World Medical Assembly (Helsinki, June 1964), and amended by the 29th World Medical Assembly (Tokyo, October 1975), the 35th World Medical Assembly (Venice, October 1983), and the 41st World Medical Assembly (Hong Kong, 1989)

Introduction

It is the mission of the physician to safeguard the health of the people. His or her knowledge and conscience are dedicated to the fulfillment of this mission.

The Declaration of Geneva of the World Medical Association binds the physician with the words, "The health of my patient will be my first consideration," and the International Code of Medical Ethics declares that, "A physician shall act only in the patient's interest when providing medical care which might have the effect of weakening the physical and mental condition of the patient."

The purpose of biomedical research involving human subjects must be to improve diagnostic, therapeutic, and prophylactic procedures and the understanding of the etiology and pathogenesis of disease.

In current medical practice most diagnostic, therapeutic, or prophylactic procedures involve hazards. This applies especially to biomedical research.

Medical progress is based on research which ultimately must rest in part on experimentation involving human subjects.

In the field of biomedical research a fundamental distinction must be recognized between medical research in which the aim is essentially diagnostic or therapeutic for a patient, and medical research the essential object of which is purely scientific and without implying direct diagnostic or therapeutic value to the person subjected to the research.

Special caution must be exercised in the conduct of research which may affect the environment, and the welfare of animals used for research must be respected.

Because it is essential that the results of laboratory experiments be applied to human beings to further scientific knowledge and to help suffering humanity, the World Medical Association has prepared the following recommendations as a guide to every physician in biomedical research involving human subjects. They should be kept under review in the future. It must be stressed that the standards as drafted are only a guide to physicians all over the world. Physicians are not relieved from criminal, civil, and ethical responsibilities under the laws of their own countries.

I. Basic Principles

1. Biomedical research involving human subjects must conform to generally accepted scientific principles and should be based on adequately performed laboratory and animal experimentation and on a thorough knowledge of the scientific literature.

2. The design and performance of each experimental procedure involving human subjects should be clearly formulated in an experimental protocol which should be transmitted for consideration, comment, and guidance to a specially appointed committee independent of the investigator and the sponsor, provided that this independent committee is in comformity with the laws and regulations of the country in which the research experiment is performed.

3. Biomedical research involving human subjects should be conducted only by scientifically qualified persons and under the supervision of a clinically competent medical person. The responsibility for the human subject must always rest with a medically qualified person and never rest on the subject of the research, even though the subject has given his or her consent.

4. Biomedical research involving human subjects cannot legitimately be carried out unless the importance of the objective is in proportion to the inherent risk to the subject.

5. Every biomedical research project involving human subjects should be preceded by careful assessment of predictable risks in comparison with foreseeable benefits to the subject or to others. Concern for the interests of the subject must always prevail over the interests of science and society.

6. The right of the research subject to safeguard his or her integrity must always be respected. Every precaution should be taken to respect the privacy of the subject and to minimize the impact of the study on the subject's physical and mental integrity and on the personality of the subject.

7. Physicians should abstain from engaging in research projects involving human subjects unless they are satisfied that the hazards involved are believed to be predictable. Physicians should cease any investigation if the hazards are found to outweigh the potential benefits.

8. In publication of the results of his or her research, the physician is obliged to preserve the accuracy of the results. Reports of experimentation not in accordance with the principles laid down in this Declaration should not be accepted for publication.

9. In any research on human beings, each potential subject must be adequately informed of the aims, methods, anticipated benefits, and potential hazards of the study and the discomfort it may entail. He or she should be informed that he or she is at liberty to abstain from participation in the study and that he or she is free to withdraw his or her consent to participation at any time. The physician should then obtain the subject's freely given informed consent, preferably in writing.

10. When obtaining informed consent for the research project, the physician should be particularly cautious if the subject is in a dependent relationship to him or her or may consent under duress. In that case the informed consent should be obtained by a physician who is not engaged in the investigation and who is completely independent of this official relationship.

11. In case of legal incompetence, informed consent should be obtained from the legal guardian in accordance with national legislation. Where physical or mental incapacity makes it impossible to obtain informed consent, or when the subject is a minor, permission from the responsible relative replaces that of the subject in accordance with national legislation. Whenever the minor child is in fact able to give a consent, the minor's consent must be obtained in addition to the consent of the minor's legal guardian.

12. The research protocol should always contain a statement of the ethical considerations involved and should indicate that the principles enunciated in the present Declaration are complied with.

II. Medical Research Combined with Professional Care (Clinical Research)

1. In the treatment of the sick person, the physician must be free to use a new diagnostic and therapeutic measure, if in his or her judgment it offers hope of saving life, reestablishing health, or alleviating suffering.

2. The potential benefits, hazards, and discomfort of a new method should be weighed against the advantages of the best current diagnostic and therapeutic methods.

3. In any medical study, every patient—including those of a control group, if any—should be assured of the best proven diagnostic and therapeutic method.

4. The refusal of the patient to participate in a study must never interfere with the physician-patient relationship.

5. If the physician considers it essential not to obtain informed consent, the specific reasons for this proposal should be stated in the experimental protocol for transmission to the independent committee (I, 2).

6. The physician can combine medical research with professional care, the objective being the acquisition of new medical knowledge, only to the extent that medical research is justified by its potential diagnostic or therapeutic value for the patient.

III. Nontherapeutic Biomedical Research Involving Human Subjects (Nonclinical Biomedical Research)

1. In the purely scientific application of medical research carried out on a human being, it is the duty of the physician to remain the protector of the life and health of that person on whom biomedical research is being carried out.

2. The subjects should be volunteers—either healthy persons or patients for whom the experimental design is not related to the patient's illness.

3. The investigator or the investigating team should discontinue the research if in his/her or their judgment it may, if continued, be harmful to the individual.

4. In research on man, the interest of science and society should never take precedence over considerations related to the well-being of the subject.

(Reprinted by permission.)

Proposed International Guidelines for Biomedical Research Involving Human Subjects

Council for International Organizations of Medical Sciences and World Health Organization, 1982

Preamble

All advances in medical practice are dependent upon an understanding of relevant physiological and pathological processes and must necessarily, in the last resort, be tested for the first time on human subjects. It is in this sense that the term "research involving human subjects" is used.

The context in which such research is undertaken is wide and includes:

- [ ] studies of a physiological, biochemical, or pathological process, or of the response to a specific intervention—either physical, chemical, or psychological—in healthy subjects or patients under treatment;
- [ ] prospective controlled trials of diagnostic, prophylactic, or therapeutic measures in larger groups of patients, with a view to demonstrating a specific response against a background of individual biological variation;
- [ ] studies in which the consequences of specific prophylactic or therapeutic measures are determined within communities.

Research involving human subjects is thus defined for the purposes of these guidelines as any study involving human subjects, and directed to the advancement of biomedical knowledge, that cannot be regarded as an element in established clinical management or public health practice, and that involves either:

☐ physical or psychological intervention or assessment, or
☐ generation, storage, and analysis of records containing biomedical information referable to identifiable individuals.

Such studies include not only planned interventions on human subjects but research in which environmental factors are manipulated in a way that could place incidentally exposed individuals at risk.

The terms of reference are framed broadly, in order to embrace field studies of pathogenic organisms and toxic chemicals under investigation for medical purposes. Analogous risks are recognized to arise in research directed to other objectives, but nonmedical research does not fall within the scope of this document.

Research involving human subjects should be carried out only by appropriately qualified and experienced investigators in accordance with an experimental protocol that clearly states: the aim of the research; the reasons for proposing that it should be undertaken on human subjects; the nature and degree of any known risks; the sources from which it is proposed that subjects should be recruited; and the means proposed for ensuring that their consent is adequately informed. The protocol should be scientifically and ethically appraised by a suitably constituted review body independent of the investigators.

The guidelines proposed below will offer some countries nothing that is not already in force in one form or another. They have been framed with special reference to the requirements of developing countries and elaborated in the light of replies to a questionnaire received from 45 national health administrations and 91 medical faculties in countries in which medical research involving human subjects is as yet undertaken on a limited scale and/or in the absence of ex-

plicit national criteria for protecting such subjects from involuntary abuse. The replies were received from a total of 60 developing countries.

International Declarations

1. The first international declaration on research involving human subjects was the Nuremberg Code of 1947, which was a by-product of a trial of physicians for having performed cruel experiments on prisoners and detainees during the Second World War. The Code lays particular stress on the "voluntary consent" ("informed consent" is now the usual term) of the subject, which is stated to be "absolutely essential."

2. In 1964, the World Medical Association (WMA), at its 18th World Medical Assembly, adopted the Declaration of Helsinki ("Helsinki I"), which was a set of rules to guide physicians engaged in clinical research, both therapeutic and nontherapeutic. At its 29th World Medical Assembly in 1975, the WMA revised this Declaration ("Helsinki II"), broadening its scope to include "biomedical research involving human subjects." Some important new provisions in the revised Declaration were that experimental protocols for research involving human subjects "should be transmitted to a specially appointed independent committee for consideration, comment and guidance" (article I, 2); that such protocols "should always contain a statement of the ethical considerations involved and should indicate that the principles enunciated in the present Declaration are complied with" (article I, 12); and that reports on "experimentation not in accordance with the principles laid down in this Declaration should not be accepted for publication" (article I, 8).

3. Both the Nuremberg Code and the original Declaration of Helsinki of 1964 have been superseded by "Helsinki II," the full text of which is appended.[3] This is the basic document in its field, and has been widely accepted as such.

---

[3]See pages 218–220 in this volume.

4. These guidelines take account of the distinction made in "Helsinki II" between medical research combined with professional care (clinical research) and nontherapeutic (nonclinical) biomedical research.

5. While the general principles laid down in "Helsinki II" may be regarded as of universal validity, their modes of application in various special circumstances must necessarily vary. The purpose of the present guidelines is, therefore, not to duplicate or amend these principles, but to suggest how they may be applied in the special circumstances of many technologically developing countries. In particular, the limitations of the informed consent procedure are emphasized, and issues specific to research involving communities rather than individual subjects are addressed.

Consent of Subjects

6. "Helsinki II" requires (article I, 9) that human subjects should not be used in medical research unless "freely given informed consent" has been elicited after having been adequately informed of the "aims, methods, anticipated benefits, and potential hazards" of the experiment and informed that they are free to abstain or to withdraw from participation at any time. Of itself, however, informed consent offers an imperfect safeguard to the subject, and it should always be complemented by independent ethical review of research proposals. Moreover, there are many individuals, including children, adults who are mentally ill or defective, and those who are totally unfamiliar with modern medical concepts, who are incapable of giving adequate consent and from whom consent implies a passive and uncomprehending participation. For such groups, in particular, independent ethical review is imperative.

Children

7. It is axiomatic that children should never be the subjects of research that might equally well be carried out on adults. However, their participation is indispensable for research on diseases of childhood and conditions to which children are particularly susceptible. The consent of a parent or other legal guardian, after a full explanation of the aims of the experiment and of possible hazards, discomfort, or inconvenience, is always necessary.

8. To the extent that is feasible, which will vary with age, the willing cooperation of the child should be sought, after he or she has been frankly informed of any possible discomfort or inconvenience. Older children may be assumed to be capable of giving informed consent, preferably also with the consent of the parent or other legal guardian.

9. Children should in no circumstances be the subjects of research holding no potential benefit for them unless with the objective of elucidating physiological or pathological conditions peculiar to infancy and childhood.

Pregnant and Nursing Women

10. While no special problems of eliciting informed consent exist in the case of pregnant and nursing mothers as such, they should in no circumstances be the subjects of nontherapeutic research that carries any possibility of risk to the fetus or neonate, unless this is intended to elucidate problems of pregnancy or lactation. Therapeutic research is permissible only with a view to improving the health of the mother without prejudice to that of the fetus or nursling, to enhancing the viability of the fetus, or to aiding the nursling's healthy development or the ability of the mother to nourish it adequately.

Research directed to induced termination of pregnancy, or undertaken in anticipation of termination, is an issue that is dependent upon national legislation and religious and cultural precepts, and, therefore, does not lend itself to an international recommendation.

Mentally Ill and Mentally Defective Persons

11. Substantially similar ethical considerations apply to the mentally ill and the mentally defective as to children. They should never be the subjects of research that might equally well

be carried out in adults in full possession of their intellectual faculties, but they are clearly the only subjects available for research into the origins and treatment of mental disease or disability.

12. The agreement of the immediate family—whether spouse, parent, adult offspring, or sibling—should be sought, but is sometimes of doubtful value, especially as mentally deranged or defective patients are sometimes regarded by their families as an unwelcome burden. Where a subject has been compulsorily committed to an institution by a court order, it may be necessary to seek legal sanction before involving the subject in experimental procedures.

Other Vulnerable Social Groups

13. The quality of the consent of candidate subjects who are junior or subordinate members of a hierarchically structured group requires careful consideration, as willingness to volunteer may be unduly influenced by the expectation, whether justified or not, of adventitious benefits. Examples of such groups are medical and nursing students, subordinate laboratory and hospital personnel, employees of the pharmaceutical industry, and members of the armed forces.

Subjects in Developing Communities

14. Rural communities in developing countries may not be conversant with the concepts and techniques of experimental medicine. It is in these communities that diseases not endemic in developed countries exact a heavy toll of illness, incapacity, and death. Research on the prophylaxis and treatment of such diseases is urgently required, and can be finally carried out only within the communities at risk.

15. Where individual members of a community do not have the necessary awareness of the implications of participation in an experiment to give adequately informed consent directly to the investigators, it is desirable that the decision whether or not to participate should be elicited through the intermediary of a trusted community leader. The intermediary should make it clear that participation is entirely voluntary, and that any participant is free to abstain or withdraw at any time from the experiment.

Community-based Research

16. Where research is undertaken on a community basis—for example, by experimental treatment of water supplies, by health services research, or by large-scale trials of new insecticides, of new prophylactic or immunizing agents, and of nutritional adjuvants or substitutes—individual consent on a person-to-person basis may not be feasible, and the ultimate decision to undertake the research will rest with the responsible public health authority.

17. Nevertheless, all possible means should be used to inform the community concerned of the aims of the research, the advantages expected from it, and any possible hazards or inconveniences. If feasible, dissenting individuals should have the option of withholding their participation. Whatever the circumstances, the ethical considerations and safeguards applied to research on individuals must be translated, in every possible respect, into the community context.

Review Procedures

18. The provisions for review of research involving human subjects are influenced by political institutions, the organization of medical practice and research, and the degree of autonomy accorded to medical investigators. Whatever the circumstances, however, a dual responsibility exists within society to ensure that:

☐ all drugs and devices under investigation in human subjects meet adequate standards of safety;

☐ the provisions of "Helsinki II" are applied in all biomedical research involving human subjects.

Assessment of Safety

19. Authority to assess the safety and quality of new medicines and devices intended for use in

man is most effectively vested in a multi-disciplinary advisory committee operative at the national level. Clinicians, clinical pharmacologists, pharmacologists, toxicologists, pathologists, pharmacists, and statisticians have important contributions to offer to these assessments. Many countries at present lack resources to undertake independent assessments of technical data according to procedures and standards now considered mandatory in many highly developed countries. Improvement in their capability to subserve this function is dependent, in the short term, on more efficient exchange of relevant information internationally.

Ethical Review Committees

20. It is not possible to draw a clear dividing line between scientific review and ethical review, for an experiment on human subjects that is scientifically unsound is *ipso facto* unethical, in that it may expose the subjects to risk or inconvenience to no purpose. Normally, therefore, ethical review committees consider both scientific and ethical aspects. If a review committee finds a research proposal scientifically sound, it will then consider whether any known or possible risk to the subject is justified by the expected benefit and, if so, whether the proposed procedure for eliciting informed consent is satisfactory.

21. In a highly centralized administration, a national review committee may be constituted to review research protocols from both scientific and ethical standpoints. In countries where medical research is not centrally directed, protocols are more effectively and conveniently reviewed from the ethical standpoint at local or regional levels. The basic responsibilities of locally operative ethical review committees are twofold:

- [ ] to verify that all proposed interventions, and, particularly, the administration of drugs under development, have been assessed by a competent expert body as acceptably safe to be undertaken in human subjects.
- [ ] to ensure that all other ethical considera-

tions arising from a protocol are satisfactorily resolved both in principle and in practice.

22. Review committees may be created under the aegis of national or local health administrations, of national medical research councils, or of other nationally representative medical bodies. The competence of committees operating on a local basis may be confined exclusively to a specific research institution or it may extend to all biomedical research involving human subjects undertaken within a defined geographical area.

23. Local review committees act as gatherings of the investigators' peers and should be so composed as to provide complete and adequate review of the research activities referred to them. The membership may include other health professionals, particularly nurses, as well as laymen qualified to represent community, cultural, and moral values. Independence from the investigators is maintained by precluding any member with a direct interest in a proposal from participation in its assessment.

24. The requirements of review committees should be particularly stringent in the case of proposed research involving children, pregnant and nursing women, the mentally ill or mentally defective persons, members of developing communities unfamiliar with modern clinical concepts, and any invasive nontherapeutic research.

Information to be Provided by Investigators

25. Whatever may be the pattern of the procedure adopted for ethical review, it should be based on a detailed protocol comprising:

- [ ] a clear statement of the objectives having regard to the present state of knowledge and a justification for undertaking the investigation in human subjects;
- [ ] a precise description of all proposed interventions, including intended dosages of drugs and planned duration of treatment;
- [ ] a statistical plan indicating the number of

subjects to be recruited and the criteria for terminating the study;

☐ the criteria determining admission and withdrawal of individual subjects, including full details of the informed consent procedure.

26. There should also be included information to establish:

☐ the safety of each proposed intervention and of any drug or device to be tested, including the results of relevant laboratory and animal research;

☐ the presumed benefits and potential risks of participation;

☐ the means proposed to elicit informed consent or, when this is not possible, satisfactory assurance that the guardian or family will be appropriately consulted and the rights and welfare of each subject will be adequately protected;

☐ evidence that the investigator is appropriately qualified and experienced, and commands adequate facilities for the safe and efficient conduct of the research;

☐ provisions that will be made to protect confidentiality of data;

☐ the nature of any other ethical considerations involved, together with an indication that the principles enunciated in "Helsinki II" will be implemented.

Externally Sponsored Research

27. The term externally sponsored research is here used to refer to research undertaken in a host country but initiated, financed, and sometimes wholly or partly carried out by an external international or national agency with the collaboration or agreement of the appropriate authorities of the host country.

28. Such research implies two ethical imperatives:

☐ The research protocol should be submitted to ethical review by the initiating agency. The ethical standards applied should be no less exacting than they would be for research carried out within the initiating country.

☐ After ethical approval by the initiating agency, the appropriate authorities of the host country should, by means of an ethical review committee or otherwise, satisfy themselves that the proposed research meets their own ethical requirements.

Where externally sponsored research is initiated and financed by a pharmaceutical manufacturer, it is in the interest of the host country to require that it should be submitted with the comments of a responsible authority of the initiating country, such as a health administration, research council, or academy of medicine or science.

29. An important secondary objective of externally sponsored research should be the training of the health personnel of the host country to carry out similar research projects independently.

Compensation of Research Subjects for Accidental Injury

30. Reports of accidental injury to subjects volunteering to participate in therapeutic or nontherapeutic research resulting in temporary or permanent disability, or even death, are exceedingly rare. In fact, human subjects of medical research are usually in exceptionally favorable circumstances, in that they are under close and continued observation by highly qualified investigators who are alert to detect the earliest signs of untoward reactions. Such conditions are less likely to occur in routine medical practice.

31. However, any volunteer subjects involved in medical research who may suffer injury as a result of their participation are entitled to such financial or other assistance as would compensate them fully for any temporary or permanent disability. In the case of death, the dependents should be eligible for appropriate material compensation.

32. Experimental subjects should not, in giving their consent to participation, be required to

waive their rights to compensation in the case of an accident; nor should they be required to show negligence or lack of a reasonable degree of skill on the part of the investigator. Support is increasing for a system of insurance against risks, financed either by public or private funds or both, the injured party having only to show a causal relationship between the investigation and his injury. For research sponsored by pharmaceutical manufacturers, the manufacturers themselves should assume responsibility in case of accidents. This is particularly necessary in the case of externally sponsored research when the subjects are not protected by social security measures.

Confidentiality of Data

33. Research may involve the collection and storage of data relating to individuals, which, if disclosed to third parties, might cause harm or distress. Consequently, arrangements should be made by investigators to protect the confidentiality of such data, as for example by omitting information which might lead to the identification of individual subjects, by limiting access to the data, or other appropriate means.

International Guiding Principles for Biomedical Research Involving Animals

Council for International Organizations of Medical Sciences

Preamble

Experimentation with animals has made possible major contributions to biological knowledge and to the welfare of man and animals, particularly in the treatment and prevention of diseases. Many important advances in medical science have had their origins in basic biological research not primarily directed to practical ends, as well as from applied research designed to investigate specific medical problems. There is still an urgent need for basic and applied research that will lead to the discovery of methods for the prevention and treatment of diseases for which adequate control methods are not yet available—notably the noncommunicable diseases and the endemic communicable diseases of warm climates.

Past progress has depended, and further progress in the foreseeable future will depend, largely on animal experimentation which, in the broad field of human medicine, is the prelude to experimental trials on human beings of, for example, new therapeutic, prophylactic, or diagnostic substances, devices, or procedures.

There are two international ethical codes intended principally for the guidance of countries or institutions that have not yet formulated their own ethical requirements for human experimentation: the Tokyo revision of the Declaration of Helsinki of the World Medical Association (1975), and the Proposed International Guidelines for Biomedical Research Involving Human Subjects of the Council for International Organizations of Medical Sciences and the World Health Organization (1982). These codes recognize that while experiments involving human subjects are a *sine qua non* of medical progress, they must be subject to strict ethical requirements. In order to ensure that such ethical requirements are observed, national and institutional ethical codes have also been elaborated with a view to the protection of human subjects involved in biomedical (including behavioral) research.

A major requirement both of national and international ethical codes for human experimentation, and of national legislation in many cases, is that new substances or devices should not be used for the first time on human beings unless previous tests on animals have provided a reasonable presumption of their safety.

The use of animals for predicting the probable effects of procedures on human beings entails responsibility for their welfare. In both human and veterinary medicine, animals are used for behavioral, physiological, pathological, toxicological, and therapeutic research; for experimental surgery or surgical training; and for testing drugs and biological preparations. The same responsibility toward the experimental animals prevails in all of these cases.

Because of differing legal systems and cultural backgrounds, there are varying approaches to the use of animals for research, testing, or training in different countries. Nonetheless, their use should be always in accord with humane practices. The varying approaches in different countries to the use of animals for biomedical purposes, and the lack of relevant legislation or of formal self-regulatory mechanisms in some, point to the need for international guiding principles elaborated as a result of international and interdisciplinary consultations.

The guiding principles proposed here provide a framework for more specific national or institutional provisions. They apply not only to biomedical research but also to all uses of vertebrate animals for other biomedical purposes, including the production and testing of therapeutic, prophylactic, and diagnostic substances, the diagnosis of infections and intoxications in man and animals, and to any other procedures involving the use of intact live vertebrates.

1. Basic Principles

I. The advancement of biological knowledge and the development of improved means for the protection of the health and well-being both of man and of animals require recourse to experimentation on intact live animals of a wide variety of species.

II. Methods such as mathematical models, computer simulation, and *in vitro* biological systems should be used wherever appropriate.

III. Animal experiments should be undertaken only after due consideration of their relevance for human or animal health and the advancement of biological knowledge.

IV. The animals selected for an experiment should be of an appropriate species and quality, and the minimum number required to obtain scientifically valid results.

V. Investigators and other personnel should never fail to treat animals as sentient, and should regard their proper care and use and the avoidance or minimization of discomfort, distress, or pain as ethical imperatives.

VI. Investigators should assume that procedures that would cause pain in human beings cause pain in other vertebrate species, although more needs to be known about the perception of pain in animals.

VII. Procedures with animals that may cause more than momentary or minimal pain or distress should be performed with appropriate sedation, analgesia, or anesthesia in accordance with accepted veterinary practice. Surgical or other painful procedures should not be performed on unanesthetized animals paralyzed by chemical agents.

VIII. Where waivers are required in relation to the provisions of article VII, the decisions should not rest solely with the investigators directly concerned, but should be made, with due regard to the provisions of articles IV, V, and VI, by a suitably constituted review body. Such waivers should not be made solely for the purposes of teaching or demonstration.

IX. At the end of, or, when appropriate, during an experiment, animals that would otherwise suffer severe or chronic pain, distress, discomfort, or disablement that cannot be relieved should be painlessly killed.

X. The best possible living conditions should be maintained for animals kept for biomedical purposes. Normally, the care of animals should be under the supervision of veterinarians having experience in laboratory animal science. In any case, veterinary care should be available as required.

XI. It is the responsibility of the director of an institute or department using animals to ensure that investigators and personnel have appropriate qualifications or experience for conducting procedures on animals. Adequate opportunities shall be provided for in-service training, including the proper and humane concern for the animals under their care.

2. Special Provisions

Where they are quantifiable, norms for the following provisions should be established by a national authority, national advisory council, or other competent body.

2.1 Acquisition
Specialized breeding establishments are the best source of the most commonly used experimental animals. Nonspecifically bred animals may be used only if they meet the research requirements, particularly for health and quality, and their acquisition is not in contradiction with national legislation and conservation policies.

2.2 Transportation
Where there are no regulations or statutory requirements governing the transport of animals, it is the duty of the director of an institute or department using animals to emphasize to the supplier and the carrier that the animals should be transported under humane and hygienic conditions.

2.3 Housing
Animal housing should be such as to ensure that the general health of the animals is safeguarded and that undue stress is avoided. Special attention should be given to the space allocation for each animal, according to species, and adequate standards of hygiene should be maintained as well as protection against predators, vermin, and other pests. Facilities for quarantine and isolation should be provided. Entry should normally be restricted to authorized persons.

2.4 Environmental Conditions
Environmental needs such as temperature, humidity, ventilation, lighting, and social inter-action should be consistent with the needs of the species concerned. Noise and odor levels should be minimal. Proper facilities should be provided for the disposal of animals and animal waste.

2.5 Nutrition
Animals should receive a supply of foodstuffs appropriate to their requirements and of a quality and quantity adequate to preserve their health, and they should have free access to potable water, unless the object of the experiment is to study the effects of variations of these nutritional requirements.

2.6 Veterinary Care.
Veterinary care, including a program of health surveillance and disease prevention, should be available to breeding establishments and to institutions or departments using animals for biomedical purposes. Sick or injured animals should, according to circumstances, either receive appropriate veterinary care or be painlessly killed.

2.7 Records.
Records should be kept of all experiments with animals and should be available for inspection. Information should be included regarding the various procedures which were carried out and the results of postmortem examination if conducted.

3. Monitoring of the Care and Use of Animals for Experimentation

3.1. Wherever animals are used for biomedical purposes, their care and use should be subject to the general principles and criteria set out above as well as to existing national policies. The observance of such principles and criteria should be encouraged by procedures for independent monitoring.

3.2. Principles and criteria and monitoring procedures should have as their objectives the avoidance of excessive or inappropriate use of experimental animals and should encourage appropriate care and use before, during, or after experimentation. They may be established by specific legislation laying down standards and providing for enforcement by an official inspectorate; by more general legislation requiring biomedical research institutions to provide for peer review in accordance with defined principles and criteria, sometimes with informed lay participation; or by voluntary self-regulation by the biomedical community. There are many possible variants of monitoring systems, according to the stress laid upon legislation on the one hand, and voluntary self-regulation on the other.

4. Methods Not Involving Animals: "Alternatives"

4.1. There remain many areas in biomedical research which, at least for the foreseeable future, will require animal experimentation. An intact live animal is more than the sum of the responses of isolated cells, tissues, or organs; there are complex interactions in the whole animal that cannot be reproduced by biological or nonbiological "alternative" methods. The term "alternative" has come to be used by some to refer to a replacement of the use of living ani-

mals by other procedures, as well as methods which lead to a reduction in the numbers of animals required or to the refinement of experimental procedures.

4.2. The experimental procedures that are considered to be "alternatives" include nonbiological and biological methods. The nonbiological methods include mathematical modeling of structure-activity relationships based on the physicochemical properties of drugs and other chemicals, and computer modeling of other biological processes. The biological methods include the use of microorganisms, *in vitro* preparations (subcellular fractions, short-term cellular systems, whole organ perfusion, and cell and organ culture), and, under some circumstances, invertebrates and vertebrate embryos. In addition to experimental procedures, retrospective and prospective epidemiological investigations on human and animal populations represent other approaches of major importance.

4.3. The adoption of "alternative" approaches is viewed as being complementary to the use of intact animals, and their development and use should be actively encouraged for both scientific and humane reasons.

Patients' Bills of Rights

Declaration of Lisbon on the Rights of the Patient

Adopted by the 34th World Medical Assembly (Lisbon, September/October 1981)

Recognizing that there may be practical, ethical, or legal difficulties, a physician should always act according to his/her conscience and always in the best interest of the patient. The following Declaration represents some of the principal rights which the medical profession seeks to provide to patients.

Whenever legislation or government action denies these rights of the patient, physicians should seek by appropriate means to assure or to restore them.

a) The patient has the right to choose his physician freely.

b) The patient has the right to be cared for by a physician who is free to make clinical and ethical judgments without any outside interference.

c) The patient has the right to accept or to refuse treatment after receiving adequate information.

d) The patient has the right to expect that his physician will respect the confidential nature of all his medical and personal details.

e) The patient has the right to die in dignity.

f) The patient has the right to receive or to decline spiritual and moral comfort including the help of a minister of an appropriate religion.

(Reprinted by permission.)

A Patient's Bill of Rights

Approved by the American Hospital Association House of Delegates, 6 February 1973

The American Hospital Association presents a Patient's Bill of Rights with the expectation that observance of these rights will contribute to more effective patient care and greater satisfaction for the patient, his physician, and the hospital organization. Further, the Association presents these rights in the expectation that they will be supported by the hospital on behalf of its patients, as an integral part of the healing process. It is recognized that a personal relationship between the physician and the patient is essential for the provision of proper medical care. The traditional physician-patient relationship takes on a new dimension when care is rendered within an organizational structure. Legal precedent has established that the institution itself also has a responsibility to the patient. It is in recognition of these factors that these rights are affirmed.

1. The patient has the right to considerate and respectful care.

2. The patient has the right to obtain from his physician complete current information concerning his diagnosis, treatment, and prognosis in terms the patient can be reasonably expected to understand. When it is not medically advisable to give such information to the patient, the information should be made available to an appropriate person in his behalf. He has the right to know, by name, the physician responsible for coordinating his care.

3. The patient has the right to receive from his physician information necessary to give informed consent prior to the start of any procedure and/or treatment. Except in emergencies, such information for informed consent should include but not necessarily be limited to the specific procedure and/or treatment, the medically significant risks involved, and the probable duration of incapacitation. Where medically significant alternatives for care or

treatment exist, or when the patient requests information concerning medical alternatives, the patient has the right to such information. The patient also has the right to know the name of the person responsible for the procedures and/or treatment.

4. The patient has the right to refuse treatment to the extent permitted by law and to be informed of the medical consequences of his action.

5. The patient has the right to every consideration of his privacy concerning his own medical care program. Case discussion, consultation, examination, and treatment are confidential and should be conducted discreetly. Those not directly involved in his care must have the permission of the patient to be present.

6. The patient has the right to expect that all communications and records pertaining to his care should be treated as confidential.

7. The patient has the right to expect that within its capacity a hospital must make reasonable response to the request of a patient for services. The hospital must provide evaluation, service, and/or referral as indicated by the urgency of the case. When medically permissible, the patient may be transferred to another facility only after he has received complete information and explanation concerning the needs for and alternatives for such a transfer. The institution to which the patient is to be transferred must first have accepted the patient for transfer.

8. The patient has the right to obtain information as to any relationship of his hospital to other health care and educational institutions insofar as his care is concerned. The patient has the right to obtain information as to the existence of any professional relationships among individuals, by name, who are treating him.

9. The patient has the right to be advised if the hospital proposes to engage in or perform human experimentation affecting his care or treatment. The patient has the right to refuse to participate in such research projects.

10. The patient has the right to expect reasonable continuity of care. He has the right to know in advance what appointment times and physicians are available and where. The patient has the right to expect that the hospital will provide a mechanism whereby he is informed by his physician or a delegate of the physician of the patient's continuing health care requirements following discharge.

11. The patient has the right to examine and receive an explanation of his bill, regardless of source of payment.

12. The patient has the right to know what hospital rules and regulations apply to his conduct as a patient.

No catalog of rights can guarantee for the patient the kind of treatment he has a right to expect. A hospital has many functions to perform, including the prevention and treatment of disease, the education of both health professionals and patients, and the conduct of clinical research. All these activities must be conducted with an overriding concern for the patient, and, above all, the recognition of his dignity as a human being. Success in achieving this recognition assures success in the defense of the rights of the patient.

(Reprinted with permission of the American Hospital Association, copyright 1972.)

A Human Right to Health
under International Law

The right to health and the corresponding responsibilities for it are enshrined in the constitutions of both the World Health Organization and the Pan American Health Organization. There is also explicit or implicit recognition of the right to health and its concomitant responsibilities in the following international instruments on human rights: the Universal Declaration of Human Rights; the International Covenant on Economic, Social, and Cultural Rights; the International Covenant on Civil and Political Rights; the International Convention on the Elimination of All Forms of Racial Discrimination; the American Declaration of the Rights and Duties of Man; and the American Covenant on Human Rights (Pact of San José, Costa Rica). The provisions of these international texts demand close attention, as they form a starting point for a legal analysis of health-related precepts in the national constitutions.

Constitution of the World Health Organization

The WHO Constitution sets forth most clearly both the modern definition of a right to health and the responsibility of the State in promoting the physical and mental health of its people. The Preamble to the Constitution declares nine Basic Principles:

The States Parties to this Constitution declare, in conformity with the Charter of the United Nations, that the following principles are basic to the happiness, harmonious relations, and security of all peoples:

Health is a state of complete physical, mental, and social well-being and not merely the absence of disease or infirmity.

The enjoyment of the highest attainable standard of health is one of the fundamental rights of every human being without distinction of race, religion, political belief, or economic or social condition.

The health of all peoples is fundamental to the attainment of peace and security and is dependent upon the fullest cooperation of individuals and States.

The achievement of any State in the promotion and protection of health is of value to all.

Unequal development in different countries in the promotion of health and control of disease, especially communicable disease, is a common danger.

Health development of the child is of basic importance; the ability to live harmoniously in a changing total environment is essential to such development.

The extension to all peoples of the benefits of medical, psychological, and related knowledge is essential to the fullest attainment of health.

Informed opinion and active cooperation on the part of the public is of the utmost importance in the improvement of the health of the people.

Governments have a responsibility for the health of their peoples which can be fulfilled only by the provision of adequate health and social measures.

Constitution of the Pan American Health Organization

The PAHO Constitution states in its first article that the fundamental purposes of the Organization shall be

to promote and coordinate efforts of the countries of the Western Hemisphere to combat disease, lengthen life, and promote the physical and mental health of the people.

Universal Declaration of Human Rights

United Nations, 1948

The Universal Declaration of Human Rights sets forth in Article 25 that

1. Everyone has the right to a standard of living adequate for the health and well-being of himself and his family, including food, clothing, housing and medical care and necessary social services, and the right to security in the event of unemployment, sickness, disability, widowhood, old age or other lack of livelihood in circumstances beyond his control.
2. Motherhood and childhood are entitled to special care and assistance. All children, whether born in or out of wedlock, shall enjoy the same social protection.

International Covenant on Economic, Social, and Cultural Rights

The International Covenant on Economic, Social, and Cultural Rights acknowledges the right to health in its Article 12:

1. The States Parties to the present Covenant recognize the right of everyone to the enjoyment of the highest attainable standard of physical and mental health.
2. The steps to be taken by the States Parties to the present Covenant to achieve the full realization of this right shall include those necessary for:
    a) the provision for the reduction of the still-birth rate and of infant mortality and for the healthy development of the child;
    b) the improvement of all aspects of environmental and industrial hygiene;
    c) the prevention, treatment, and control of epidemic, endemic, occupational, and other diseases;

d) the creation of conditions which would assure to all medical service and medical attention in the event of sickness.

International Covenant on Civil and Political Rights

With regard to the protection of health, the International Covenant on Civil and Political Rights states that:

Every human being has the inherent right to life. This right shall be protected by law. No one shall be arbitrarily deprived of his life. . . . (Article 6, Paragraph 1.)

No one shall be subject to torture or to cruel, inhuman or degrading treatment or punishment. In particular, no one shall be subject without his free consent to medical or scientific experimentation. (Article 7)

International Convention on the Elimination of all Forms of Racial Discrimination

Article 5 (e) of the International Convention on the Elimination of All Forms of Racial Discrimination recognizes among the economic, social, and cultural rights that the States Parties should guarantee to everyone without discrimination as to race, color, nationality, or ethnic origin:

(IV) the right to public health, medical care, and social security and social services.

American Declaration of the Rights and Duties of Man

The American Declaration of the Rights and Duties of Man recognizes the following:

Article I. Every human being has the right to life, liberty, and the security of his person.

233

Article VI. Every person has the right to establish a family, the basic element of society, and to receive protection therefor.

Article VII. All women, during pregnancy and the nursing period, and all children have the right to special protection, care, and aid.

Article XI. Every person has the right to the preservation of his health through sanitary and social measures relating to food, clothing, housing, and medical care, to the extent permitted by public and community resources.

Article XVI. Every person has the right to social security which will protect him from the consequences of unemployment, old age, and any disabilities arising from causes beyond his control that make it physically or mentally impossible for him to earn a living.

Article XXVIII. The rights of man are limited by the rights of others, by the security of all, and by the just demands of the general welfare and the advancement of democracy.

Article XXIX. It is the duty of the individual so to conduct himself in relation to others that each and every one may fully form and develop his personality.

Article XXX. It is the duty of every person to aid, support, educate, and protect his minor children, and it is the duty of children to honor their parent always and to aid, support, and protect them when they need it.

Article XXXV. It is the duty of every person to cooperate with the State and the community with respect to social security and welfare, in accordance with his ability and with existing circumstances.

American Convention on Human Rights

The American Convention on Human Rights (Pact of San José, Costa Rica) recognizes implicitly that health is a human right:

Article 4. Right to Life: 1. Every person has the right to have his life respected. This right shall be protected by law and, in general, from the moment of conception. No one shall be arbitrarily deprived of his life.

Article 5. Right to Humane Treatment: 1. Every person has the right to have his physical, mental, and moral integrity respected.

Article 17. Rights of the Family: 1. The family is the natural and fundamental group unit of society and is entitled to protection by society and the State.

Article 19. Rights of the Child: Every minor child has the right to the measures of protection required by his condition as a minor on the part of his family, society, and the State.

Article 24. Right to Equal Protection: All persons are equal before the law. Consequently, they are entitled, without discrimination, to equal protection of the law.

Article 32. Relationship between Duties and Rights: 1. Every person has responsibilities to his family, his community, and mankind. 2. The rights of each person are limited by the rights of others, by the security of all, and by the just demands of the general welfare, in a democratic society.

• • •

These principles are almost universally accepted. Every sovereign nation on earth is a member of WHO, and has thus formally agreed to its clear and complete constitutional Declaration of Principles. On a regional level, the same may be said about PAHO, as the specialized organization for health in the Americas. The Universal Declaration of Human Rights has become, as was the intention at its drafting in 1948, "the common standard for achievement for all peoples and nations." The international covenants on Economic, Social, and Cultural Rights and on Civil and Political Rights are recognized as codifying rights that, as stated in their preambles, "derive from the inherent dignity of the human person." The International Convention on the Elimination of All Forms of Racial Discrimination is the means "to implement the principles embodied in the United Nations Declaration on the Elimination of All Forms of Racial Discrimination and to secure the earliest adoption of practical measures to that end." The American Declaration and the American Covenant are the traditional means of guaranteeing the protection of human rights in the Inter-American System.

In summary, there can be no doubt that in the modern world a right to health is a basic human right or, to reiterate the WHO Constitution: "The enjoyment of the highest attainable standard of health is one of the fundamental rights of every human being, without distinction of race, religion, political belief, economic or social condition." In the WHO system and according to modern public health and medical thought, "health is a state of complete physical, mental, and social well-being and not merely the absence of disease or infirmity." There is virtually no country in the world that does not accept at least some governmental responsibility for the public and individual health of its people, thereby recognizing the pledge made upon ratification of the WHO Constitution, that "Governments have a responsibility for the health of their people which can be fulfilled only by the provision of adequate health and social measures."

Contributors

Francesc Abel
Borja Institute of Bioethics, Sant Cugat del Vallès, Barcelona, Spain

Teresa Asnariz
Human Genetics Association of Mar del Plata, Mar del Plata, Argentina

Ronald Bayer
Columbia University, American Foundation for AIDS Research, United States of America

Natalia Biló
Institute of Legal Philosophy, College of Lawyers, Judicial Department of Mar del Plata, Buenos Aires Province, Argentina

Héctor Brunamontini
National University of Mar del Plata, Rectorate, Mar del Plata, Argentina

Isabel Bustos D.
Pontificia Universidad Católica, School of Nursing, Santiago, Chile

Daniel Callahan
The Hastings Center, New York, United States of America

Orlando Calo
National University of Mar del Plata, Rectorate, Mar del Plata, Argentina

Courtney S. Campbell
The Hastings Center, Associate for Religious Studies, New York, United States of America

Susan Scholle Connor
Pan American Health Organization, Legal Consultant, Washington, DC, United States of America

Gabriel de la Escosura
General Hospital of Mexico, Pneumology Unit, Mexico City, Mexico

Juan Ramón de la Fuente
Autonomous National University of Mexico, Mexico City, Mexico

Bernard M. Dickens
University of Toronto, Faculty of Law, Faculty of Medicine, Toronto, Canada

Cristina Di Domenico
National University of Mar del Plata, School of Psychology, Mar del Plata, Argentina

James F. Drane
Edinboro University of Pennsylvania, Department of Philosophy, Russell B. Roth Professor of Clinical Ethics, Pennsylvania, United States of America

Hernán L. Fuenzalida-Puelma
Pan American Health Organization, Legal Affairs Office, Washington, DC, United States of America

Eliana Gaete Q.
Pontificia Universidad Católica, School of Nursing, Santiago, Chile

Laura Golpe
National University of Mar del Plata, School of Psychology, Mar del Plata, Argentina

Larry Gostin
American Society of Law and Medicine and Harvard University, School of Public Health, Boston, United States of America

Diego Gracia
Complutense University, Department of Public Health and History of Science, Madrid, España

Cristina Gurrea
National University of Mar del Plata, Rectorate, Mar del Plata, Argentina

Pedro Hooft
Institute of Legal Philosophy, College of Lawyers, Judicial Department of Mar del Plata, Buenos Aires Province, Argentina

José Kuthy Porter
Anáhuac University, School of Medicine, Mexico City, Mexico

María del Carmen Lara
Mexican Institute of Psychiatry, Mexico City, Mexico

Diana Serrano LaVertu
Pan American Health Organization, Legal Affairs Office, Washington, DC, United States of America

Ana María Linares
Pan American Health Organization, Program of Evaluation of the Health, Situation and Trends, Washington, DC, United States of America

Fernando Lolas
University of Chile, School of Medicine, Psychophysiology Unit, Santiago, Chile

Alfonso Llano Escobar
Colombian Association of Medical Faculties (ASCOFAME), Bogotá, Colombia

Robert Llanos Zuloaga
Sacred Heart University for Women, Department of Psychology; Cayetano Heredia University; Ricardo Palma Clinic, Lima, Peru

José Alberto Mainetti
Universidad Nacional de La Plata, Chair for Postgraduate Medical Humanities; and Institute of Medical Humanities and Center for Bioethics, Dr. José María Mainetti Foundation, Buenos Aires, Argentina

Jorge Manzini
Private Community Hospital, Mar del Plata, Argentina

María I. Pacenza
National University of Mar del Plata, School of Psychology, Mar del Plata, Argentina

Edmund D. Pellegrino
University of Georgetwon, Center for the Advanced Study of Ethics, and John Carroll Professor of Medicine and Medical Humanities, Washington, DC, United States of America

Emilia Pepa
Dr. Juan H. Jara National Institute of Epidemiology, National Ministry of Health and Social Action, Mar del Plata, Argentina

Hélio Pereira Dias
Ministry of Health, Brasílla, DF, Brazil

Ana María Petriella
National University of Mar del Plata, Faculty of Exact and Natural Sciences, Mar del Plata, Argentina

M. Angélica Piwonka de A.
Pontificia Universidad Católica, School of Nursing, Santiago, Chile

Fernando Sánchez-Torres
National University of Colombia, National Tribunal for Medical Ethics, and Colombian Institute for Bioethical Studies, Bogotá, Colombia

Hans-Martin Sass
Georgetown University, Kennedy Institute of Ethics, Washington, DC, United States of America

Orlanda Señoriño
National University of Mar del Plata, Rectorate, Mar del Plata, Argentina

Juan Carlos Tealdi
Universidad Nacional de La Plata, Chair for Postgraduate Medical Humanities; and Institute of Medical Humanities and Center for Bioethics, Dr. José María Mainetti Foundation, Buenos Aires, Argentina

Mila Urrutia B.
Pontificia Universidad Católica, School of Nursing, Santiago, Chile

Francisco Vilardell
School of Gastroenterology, Hospital de la Santa Cruz y San Pablo, Barcelona, and Council for International Organizations of Medical Sciences, Barcelona, España

Justo Zanier
National University of Mar del Plata, Rectorate, Mar del Plata, Argentina